AIDS:
Individual, Cultural and Policy Dimensions

AIDS:
Individual, Cultural and
Policy Dimensions

Edited by
Peter Aggleton, Peter Davies and Graham Hart

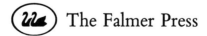 The Falmer Press

(A member of the Taylor & Francis Group)
London • New York • Philadelphia

UK   The Falmer Press, Rankine Road, Basingstoke, Hampshire, RG24 0PR

USA   The Falmer Press, Taylor & Francis Inc., 1900 Frost Road, Suite 101, Bristol, PA 19007

First published 1990

British Library Cataloguing in Publication Data
AIDS: individual, cultural and policy dimensions.
  1. Man. AIDS. Social aspects
  I. Aggleton, Peter *1952–* II. Davies, Peter III. Hart, Graham *1957–*
  362.1' 042
  ISBN 1–85000–763–2

Library of Congress Cataloging-in-Publication Data
AIDS: individual, cultural, and policy dimensions/edited by Peter
  Aggleton, Peter Davies and Graham Hart.
          p.   cm.
  Some papers originally presented at the 3rd UK Conference on
  Social Aspects of AIDS, held at South Bank Polytechnic in February
1989.
  ISBN 1–85000–763–2: — ISBN 1–85000–764–0 (pbk.)
  1. AIDS (Disease)—Social aspects—Congresses. I. Aggleton, Peter.
II. Davis, Peter. III. Hart, Graham. IV. UK Conference on Social
Aspects of AIDS (3rd: 1989: South Bank Polytechnic)
  RC607.A26A347424 1990
  362.1' 969792—dc20

Jacket design by Caroline Archer

Typeset in 11/13 Bembo by
Chapterhouse, The Cloisters, Formby L37 3PX

Printed and bound in Great Britain by
Taylor & Francis (Printers) Ltd.
Basingstoke

Contents

Preface

In February 1989 the third conference on Social Aspects of AIDS took place at South Bank Polytechnic in London. Social researchers working in psychology, sociology, history, anthropology and education were represented, along with health care workers and members of statutory and voluntary organizations. The conference's themes emphasized the individual, cultural and policy dimensions of HIV disease, and under these broad headings a wide range of papers was given.

As with previous volumes in this series (P. Aggleton and H. Homans, eds, *Social Aspects of AIDS*, Falmer, 1988 and P. Aggleton, G. Hart and P. Davies, eds, *AIDS: Social Representations, Social Practices*, Falmer, 1989), this book contains many of the papers given at the conference as well as additional contributions. In editing it, our concern has been to identify the range of research that is currently under way. Some of the chapters are empirical in their emphasis, some are more concerned with the cultural dynamics that surround HIV disease, some with reporting on particular health education and health policy interventions, and a few begin to develop a critique of some of the assumptions that operate in and around contemporary research agendas.

We would like to thank all who attended the conference for their readiness to engage in sometimes painful but nevertheless important debates. We owe a special debt to Paul Broderick, Andrew Hunt, Vijay Kumari, Paul Simpson, Gary Stevens, Ian Warwick and Gary Wych, who played a key role in organizing the pre-conference publicity as well as arrangements on the day; and to Adrian Coyle for his work throughout the year. We are grateful to the Economic and Social Research Council (ESRC) for financial support. Finally, we must thank Helen Thomas who, with consummate skills, prepared the manuscript for publication.

Peter Aggleton, Peter Davies and Graham Hart
August 1989

Chapter 1

What Science Knows: Formations of AIDS Knowledges

Cindy Patton

In private conversations and in public health campaigns, knowledge is promoted as the essential ingredient in the effort to halt HIV. To the fearful, knowledge means information that will prove that they will not develop AIDS. To the far right, knowledge means information that promotes homosexuality and promiscuity — carnal knowledge — and, therefore, dangerous knowledge. To health officials and many concerned activists, knowledge means neutral information with the magic power to change attitudes and behaviours by 'empowering' people to make what seem to be self-evidently wise decisions.

But despite the obvious differences in the meaning of the term 'knowledge', all of these usages attempt to shore up the idea that there is some centrally effective knowledge with a privileged access to reality, a knowledge which at the most needs sensitive translation into everyday languages. In the legitimated AIDS discourse, knowledge inevitably refers back to the knowledge of science, the master administrative discourse of all other discourses. But there is a whole range of important knowledges, which come from different places within the social and imaginary worlds. These knowledges arise and compete with one another, but *science* anchors the power relations which determine *whose* knowledge is most relevant in public policy debate.

A tremendous political and social backlash is occurring through the increasing bureaucratization of the dispensing of AIDS knowledge. From workshops to pamphlets to HIV antibody tests to public service announcements, there is apparently more AIDS knowledge and there are more people knowledgeable about AIDS. But by constructing AIDS knowledge as based in science, the most important forms of information construction and movement within and between communities are being foreclosed in two ways. First, promoting science-logic over complex folk-logics makes people dependent on the medical bureaucracy and leads to the idea that more information *by itself* is efficacious in producing behaviour change. Second, by asserting the 'correctness' of science over community, policies like the Helms Amendment in the US[1] and Section 28 of the 1988 Local Government Act in Britain[2] make it illegal or unfundable to couch messages in dissident vernaculars.[3] The new scientific knowledges associated with AIDS research almost perfectly rationalize the systems of social control which predate them, especially those which silence or distort the speech and culture of 'minority communities'.[4]

But this rise in the credibility of scientific explanation is ironic. Despite highly publicized stories alleging that Bob Gallo stole the virus from Luc Montagnier,[5] the recent revelations that Burroughs-Wellcome lost track of over 1000 (nearly a quarter) of the compassionate-release AZT trial subjects,[6] despite the inability of seven years of international research to turn up anti-virals that predictably or substantially improve anyone's life, despite the apparent failure of tens of thousands of scientists to make meaningful headway against HIV infection, *science* as an ideal has increased its stature and successfully claimed itself to be above politics.

The comforting causal-logic knowledge of science, ineffective even on its own terms, has increasingly become the basis for expanding discrimination and surveillance. The effectiveness of science-logic in policing society has both reified science-logic and inured us to science's inability to solve the problems it sets itself. Discoveries are haphazard when they happen, but accounts of them revise the scientific process to make them appear like the outcome of rational and methodical enquiry. The categories of science, particularly the conjuncture of epidemiology and virology, have placed a barely invisible *cordon sanitaire* around minority communities, deviant individuals, and perhaps around an entire subcontinent. We no longer need camps or border passes, although several countries have used them in an effort to prevent the spread of HIV. The ideologies encoded in AIDS research have laid a more sublime foundation for selecting groups of people for detention and destructions. The mechanism for this is, ironically, an education strategy which separates the 'general public' from 'communities'.

Dominant AIDS discourse redraws the line of social and personal responsibility, making present police and public health systems infinitely more able to exert their forms of social control. Indeed, it has never been part of the *logic* of science actually to stop the epidemic, only to sculpt its path to a 'final solution'. Science must indeed be very ambivalent about halting transmission. Under current research methods, vaccine trials require some group of people efficiently transmitting the micro-organism the vaccine is to protect against. Moreover, the idea that it is through sex that HIV is passed makes it quite easy to claim that safer sex education has found some group of people recalcitrant, and that they thus constitute a prime target for vaccine trials. Although Phase One trials are under consideration in Britain at the present, most markers point to Africa as the likely site of Phase 2 vaccine trials where the ideologies of sexually permissive and uneducable 'Africans' collide with and bolster the idea that

AIDS is already wildly out of control throughout the continent — more out of control and more dangerous, that is, than in the US, still the country hardest hit numerically in the world. Together, the images of 'African sexuality' and 'African poverty' create the conditions for recreating the US Tuskegee syphilis experiments on a continental scale:[7] the West is gearing up to believe that it can in good conscience conduct unethical vaccine trials on the pretext of actually 'helping Africans'.

If this seems far-fetched or a reflection of antiquated methods now properly supervised by review boards, let us recall that some 10,000 gay men in the US and several thousand more from northern European capitals were the willing subjects of the hepatitis B vaccine trials between 1978 and 1982. Here hepatitis was taken as a fact of sexual life in the most dense and active gay male communities. Depicted as compliant and helpful altruists (an image of gay male research subjects that has persisted until recently, and one that resonates uncomfortably with contemporary depictions of the cheerful subjects of Tuskegee), we must wonder why these men were never told to use condoms, why condoms were not tested for efficacy against hepatitis B, HIV and a wide range of other STDs until 1986.

It was only 1982, with the emergence of AIDS, that gay men in significant numbers began to practise generalized preventive sex education, despite efforts of a small gay health movement in the 1970s. Inside the gay community, the tremendous effort directed towards liberating men from psychological stigma obscured, for a time, the link between closet and decreased access to preventive medical care. It was a historic step to have homosexuality changed from a medical anomaly to a psychological impairment in the early part of the century, and an equally significant step to have homosexuality removed from DSM-3 and ICD-9 in the early 1970s and later 1980s. Moreover, to understand gay life as having a medical dimension was barely possible with the 'gay is good' rhetoric of the 1970s. Lesbians and gay men had risked their careers and safety to have their sexuality declared 'healthy'. It is perhaps no surprise that STDs were considered a minor inconvenience of gay male life. Until about 1986, after the 'heterosexual' AIDS scare, gay men worked without the help of mainstream researchers or health educators to develop the concept and pedagogy of safe sex.

It is important to recognize here that safer sex was above all a form of resistance developed by gay men acting in micro-networks linked by their own newspapers in an imagined national and international community.[8] Safer sex was a community-based response, not one promoted at the time by 'science', nor one supported by the mainstream doctors and epidemiologists who had a more 'objective' and global view of gay male sexually transmitted disease rates. Most importantly, safer sex minimized the risk of further HIV infection in major portions of the gay male community before there was any official response (Aggleton, Coxon and Weatherburn, 1989). If all this seems like an accident of historical oversight, we might recall that at the First International Conference on AIDS (1985) in Atlanta, Georgia, a key Centre for

Disease Control (CDC) official — complete with charts and graphs — suggested that all gay men should take the then new antibody test and have sex only with people of like status. He saw no reason why HIV seropositive men should not continue to engage in transmission behaviours. He saw nothing wrong with creating a sexual apartheid based on HIV serostatus, instead of promoting the universal adoption of non-transmitting practices. At the 1988 Fourth International Conference on AIDS in Stockholm, an American researcher argued from the audience that the few remaining asymptomatic, long-term HIV seropositive men from San Francisco hepatitis-cum-HIV cohort be denied any early intervention treatments so that scientists could see what the natural history of HIV infection would ultimately be.[9]

The uneven success of AIDS health educational campaigns has not led to a re-evaluation of strategies. Rather, it is often suggested that the reasonable have been educated and all that remains are a hard core, hard to reach population. 'Hard to reach' in this context encodes deviance: they are hard to reach because of social attitudes towards their risk behaviour, not due to, for instance, intransigence of mental attitude. If we applied that latter criterion, we must with justice consider Senator Jesse Helms and the Right Honourable Margaret Thatcher as members of the 'hard core, hard to reach population'.

Most educational efforts so far have been directed either towards a general public thought to be ignorant of the fact that HIV cannot be transmitted via door knobs (cathecting strange sexual phantasies, no doubt), or towards 'communities' in which the so-called risk behaviours are believed to occur recalcitrantly. This division of educational strategy, and the illusory epidemiology on which it is based, constitutes the terrain in which legal and social discriminations occur. The targeting of education, anchored by the mobile metaphor of the HIV antibody test, enables, rather than decreases, discrimination. The more we educate under this ideological division of labour, the more we inscribe the system of discrimination against people associated with AIDS. The mere idea of a test — regardless of what it actually detects, and regardless of its reliability and validity — means the individuals *could* know their status, and that a policing public health system *could* find it out. This displaces all responsibility onto the putatively or provably HIV seropositive individual, and implies that there can be no such thing as consent to unsafe sex with an HIV seropositive person. This does not dismiss our concern for the rationales for such 'consent': few people will be consenting to transmission. The meaning of engaging in an act — even one deemed unsafe by science — may be more powerful than the recognition of risk. Implicitly, a sexual act becomes unsafe sex simply because of the HIV serostatus of a partner, not according to whether the practice itself could be transmitting or not.

This view is explicit in Swedish law where it is illegal for a person who knows they are HIV seropositive to have sex of any sort with a person who knows they are seronegative. Lest the problem be circumvented by avoiding testing altogether, Swedish law also requires anyone who has reason to believe they have been exposed to

HIV or any STD to present themselves for testing. Anyone who is named as a partner of an HIV seropositive person who does not voluntarily come forward for testing may be arrested on medical grounds. Increasingly, in the US, HIV seropositive individuals are being brought up on criminal charges for engaging in sex with seronegative individuals, regardless of whether or not the individual consented to the act and regardless of whether or not the act results in transmission, ignoring all the problems with attributing HIV seroconversion to a particular exposure.

The Discourse of Science and the Practice of Education

Traditionally, science is seen as having privileged access to reality through its special technologies and its reasoning system. Scientific knowledge is popularly believed to be accumulated in a pure, unmotivated fashion. 'Theoretical' knowledge is weeded out, and 'practical' information watered down into lay terms for everyday application. Health educators and clinicians are typically viewed as conduits in this process, receiving scientific knowledge at one step removed and passing it on to their 'clients' or 'audiences' after paring down the information again. Evaluation of whether the knowledge has been correctly conveyed can be accomplished by objectively testing the recipient and by obtaining measures of the educator's ability to remain neutral, consistent and legitimate in the eyes of the recipient. This system of information conveyance is thought to work best when the intermediaries add as little to the 'knowledge' as possible, while convincing the audience that they 'know what they are talking about.' This is a performance of scientific legitimation, overlayed with theatrical competence.

This conception of knowledge as an inverted pyramid transforming knowledges from pure sciences to popular understandings and bounded by a single logical construction has become standard social mythology. After Kuhn's (1962) *The Structure of Scientific Revolutions*, people with any passing exposure to popular science have come to view knowledge as coherent only within a given framework or paradigm. Hard science is at the leading edge of these knowledge formations. Ideas compete, explanatory schemes win out and science progresses within the turf defined. Clearly, the newness of retroviral research and the association of a newly identified disease with social stigma argues, in Kuhnian terms anyway, that we ought to be in the middle of a paradigm shift. A Kuhnian analysis also suggests that where there are problems with existing explanatory frameworks, the fittest theory will eventually win out over others. This particular account, however, obscures the power relations between science and public policy in three ways. First, it ignores the role of social ideologies in directing research programmes. Second, it incorrectly describes and, in effect, erases the local knowledge of social and health practices which are essential to minimizing HIV transmission. Third, it reifies science-logic over folk interpretive processes.

This positivist view of knowledge is fatal to people in danger of HIV infection and is catastrophic for the communities and nations in the developing world which are currently and inextricably the objects of scientific research. To clarify these processes, I will propose here a more constructionist view of the role and rise of knowledge about HIV and AIDS and suggest how this view may alter research and educational strategies. In doing this, I am not suggesting that there is any one 'perfect' educational strategy. Rather, we must be more sophisticated in our understanding of the mix of intended and unintended consequences that may arise from particular combinations of health education interventions and media initiatives. We cannot assume that any one approach will necessarily be more effective than another in promoting health or in challenging vernacular logical processes.

In crude terms, the traditional model of health education locates 'unhealthy' behaviours in the individual, and relates them either to ignorance or to an inability to overcome drives. The solution in this model is to provide information and individual therapy, on the assumption that information changes attitudes, which increase intentions to engage in healthy behaviours, which result in changed behaviour. Those who do not respond as predicted are described as 'deficient' or 'compulsive'. Behaviours therefore are acts that arise from an unconscious which may be overcome by will. Most important, this model frequently views the social aspects of a behaviour in terms of peer pressure, a sort of externalized will or group contract to suppress the bad drives.

According to this model, the lay person is not thought capable of understanding 'science', which requires specialized training. The health educator must therefore act as a translator, taking their best understanding of science and putting it into 'everyday' terms. Most usually common people are assumed to need metaphors for the scientific, there being an assumption that if the right, culturally sensitive metaphors are found, the information given to the common person will be roughly equivalent, at least in its practical effects, to that produced by science. In this account, the role of the health educator is to pare down and simplify a supposedly objective scientific knowledge.

'What Science Knows about AIDS'

The October 1988 issue of *Scientific American* had a rather astonishing cover. Burned in white type over a typically elegant reproduction of a budding virus were the words, 'What Science Knows about AIDS'; not, it should be noted, 'The Progress of Science towards a Vaccine or Cure' or 'What Scientists Have Learned about AIDS'. Two semantic elements in this title give the game away: *science*, as opposed to non-science and commonsense ideas; and *knows*, as opposed to posits, imagines or thinks. This same issue is filled with photographs and diagrams of HIV and advertisements for companies producing test and imaging systems. Science can, after all, *see* the virus, whereas you and I have access only to their pictures.

In the same issue, we are presented with romantic, tragic photos of the 'real people' with AIDS — a white, North American family in which the father is a haemophiliac. We also see people said to be affected as a group — those who stand for communities, perhaps even for a whole continent, that we are invited to imagine is potentially waiting to be destroyed by the slow-ticking bomb of HIV. Of course, sophisticated readers know that you cannot tell whether an individual is infected by looking at them, but at the same time, readers are presented with a powerful image of what it looks like to 'have AIDS'.

In this process of 'putting a face on AIDS' the illness has been concretized but also romanticized: the health and vulnerability of certain groups of people being valorized at the expense of demonizing others. It is the encodings of these 'real people' images more than the cool logic of policy debate which makes it increasingly possible to see wholesale discrimination as uncomfortable but in the public interest, and to see the placebo trials for vaccines planned for the third world as noble, and not as genocide. Of course, all knowledge is much like the picture of the virus — mediated, enlarged colorized and stylized. Scientific knowledge itself is produced through and around tropes of cultural symbols: the ideas of science come as much from the demands of the popular imagination as they come pristine from the great minds of science.

A better understanding of the movement of information from science to people can be attained via a negotiation model. Here the health educator, the common person, and the scientist are each conceptualized as 'coming from' linguistic and symbolic systems rich in personal and social meaning. None has a privileged access to a a fixed and pre-given reality. Each arena contains its own specialized knowledge and has a set of logics for incorporating 'news' — that is, ideas that are designated as coming from another realm or coming via revelation or reframing from within that same realm. This has been discussed in other work in terms of 'exoteric and esoteric' knowledge (see, for example Fleck, 1978), or as vernaculars.

In this social constructionist model, a group decides to access 'news' or takes it on itself to deliver 'news' to another realm. This produces a motivation (or an intention in the sense of movement relative to an another) to 'communicate'. Rather than a translation model that never calls attention to motives as politics or power relations, a negotiation model suggests that in the process of moving 'news' across the limits of a realm of knowledge, a great deal of violence is done. But this violence does not simply take the form of distortion (which assumes metaphor can, at least in the abstract, approach a state of one-to-one correspondence with meaning). Rather, it is embedded in the power relations co-created or imposed through the hierarchical valuation of forms of knowledge. This form of power may be hegemonic if a group, strongly needs 'news' from a more socially powerful group, as may be the case when people with HIV and AIDS become complicit with unethical medical practices as a result of their desire to seek treatment. Alternatively, it may be overtly coercive, as in the loss of civil rights when an HIV-related diagnosis is confirmed.

Health educators can have a range of motives for taking on the scientific 'news' about HIV infection and AIDS — helping others, self-improvement, a desire to become a scientist, social role conformity and so on. These motives provide the context for their involvement in the reconstruction and mediation of AIDS knowledge. For example, health educators in the AIDS context may wish to bring about specific behaviour changes, and may be schooled in certain assumptions about behaviour. These health educators interface with the science-news to decide what the 'problem' is and which disciplinary techniques to apply to the 'problem' as defined within the pre-figurative logic of their discipline. The pre-figurative ideologies and the immediate motives of the health educator may thereafter bracket consideration of power relations in negotiative interactions. Thus the educator described above may fail to question the basis of behaviourism, and may co-create systems of meanings with the scientist which are mutually consistent with pre-existing frameworks. Likewise, the health educator's motives and those of individuals falling in the path of education co-create a further set of meanings which link what was mutually consistent from the science/educator co-creation. To the extent that these cannot be reconciled, either the more socially powerful knowledge system will be accepted ('Well, that's what the studies show') or a profound scepticism will emerge ('The science is all lies') which both revert to a reality-based model of meaning.

Virology and Immunology: Cultural Tropes/Scientific Pursuits

The rise of virological and immunological explanations of AIDS suggests how cultural metaphors direct scientific thinking. In 1981, when the first cases of what we now know as AIDS were described, immunology was a cutting-edge scientific discipline. The syndrome was first called GRID — Gay Related Immune Deficiency — a name considered blatantly prejudicial and one soon changed. But it was an entirely logical name within the premises of immunology, and the legacy of immunological thinking was retained in the subsequent name, Acquired Immune Deficiency Syndrome (AIDS), which many now argue should be called HIV disease. These two names — AIDS and HIV disease — represent in relief the style of thinking within each subdiscipline. The tension between these two ways of thinking about this disease phenomenon are duplicated in education strategies, treatment trials and public policy. In 1981 virology was evidencing some important technological breakthroughs, but it was at that time considered a highly specialized science, not one capable of generating wide ranging explanations for disease processes. Today several broadly defined ailments — arthritis, multiple sclerosis and the elusive chronic fatigue syndrome — are being broken into aetiological subcategories, with some forms now being attributed to retroviruses. Recently, scientific controversy broke out over the discovery of a 'virus-like particle' (VLP) correlated with clinical AIDS.[10] Virology and now retrovirology and 'virus-like'-ology vie as more precise explainers of disease.

Immunology had won its place from endocrinology, which had had a brief career as master science after bacteriology had dominated for the early part of the twentieth century. On one hand, the changes in master science reflect the progressive solving of discrete problems. But this does not explain why subdisciplines gain the power to control the metaphors that provide the context for, or enmesh themselves in, larger cultural explanations of diseases and remedies. Why did immunology provide such an appealing narrative between the late 1960s and the early 1980s? This is a complex question, but several answers suggest themselves.

Immunology developed at a time when holistic models of health were re-emerging in the US. The idea of a delicately balanced internal ecology nicely mirrored the growing perception of the human being precariously perched in a world ecology. Immunology met the cultural needs of an 'America' fascinated by a return to homeopathic ideas, but unwilling to abandon the miracles of modern medical technology. Moreover, immunology had radical implications for how people were encouraged to understand their bodies. Where the bacteriological body had been static before and after the assault by germs; and the endocrinological body ran hot and cold, oily and dry, in essence, mapping gendered and emotional tropes; the immunological body was more gracefully fluid and fragile, like a dancer in a delicately balanced environment in which it was placed almost without boundaries. Inside and outside broke down as imaging technologies produced new views of 'natural' parasites rivalling 1950s B-movie monsters. Simultaneously it was revealed that there were 'good' bacteria, which made our favourite cheeses and which made our digestive systems work, and 'bad' bacteria which made us sick. According to both holistic and immunological accounts, it was our own bodies and not outside invaders that were the problem in a pathology, and our bodies were increasingly inscribed within a futuristic scenario of massive environmental stress. The chief evil was a modern society that wore our bodies down: we were breaking ourselves down from within. The very structure of modern life thereby became the locus for negotiating health logic. Health in the immunological body was sustained by careful management: management science and terminology in the late 1970s converge with the metaphors of self-care health-logic.

Immunology shifted dominant metaphors of disease from offence to defence. Increasing concern with domestic unrest and lingering Cold War paranoia demanded that our immune systems should conform to a policing and confessional ideology which suggested that it was *not* that the Commies had got through the doors, rather that there was a more general weakness in the body politic. Immunology was about making fine distinctions between self and barely distinguishable other. It was not so much about Other with a capital O as about the marginally different that had already been admitted to close proximity, people who became pathological once the tolerant host had diminished in capacity. Immunology provided the ideal discourse within which pathologically to discuss homosexuality and masculinity which in the 1940s and 1950s had been inscribed by hormonal theories. The 1980s would be rife with an undercurrent of accusations of 'wimpiness' which mapped allegations of political decisiveness as effectively as they mapped allegations of medical risk.

Rapidly improving imaging technology coincided with an era described as unprecedented world peace. People could now visualize their bodies as filled with tiny defending armies in a quest to return the 'self' to a normal state of health. But this tacitly made the individual responsible for the success of these little wars on pathology: if you failed to defend against germs, failed to cope, it was because you did not personally manage your army well.

Immunology is only the most recent contender in a classic competition between sin versus demon understandings of pathology in the Western imagination. Both tropes co-exist and both are non-dialectical, with each providing a different logic of relationship between the 'body' and systems of power. While one or the other generally predominates at a given point, culturally, most micro-networks and individuals employ combinations or alternations between the prevailing metaphors of health that encircle each logic. Indeed, the coincidence of community health movements with liberation movements in the 1960s and 1970s used particular understandings of the political relationships enacted in health care and health surveillance to de-pathologize and limit the power of pathological metaphors related to race, gender and sexuality. The complexity of incorporating liberationist health logics, and the contradictions of race, gender and sexuality they contain, accounts for the conflict between community-based groups over issues like needle exchange, evolving sexual-relational norms, and interfacing with clinical medical systems. The rise of recent AIDS community research initiatives is an outcome of this convergence.[11]

Scientific accounts of the successes attributable to AIDS research are completely contradictory yet they demonstrate the workings of each system's logic. In the early 1980s immunological interpretations of AIDS emphasized the relationship between environmental management and internal bodily breakdown. These early studies were cited as evidence of a failure to thrive in a given lifestyle of a wilful straying from the ideal of health. Thus immunological explanations of AIDS emphasized immune overload due to drugs, 'fast' living, an excessive exposure to semen (which was said to cause a bizarre rejection of 'self' in men), or simply too much sex.

Later virological schemes, waiting in the wings to become the new demonological explanation, and applied to the same hastily conducted epidemiological studies, fuelled the idea that AIDS might be caused by a single, transmissible pathogen. Modern medicine had until this point considered the immune system and the aetiological agent as phenomena in two different, if interactive, realms. Never before had a pathogenic disease of the immune system been conceptualized, and the competing explanations offered made peace in a theoretical compromise. The continued co-existence of immunological and virological explanations — despite the implications for the political economy of research and for education policies — in themselves argue against the strictly Kuhnian position. No new paradigm was realized between these two incommensurate scientific schemes. Neither ultimately wins full explanatory power, and both must account for the logic of the other.

This conceptual crisis came to be played out dramatically in the modelling of treatment trials. Early treatments for opportunistic infections, based on immunological models, advocated megadoses of known drugs specific to the particular infections. These toxic regimes may well have killed as many patients as they helped. It is important to recognize here that virology and immunology understand 'side effects' in very different terms: for virology, if the treatment kills the virus without killing the patient, it is a success; for immunology, the balanced well-being of the person is the ultimate criterion of success. Generally, immunology is concerned both with enhancing the natural immune response and with reducing the symptoms of the underlying disorder, symptoms which in AIDS are conceptualized as diseases in themselves.

Once a virus was identified, however, immune system support therapy was almost totally abandoned to holistic non-Western interventions, and bio-medical research was directed toward finding a 'magic bullet' along the lines of AZT. Only since 1987 has research into combination therapies for virus-blocking and immune-boosting been legitimated by the major researchers. Now Chinese herbs are licensed as research 'drugs' for investigation, and holistic therapies including meditation are considered researchable within scientific protocols. However, only the use of 'real drugs', as traditionally defined, is used as a criterion for excluding people from drug company protocols, that is, one cannot be on AZT if one wishes to enrol in the Peptide T trial. However, one may mediate, or take herbs, treatments which many claim have demonstrable effects.

Virology's assumption that a virus could simply be eliminated or blocked misdirected research efforts for nearly three years, denying thousands of patients potential therapies which might have improved their lives. The rise of black market research into both virus blockers and into immune boosting agents was not simply a function of the slowness of the research empire: it was a challenge to cultural concepts of patient, researcher and science. People living with HIV illnesses organized with sympathetic clinicians and researchers to form community research initiatives which investigated simple, often natural, organic compounds to improve morbidity. Working within an ecological/immunological framework, they confronted head-on the highly individualistic and single-response oriented research establishment as well as the cultural metaphors on which it rests.

Metaphor and Public Policy

The dominance of virological thinking has had several effects on the evolving risk reduction strategies in the US, especially since 1985 when virology and behaviourist health education each came to power in their respective venues, usurping agenda control from the community-based initiatives which had hitherto been coping with the crisis. First, virology promotes the idea that there can be a 'cure' and a 'vaccine' for HIV infection. This conveys the idea that any behavioural changes are simply stop gap measures, only necessary until science 'puts things right'. This obviously sells out on those currently infected, or on those who will become infected until virology accomplishes its feat. Moreover, it implicitly makes HIV infection a matter of moral culpability now, but a matter of chance error on a par with syphilis once there is a 'cure' or 'vaccine'. In addition, it marks AIDS as the fate of deviance, and prevents the self-identified mainstream from perceiving any need to change their behaviour, thereby preventing them from seeing their culpability for failing to change by circumscribing some sexual acts (but not others) into a danger zone.

Ultimately, identifying a cure or a vaccine depends on locating a single agent with a highly predictable outcome. HIV apparently requires some set of co-factors to produce its various chronic or fatal sequelae. Not only have at least three major forms of HIV been discovered, even within these types the virus may be such a sloppy replicator that it produces multiple variants in a single person. Moreover, because there is no clear-cut relationship between HIV infection, ARC or AIDS, HIV, like the variants of hepatitis, may not be best understood as a single pathogen at all. The mutation rate of HIV is so high that it is virtually forcing a reconceptualization of viruses in general. Viruses had previously been conceptualized as stable, not 'alive' — they replicated rather than reproduced. HIV's relative unpredictability in this respect may be the reason for its tending to elude immune response. It thereby presents a challenge to the work of virology over the past decade, in which viruses were hypothesized as non-evolutionary, unlike bacteria, which evolve to outwit the bacteriologists' drugs. These events have forced scientists to reconceptualize what is meant by 'living matter', partial hunks of DNA or RNA.

Second, the thought style of virology ignores the historical consequences of curative rather than preventive approaches to sexually transmitted disease, duplicating in this respect some of the clinical blindspots of bacteriology. These understandings enabled the particular patterns of HIV spread in the first place. But more insidiously, virology thinking, which offers a demon-invader theory of disease, implies that there is little one can do for oneself. By collapsing together HIV infection and AIDS, a move which is highly consistent with the concerns and logic of virology, both infection and the subsequent development of sequelae are lent a kind of randomness. 'Catching it' or 'avoiding it' seem to be a matter of luck rather than a matter of adopting safer sex and safer injecting practices.

The foregrounding of a virus over the array of contextual facts in individuals' lives continually anchors AIDS education to testing: it little matters what the test is for, as long as it can serve in some ideologically coherent ways to separate one social group from another. The history of HIV antibody testing is not one of technological improvement, but one of refining the method of interpreting results so as to maintain a system of meaningful difference between those who test negative and those who test postive. The test, by appearing objective rather than interpretive, has enabled repressive ideologies about sex and drug use to re-group and re-form under the guide of public safety.

'You Don't Have AIDS'

The consequences of test-backed public health interventions are both an inability to reduce overall patterns of transmission and an increase in mechanisms of discrimination. The chief mechanism for representing to the public the plausibility of AIDS science is in the HIV antibody test. A large poster currently appears on the walls of several New York City subway stations in which stark white type appears against a black background and reads, 'You don't have AIDS. Now prove it.' This is followed by the number of a testing service sponsored by a hospital. The New York City AIDS Discrimination Unit is suing to have the posters removed.[12]

The original AIDS educational message was straightforward enough, 'You cannot get HIV through casual contact, but you can become infected by receiving HIV-infected semen in anus or vagina, or by injecting HIV infected blood.' But for reasons having to do with the political economy of AIDS in the US this message was bifurcated after the 'no one is safe' media hype that followed Rock Hudson's death in 1985. Who we were to read as the 'no one', and how we were to undertand 'safety' were obscured by the science-logic which views AIDS as an absolute phenomenon and describes risk categories as fixed. AIDS education was radically altered in 1986 with the incursion of government censorship and under the influence of health education professionals largely ignorant of the social history of the AIDS. Education became divided into public versus community-targeted projects, a division which has been retained in some form uncritically in nearly every US AIDS agency. With this division in place, a new set of messages began to emerge, pared down to: 'You can't get AIDS' and 'You can get AIDS.' The problem now faced by the subject of education was not how do I avoid this virus, but which of these 'You's' am I. Am I a member of the public, or a member of a community 'at risk'? In this context, public came rapidly to mean those not at risk, and community those 'at risk', thereby encoding a system of social differences which conflates deviance and risk. But all this rests on a quite inadequate view of how identities are constucted. It implies that we each have only one relevant aspect of identity and that we consciously acknowledge it. Splitting identities and targeting messages induce a fatal disabling of an individual's interpretive powers.

Consider a gay man who is a nurse: at work he is told he cannot get AIDS, whereas at the bar or in the clubs he is told that unless he takes extraordinary precautions he will get AIDS. In the context socially constructed as 'work', he is assured that saliva cannot transmit the virus, whereas in contexts socially constructed as 'dangerous venues of sexual possibility' he is told not to 'deep kiss' his lover for fear of contracting the virus. Or take the case of young people. They are told that good citizens do not fear people with AIDS, even though it may be suggested that once upon a time 'they did'. At the same time, they are given virtually no practical information about HIV transmission in relation to the practice of sex or drugs in their own lives. The benevolence they are asked to bestow on people with AIDS is thereby directly contingent on their understanding of such people as irrevocably 'others', based on a set of sex or drug practices which intrinsically encodes deviance. Reciprocally, young people's ability to access meaningful risk reduction information is contingent on identifying with the 'other', thereby disrupting the logic of self-disengaged altruism.

The silence surrounding safer sex education for youth (except for 'hardcore, hard to reach' street youth) leaves many young people with the idea that only dangerous people need to know about safer sex. My own experience now suggests that 'dangerous' people, to those youth, are adults of approximately yuppy lifestyles. Few young people identify even 'hardcore, hard-to-reach' street youth as those who might have been infected. Few young people seem to label themselves or their peers dangerous, and thus they believe they may proceed without any special knowledge or techniques. They are smart enough to realize that there is something wrong here, but unfortunately, many are too terrified to seek proper information on their own. If asking for birth control were an admission of planning for sex, asking for safer sex information must seem like an intention to court death. The silence surrounding applied sexual and drug behaviour information for young people is as morally bankrupt as it is lethal, something which new epidemiology from the major urban areas of the US now reveals.[13] Thus differences in access to information by class, ethnicity, gender and sexuality make HIV pedagogic practices complicit in public health policing through maintaining stigmatized people in relative ill-health.

But the problem does not end here. There is a hidden ethical structure underlying information-giving models of health education which directs different strategies at what are perceived as 'high risk' and 'low risk' audiences. This is especially true of messages emanating from government agencies, with their huge investment in the research and medical power structures. Even though both sets of people are getting fact-based messages, mainstream people are given facts on the assumption that they have a *right to know*, that is, a right to protect themselves, while 'high risk' people have an *obligation* to know and act appropriately. Even if there is some awareness here that not everyone in a 'high risk' population is infected, and that increasing numbers of people in the 'general population' may be, the two groups are nevertheless defined as audiences with different reasons for needing to know the 'facts about AIDS'. Because of this hidden loading, the information giving model, at least as currently used, cannot break down the dubious idea that it is risk group susceptibilities rather than how one engages in specific sexual and drug related acts that create the possibility of HIV transmission.

The hidden moral judgment in the mode of address to the 'general population' versus 'risk groups' (or even to venues or neighbourhoods thought likely to be the sites of 'risk behaviours') means that most people engaging in risk behaviours who do not already self-identify with a subculture will not be able to apply safer sex information to themselves. They may instead seek HIV antibody testing as the means of deciding risk and determining whether they need more education. The outcry among middle-class heterosexuals, especially evident in women's magazines, mainstream newspapers and recent popular texts against practising safe sex,[14] hinges on the inherent contradiction between the right to know versus the responsibility to know encoded in numerous information-giving initiatives.

Nowadays, ordinary people are often thought ignorant when they fail to absorb the fact that 'they can't get AIDS from a doorknob' (a phrase constructed in a way that confuses the issues from the start). Gay men, prostitutes and injecting drug users are also widely believed morally derelict for refusing to be tested for HIV antibodies, even if they have been practising safer sex and needle hygiene. Thus intransigently stereotyped 'high risk' people — gay men, prostitutes, drug users, prisoners — are increasingly held legally accountable for failing to find out their HIV antibody status when they knew, or should have known, they were 'at risk'. Thus, even under the rubric of 'risk behaviours' not 'risk people', identity is collapsed with acts, even though there is no necessary correlation between them. The language of HIV epidemiological reporting continues to reinforce the equation of acts with identity, rather than suggesting that identity and community constitute a close dyad, and that it is the separateness of minority communities from the mainstream, rather than the incidence of deviant acts, that accounts for the apparent concentration of HIV among certain 'communities'. Only South Africa acknowledges the social construction of the differences which account for the uneven distribution of HIV in its use of categories such as 'white AIDS' and 'black AIDS', but this is because this regime is already aware of the ways and extent to which apartheid enhances efforts to police public health.[15]

Conclusions

In this chapter, I have emphasized the hidden power of scientific thinking because I have grown increasingly concerned about the simplistic suggestions idea that we should simply 'empower people to make decisions'. While I agree with increasing individual autonomy, it is critical to understand that we do not educate in a neutral environment. Not only are prejudice and misinformation rife, but the very educational system in which we operate implicitly loads some information with liabilities, while leaving much ignorance tolerated. And critically, the tropes and logics of science anchor this educational system, making it virtually impossible to escape certain ideas — like the notion that some people are intrinsically 'at risk' because of who they are.

People have more than a responsibility to know, more than a right to choose. People have a right to understand the ideologies of science education as processes to which they are subjected. Such a view insists that HIV/AIDS education must always be political: in the service either of the status quo which is best understood as a hegemony of sexual, class and racial ideologies shot through with moral and scientific logics, or in service of disrupting anticipated hierarchical formations of knowledge.

Notes

1 The first federal funding for AIDS education came in late 1985 and was less than $500,000. This initial funding came with a provision that federally funded education would be adjunct to HIV antibody testing and that materials should be acceptable according to 'community standards', the same language used in obscenity law. In each subsequent year, conservative North Carolina Senator Jesse Helms tried to have riders attached to funding bills which would prohibit expenditure of federal funding on any education that 'promoted homosexuality'. In 1988 the federal government finally passed a standing law which set the formula for AIDS funding, so that instead of passing a new AIDS funding bill each year only the overall dollar must now be set. Helms was successful in having an amendment attached to the enabling law prohibiting funding for education which promotes homosexuality or promiscuity.
2 This law prohibits local authorities spending money on activities which 'promote homosexuality'.
3 'Dissident vernaculars' seems a better term than 'culturally sensitive' as it moves away from a model of pristine ideas which need 'translation' to people lacking in the dominant culture's language skills or concepts. 'Dissident vernaculars' also implies resistance and places the health educator in a much different role: perhaps that of a technician rather than a translator.
4 The term 'minority communities' reads through to a range of micro-networks of resistance defined oppositionally by race, class, gender, sexuality and culture.
5 This story was reported widely and sensationally in the gay press beginning in 1985. What is significant is less whether Gallo 'stole' the virus from Luc Montagnier, but the way in which scientific competition was inscribed into the story of the epidemic from quite early on.
6 See John Lauritsen's article, 'On the AZT Front, Part 2,' in *New York Native*, 16 January 1988, pp. 16–17. This is a critique of the 25 November 1987 *Journal of the American Medical Association* report on the 'compassionate release' AZT trials, entitled 'Survival Experiences among Patients with AIDS on Zidovudine (AZT)' Lauritsen works from the data presented in the article and shows that 1120 patients, or 23 per cent were missing from the final report overall and 734 of the original 1043 patients enrolled in September 1986 were 'lost'.
7 This 'experiment' on the natural history of syphilis in black men was begun in the 1920s and ended only in the 1970s when journalists exposed the unethical practices in the study. The intricacies of the study are detailed in James Jones' (1980) book, *Bad Blood* (New York. Basic Books). The similarities of the ideologies apparent in the invention 'African AIDS' is further explored in Cindy Patton 'Inventing African AIDS' in *City Limits*, 15 September 1988, p. 85.
8 Benedict Anderson's (1986) book, *Imagined Communities* (London, Verso), suggests that there are

face-to-face 'communities' and then larger 'imagined communities' which may or may not correspond to national boundaries, linguistic groups, etc. Since, in the US, minority movements have had both a strong nationalistic tendency (including the gay movement with its economic infrastructure and geographic 'ghettos') and an emphasis on cultural autonomy conceived across geograhic limitations, the idea of 'imagined community' seemed important. In particular, the gay community is strongly related to an underground press which links geographically isolated gay men and lesbians. This accounts for the rapid dissemination and ease of understanding of early safer sex information within gay communities of quite divergent political and social norms.

9   This argument was offered despite the fact that in San Francsico it is quite easy to obtain black market anti-HIV trial drugs, and despite the fact that holistic measures are considered significant in reducing some symptoms of HIV infection and in staving off some stress-linked sequelae.

10   The paper, originally presented at the Fourth International AIDS Conference in Stockholm, began receiving extensive coverage in the gay press in April 1989, beginning with the often sensational *New York Native*.

11   Community research initiatives are not as uncommon US medical history as it might seem. The US has a long and rich history of 'science for the people' endeavours, some detailed in Paul Starr's (1982) controversial and ultimately liberalist *The Social Transformation of American Medicine* (New York, Basic Books). Nevertheless, they represent an important coalition of sensitive researchers and doctors and HIV activists in creatively designing treatment research protocols.

12   A major new argument in both the gay and medical press in favour of testing stems from the fact that early interventions are now available (in some cities, and for some people). Nevertheless, major educational efforts and the mass media continue to depict the test as diagnostic for AIDS, as a mechanism for proving you 'don't have it', and as a way of determining whether or not to practise 'safer sex'.

13   Centers for Disease Control figures for all but a handful of major metropolitan areas show that it is among the young, inner-city people, and largely people of colour that we find the highest increase in clinical cases of AIDS. This evidence suggests that many of these same individuals became HIV infected in their teens or early 20s.

14   See Jan Grover's chapter, 'Reading AIDS', in P. Aggleton, G. Hart and P. Davies (eds) (1989) *AIDS: Social Representations, Social Practices* (Lewes, Falmer Press).

15   Several officials from the South African government, including ones from the Ministry of Mining, presented papers at the Global Impact of AIDS economic summit in London, March 1988. The differential patterns of HIV-2 and HIV-1 were just being discussed. One official said offhandedly that the 'white AIDS' was among homosexuals and consisted of HIV-1, and 'black AIDS' was among heterosexuals and consisted of HIV-2. He said the historical state of apartheid had in this case provided an opportunity to see if the two HIVs progressed differently, ignoring the possibility of both interracial relations among gay men and homosexual relations among black men.

References

AGGLETON, P.J., COXON, A.P.M. and WEATHERBURN, P. (1989) *AIDS Health Promotion Activities Directed Towards Gay and Bisexual Men in London (UK): A Briefing Document Prepared for the World Health Organisation Global Programme on AIDS*. Geneva, WHO/GPA.

FLECK, L. (1978) *Genesis on Development of a Scientific Fact*. Chicago, Ill., University of Chicago Press.

GROVER, J.Z. (1989) 'Reading AIDS', in P. AGGLETON, G. HART and P. DAVIES (eds) *AIDS: Social Representations, Social Practices*. Lewes, Falmer Press.

KUHN, T.S. (1962) *The Structure of Scientific Revolutions*, Chicago, Ill., University of Chicago Press.

MASTERS, W., JOHNSON, V. and KOLODNY, R. (1988) *Crisis: Heterosexual Behaviour in the Age of AIDS*. Grove, New York.

Chapter 2

Safer Sex as Community Practice[1]

Simon Watney

Throughout the 1970s and 1980s many lesbians and gay men have been deeply involved in sustained and sometimes difficult debates concerning questions of sexual identity, representation and cultural politics (Watney, 1987; Altman *et al.*, 1989). In retrospect it almost seems as if we had been limbering up in advance to face the immensely complex and challenging problems raised by HIV disease, and the international 'pro-family' politics of the past decade. There can be little doubt that these debates over theory have substantially improved our understanding of much of the political and cultural hysteria that surrounds us, and have helped us plan effective strategic interventions on behalf of people living with HIV disease, and their various communities.

The formal title of the panel of the Fifth International Conference on AIDS in Montreal at which I gave a version of this chapter in mid-1989 — 'Eroticism, Safer Sex and Behaviour Change' — involves three distinct terms, two of which are fundamental, and one of which, the third, is frequently highly misleading. Day after day at major conferences on AIDS, and in literally hundreds of published articles, we have witnessed the ways in which the institutions of behavioural psychology and quantitative social science have recoded their latent racism, mysogyny and homophobia across the fields of epidemiology and health education — into which they have lately trespassed in search of sweeter funding pastures. Hence at Montreal we were invited to consider issues such as: 'Smoking as a Risk Factor for Heterosexual Transmission of HIV-1 in Haitian Women', and 'Hypermasculinity as a Predictor of Sexual Risk Behaviours in a Cohort of Gay Men', and the claim that: 'Childhood Gender Nonconformity Predicts HIV-1 Seropositivity in Homosexual Men'. It would appear from this that regardless of whether a gay teenager tries on his mother's shoes or his father's tweed jacket, he is equally doomed. Frankly, one might as well consider ownership of the 'July Garland at Carnegie Hall' double album as a predictor of HIV seropositivity, or indeed the possession of a pair of Levi 501 jeans. When considering the gay communities in which HIV was widely transmitted for at least a decade before its existence was even suspected, *any* aspect of our cultural lives might be selected as significant indicators or 'risk factors' by researchers who, by doing so, reveal only the depths of their ignorance of the diversity of gay culture. It is hardly surprising that many safer sex educators are infuriated by such inane 'research' at a time when resources for effective health promotion are so hard to come by, and when so many lives are potentially at stake.

Of the hundreds of research projects presented at the Fifth International Conference on AIDS, only three considered the role of health care providers from the perspective of clients. AIDS has evidently provided many social scientists with a hitherto unparalleled 'opportunity' to survey the behaviour of gay men. This amounts to no less than a grand recapitulation of just the type of deviance theory that originally constituted the modern 'homosexual' as an object of surveillance and 'knowledge'. It is therefore high time that we evaluate the methods and values of this disease-inflected scrutiny of our lives as exhaustively as its curious investigations of ourselves. This is especially important because behaviourism so critically lacks any theory of *desire*, for which it substitutes a mechanical and profoundly problematic notion of 'sex', taken as an a priori reality that blinds researchers to the multiple, uneven, shifting relations of desire to sexual behaviour and identities, both in the lives of individuals and desiring collectivities (Foucault, 1980).

Effective safer sex education requires a sensitive awareness of the finely nuanced variations of gay sexuality, understood as an extremely complex site of overlapping and frequently conflicting sexual desires, behaviour and identities in which irreducible and unconscious forces find expression in a multitude of specific concrete historical and cultural circumstances. Eroticism — that is, the pleasures of the body — is rooted in desire and desiring fantasy, while it is invariably articulated through practices that are intimately connected to contingent cultural forms and institutions. Located thus, eroticism cannot simply be switched on or off, or subjected to arbitrary re-direction. Indeed, one of the profoundest insights offered by psychoanalysis is the recognition that we should have little faith in any attempt finally to demarcate between what is, or is not, sexual — between what may or may not be desired, and experienced, as sexual pleasure. The main problem with casual notions of 'behaviour change' is their inability to approach this primary domain of sexual fantasy, on which the substitutions and displacements that constitute safer sex must be established and libidinized. For what does it mean to say that we 'know' that HIV exists, in the face of pleasures that precisely threaten to destabilize and dissolve the conscious knowing self? Indeed, sexual gratification *requires* the abandonment of the very levels of self-conscious awareness that behaviourism attempts to redress. While it may be easy to have safer sex on an initial encounter, how do we sustain it over time, how do we translate the shallow notion of 'behaviour modification' into actual erotic practices, consistent with the great complexity and diversity of individual and collective sexual fantasies?

As gay men, we were initially vulnerable to an increased rate of the transmission

HIV because we tend both to fuck and get fucked. This is the only 'mystery' of gay sex. At the same time, our generally marginalized position has encouraged a certain frankness and articulateness about sexual behaviour which should properly be considered as exemplary. It is one of the larger ironies of our times that HIV has coincided with an especially fierce conflict between rival definitions of sexual morality in the West, most evident in the increasing gulf between heterosexual expectations of marriage and the reality of sexual relationships. Indeed, marriage has perhaps never been more culturally idealized than in the period of no-fault divorce laws. In all of this we may observe that a fundamental conflict is being waged between a widespread and radical demand for an enlargement of culturally legitimate estimations of human social and sexual relations, and the institutions and discourses of a largely secularized, yet nonetheless potent, Christian cultural tradition. Lesbians and gay men are inevitably positioned at the very heart of this conflict, since on the one hand we represent the possibility of a more open model of sexual relationships cemented in an ethics of mutual consent, and on the other we constitute the very embodiment of all that is perceived to be most threatening to supposedly 'traditional' values, many of which are of comparatively recent origin. This is the context in which we should emphasize Crimp's (1988: 253) forceful argument that gay men's promiscuity 'should be seen instead as a positive model of how sexual pleasure might be pursued by and granted to everyone if those pleasures were not confined within the narrow limits of institutionalised sexuality.' In all such formulations it remains important to emphasize that 'gay men' do not represent a simple homogeneous social category, and that our sexuality contains the same diversity — both qualitatively and quantitatively — as that of any other population group defined by sexual object-choice.

The Origins of Safer Sex

It is vital to remember that gay men invented safer sex, long before the identification of HIV or the widespread availability of HIV antibody testing in the West (Watney, 1989a). Callen's (1983) ground-breaking *How to Have Sex in an Epidemic* offered both a theory and a practice of risk reduction that has stood the test of time remarkably well, and represents an approach to safer sex education that continues to contrast strongly with the vast majority of UK and US government funded initiatives, that might collectively be regarded under the heading: 'How to Give up Sex in an Epidemic'. Furthermore, both British and American government officials continue to claim that their interventions were responsible for the dramatic fall in new cases of HIV infection among gay men, in spite of the overwhelming epidemiological evidence that this took place on both sides of the Atlantic long before either government began their belated respective campaigns (Aggleton *et al.*, 1989; Evans *et al.*, 1989). As Evans *et al.* (1989) observe: 'The part played by the information campaign funded by the government in bringing about modifications in homosexual lifestyle seems to have been small. The most substantial changes had occurred before the campaign started.'

Since the earliest years of the epidemic, safer sex education among gay men has been most successful when rooted in the recognition that HIV is a community issue, requiring a community-based response. The motivation behind the non-government safer sex campaigns that led to the original fall in the incidence of HIV was the recognition that safer sex should be established as a practice for *all* gay men, regardless of known or perceived HIV antibody status. Such an approach contrasts strikingly with 'official' messages, generally targeted at isolated individuals who are assumed to be uninfected. Such 'official' campaigns seem to regard safer sex as if its adoption were akin to a personal decision to change one's brand of toothpaste, or perhaps to become a vegetarian. For example, in England the Health Education Authority's (HEA) first venture into the field of AIDS education for gay men early in 1989 simply exhorted us to 'Choose Safer Sex', as if this had not been a central aspect of gay culture for years. Moreover, advertisements as part of this campaign only appeared in the gay press, and thus never reached men having sex with men who have little or no gay identity.

Sustaining Safer Sex

The real issue facing safer sex educators working with gay men is how to sustain safer sex over time, especially since there is some evidence that social and other factors may combine to undermine its importance (Stall, 1989). The terrible scale of personal grief and loss must play a central role in this context for many individuals, especially those who do not have ready access to community-based support and counselling facilities. As Ben Schatz (1989), Director of the American public interest law firm *National Gay Rights Advocates*, has pointed out, we sometimes speak of the gay community's achievement in cutting down new cases of HIV infection to 'only' 2 or 3 per cent per annum, whereas we should be horrified by the potential loss of life that such statistics continue to imply.

It is painfully clear that in relation to the need for effective health education, gay men are still not officially regarded as a part of the 'general public' by the state or large sections of the press, in spite of the fact that in Europe, Australia and North America we have been far more terribly affected by HIV than any other section of the population. This places a tremendous weight of responsibility on non-government AIDS service organizations, which are largely founded and financed by gay men. We thus face the curious paradox of a situation in which the government in Britain can praise the work of organizations such as the Terrence Higgins Trust and the gay community as a whole, which in all other circumstances are not even acknowledged to exist, save as a general 'threat' to the rest of the supposedly heterosexual population (Watney, 1989a). Yet to obtain minimum funding, such non-government organizations have frequently found it convenient to turn their backs on the long-term volunteers who contributed so much to their early success. This 'de-gaying' process, as Patton (1985) has described it, does not automatically resolve the immediate problems of internal management and funding which it is ostensibly designed to address. Furthermore, the human resources of AIDS volunteers are limited in relation to the long-term stress of such work, and 'burn-out' is an increasingly serious factor across the entire field of HIV/AIDS-related volunteer work. In these grim circumstances, we must ask ourselves what exactly the state is for. Certainly official government funded AIDS 'information' campaigns throughout the West have consistently preferred the promotion of ideological and frankly moralistic nostrums to effective health promotion.

Unfortunately, Britain's ludicrous indecency and obscenity laws means that it is more or less impossible to develop the kinds of frank and sexually explicit safer sex materials that abound in more civilized countries such as Denmark or the Netherlands. This situation is complicated by the fact that the 'de-gaying' of non-government AIDS service organizations, and the power of conservative doctors within them, has guaranteed a widespread timidity in this vital area: one which is frequently reinforced by the fear of losing such relatively small sums of public money as have so far been made available, but upon which such organizations are entirely dependent. There is thus all the more reason to think about the ways in which safer sex is discussed, publicized and developed, especially since international evidence now demonstrates that effective safer sex education is invariably rooted in the development of collective community values. As I have written elsewhere, 'community development *is* effective AIDS education, in so far as worldwide evidence strongly suggests that gay pride has played a major factor in preventing HIV transmission by establishing safer sex not just as a set of techniques, but as a fundamental aspect of gay cultural practices' (Watney, 1989b: 44).

Strategies for Safer Sex Education

In the early years of the epidemic it was recognized that a sexually transmitted agent (or agents) was probably responsible for AIDS. Thus, before the isolation of HIV, gay men in the USA developed guidelines to help minimize the possible risk of infecting one another. Understandably, such guidelines initially listed almost every conceivable sexual practice in relation to possible risk factors. Hence the emergence of the familiar categories of 'high', 'medium' and 'low' risk sexual activities, which formed the model for subsequent materials after the isolation of HIV in 1983 and its public announcement the following year. Such lists have subsequently been expanded and modified in the light of changing epidemiological information, and new knowledge of the natural history of HIV and its modes of transmission. Yet the problem remains that this approach tends to regard safer sex simply as a series of *techniques*, rather than as a way of life, or as a question of collective *cultural practice*.

Hence the growing tendency to approach safer sex education in teams of three overlapping objectives. The first of these is to provide the most basic general information concerning which sexual practices are most potentially likely to facilitate HIV transmission. The second is to present this information in the context of specific, easily recognized situations, addressed to groups of gay men, and men who have sex with other men but who do not have a positive gay identity. Third, safer sex education aims to provide a level of general, collective cultural empowerment, encouraging us to be able to identify one another's needs, and to think of ourselves as a community united in response to the epidemic. Hence the significance of Patton's (1985) emphasis on the need to eroticize the process of negotiation that must always precede safer sex. As D'Eramo (1988: 72) argued in a leading US gay porn magazine:

> The idea that gay men have no option for sexual expression left is a common appraisal, but it simply is not true. Safer Sex itself cannot motivate us unless we eroticise it and make it more than a mere technique. Safer Sex, as a motivator, without self-esteem — a mix of self-love and caring (gay pride included) — is very limited at best, and, at worst, doomed to failure. The crux is *what* you do and *why*. And what you do is your choice. Abstinence doesn't work because when people abstain, they don't learn about Safer Sex . . . and when they get horny enough, they'll go out and break every rule in the book.

Individual and community empowerment is thus fundamental to effective safer sex education for gay men and lesbians, especially in countries such as Britain that so conspicuously lack strong political traditions founded in notions of civil rights. Furthermore, it is important to combat anti-gay prejudice in *all* forms of safer sex education targeted at heterosexuals, in the light of the possibility 'that anti-gay attitudes stand between media information and public knowledge and public opinion' (Stipp and Kerr, 1988: 12). American research conducted in San Francisco demonstrates that in the reporting of AIDS, the main determinants of media coverage were initially based on prior attitudes to gay men, which again raises the possibility 'that anti-gay attitudes constrain the ability of the media to effectively communicate information about risk factors and how the disease is transmitted' (*ibid*: 16). The same researchers also discovered that: 'as we expected, education was a significant predictor of knowledge about HIV transmission, but it accounted for considerably less variance . . . than attitudes towards gay rights' (*ibid*: 18). There is thus strong evidence to support the hypothesis that anti-gay, and also probably racist, attitudes tend to encourage the denial of heterosexual transmission among prejudiced individuals, and there is clearly an urgent need for cross-sectional studies of correlations between accurate HIV/AIDS knowledge, safer sex behaviour among heterosexuals and racist and anti-gay prejudice. It would also be extremely useful to devise research protocols to assess the role of homophobic and racist attitudes within and between different national media institutions, comparing television and the press, for example, in relation to levels of inaccuracy and conflicting information concerning all aspects of HIV/AIDS. This is especially important since most people gain such information as they may possess from such primary cultural sources.[2]

If, as seems highly likely, the routine provision of ambiguous, misleading and conflicting messages throughout the media puts viewers and readers at *increased* risk of HIV transmission, it is important to devise counter-strategies that might protect them. For example, effective safer sex education should actively encourage everyone to disregard in its entirety *any* HIV/AIDS education materials or information that continues to speak of the 'AIDS virus' or 'the AIDS test', and thus demonstrates its own inability (or refusal) to distinguish between HIV and AIDS. Other direct indicators of unreliability would include all references to so-called 'AIDS carriers', and a refusal to comply with the demands of the *Denver Principles* and the international principles established in the 1988 World Health Organization resolution concerning the avoidance of discrimination in relation to HIV-infected people and people with AIDS.[3] This in turn would constitute an immediate and easily achievable form of individual and collective empowerment that is the prerequisite for adopting and sustaining safer sex over time. Such an approach encourages people to read critically, and to make their own assessments of health education materials and all other sources of supposed 'information'. It recognizes that safer sex education should aim to provide not only generalized short-term information but also longer-term focused campaigns and strategies to counteract unjustified fears and anxieties that may derive from cultural sources, including politics and religious fundamentalism, which seek to legitimize prejudice. It also refuses any suggestion that sex is simply an autonomous 'behaviour', like driving or fixing one's hair. It must continualy be asserted that one does not take up, or stick with safer sex in the same way that one might choose a new car, or consider changing one's favourite brand of hair gel.

It is particularly regrettable that many governments have entrusted their national HIV/AIDS education campaigns to commercial advertising agencies, and have turned their backs on the accumulated findings of decades of research in health education and health promotion. As the distinguished medical historian Brandt (1988: 369) points out: 'The limited effectiveness of education which merely encourages fear is well-documented.' Yet this is totally ignored by many governments throughout the world. For example, in Britain the HEA has been subject to heavy state pressure in relation to all aspects of HIV/AIDS education. A recent HEA campaign included a two-page advertisement that appeared throughout the British press in the early months of 1989. It showed a very glamorous young woman, staring seductively out from the page, looking at us over her bare shoulder. She looks very much like a television actress from *Dallas* or *Dynasty*. Beneath the image there is a text which reads: 'If This Woman Had the Virus Which Leads to AIDS in a Few Years She Could Look Like the Person over the Page'. Turning the page, we find — the same photograph, but this time it appears with a caption that simply states: 'Worrying Isn't It'. There is not even a question mark here to raise any doubts about the intended meaning. As I have written elsewhere, 'Throughout the entire campaign, people with HIV infection or disease appear only as anonymous deterrents, rather than people who need to be seen as very much like any newspaper readers — as ordinary people. This is clearly because at some basic level they are not regarded in this way by the advertising agency or the HEA' (Watney, 1989a: 33). It is difficult to think of any other group of people living with long-term disease who could be considered 'worrying' because they look perfectly well!

The HEA's most recent campaigns have all shared a common by-line: 'AIDS. You're as Safe as You Want to Be'. This significantly places all responsibility for HIV transmission on the isolated individual, and clearly colludes with both the example just given and many other such advertisements, in the implication that people with HIV or AIDS constitute a threat that only the individual can avoid. Yet such campaigns never attempt to provide practical safer sex advice, beyond conflicting messages such as: 'Having fewer partners is only one way to reduce the risk. Safer sex also means using a condom, or alternatively, having sex that avoids penetration.' Encouraging people to talk about sex is at least as important as condom use, and this is especially important for population groups like many British heterosexuals, that may be characterized as hysterically modest and all but pathologically inhibited in their ability to discuss sex. One medium that might almost have been designed to meet the needs of safer sex education, domestic video, is unfortunately subject to far stricter legal controls than in any other European country except for the Republic of Ireland. Most British HIV/AIDS videos have therefore tended to be extraordinarily dreary, with little or no attention being paid to sexual desire or practice.

Homophobia, 'Lifestyles' and 'Addiction'

The underlying puritanism that determines so much British legal moralism may also be widely found in national safer sex materials, which often seem to be affected by a refusal or inability to acknowledge the diversity of sexual behaviour, even among lesbians and gay men. While it is clear that safer sex aims to minimize the transmission of HIV by preventing semen getting into the rectum or the vagina, this does *not* mean that effective sex education works by telling people not to fuck. It is certainly not helpful to pretend, for example, that many lesbians do not enjoy both anal and vaginal penetration, or that 'non-penetrative sex' is some kind of ideal goal independent of safer sex, as some feminists strongly imply. Indeed, it should be noted that safer sex education has provided an opportunity for sexual puritans of all persuasions to rush into print and workshops, whether from the perspective of revolutionary feminism or from other forms of evangelical culture. Such strongly directive approaches are only likely to encourage resistance, which can prove very dangerous. We should be very cautious of ostensible safer sex advisers and 'experts' who seem more interested in promoting their particular moral beliefs than in trying to understand and respect the full range of their clients' consensual sexual needs and pleasures.

This is especially important when many of the lesbians and gay men who developed the early models of effective safer sex education are either leaving non-government organizations as the result of burn-out, or because they feel they can no longer work within increasingly bureaucratic structures that are often more concerned with 'not rocking the boat' than meeting the needs of those constituencies most at risk from HIV. It is crucial that lesbians and gay men do not collude with such processes in desperately underfunded non-government organizations, which are often directed by boards and board members who have little or no understanding of the basic issues of safer sex education. For we have an absolute responsibility to our various lesbian and gay communities, in all their diversity, and especially to those whom no one else is prepared to support — gay teenagers, racial minorities, the elderly and the disabled. It is worth pointing out that 15 per cent of people with AIDS diagnosed in Nice are over 60.[4] While it is frequently, and correctly, pointed out that HIV has had a disproportionate impact on the black and Hispanic population of the United States, this same structure of argument is *never* employed in Britain to describe the impact of HIV on gay men. This is presumably because gay men are not regarded as proportionally comparable to heterosexuals in the first place. The sheer scale and efficiency of British homophobia often seem all but overwhelming, and insuperable. For example, the leading London weekly magazine, *Time Out*, recently compiled a long list of subjects that are supposedly 'In' and 'Out' for the summer of 1989. Thus sex, we learned, is 'In', together with comics, the singer Madonna and Batman. Food and political comedy are 'Out'. So, apparently, is AIDS: 'Do you want to be bored to death?' asked *Time Out*.[5]

Such attitudes do not lack more sophisticated exponents. For example, the same team of epidemiologists that reported the fall in new cases of HIV infection among gay men in the UK write of the epidemic from which their statistics derive in a manner that reveals an extraordinary ignorance about human sexuality. Hence their bizarre and insulting hypothesis that 'the profound consequences of HIV infection might have been expected to suppress the expression of a homosexual lifestyle in younger men' (Evans *et al.*, 1989: 217). It is precisely such 'expectations' that reveal much about the attitudes of professional social scientists and other involved in AIDS 'research'. What might the readers of the *British Medical Journal*, where their report was published, have made of the claim that 'the profound consequences of HIV infection might have been expected to suppress the expression of a *heterosexual* lifestyle in younger men'? It is the stark double-standard applied to gay men in relation to heterosexuals that is so alarming.

The key term in these and allied debates is that of 'lifestyle', which is frequently used throughout the AIDS literature to refer to gay men in such a way that it protects the unstated but underlying assumption of a 'natural' heterosexuality, from which homosexuality is regarded as a voluntary aberration. This provides an ostensibly 'scientific' legitimation for any amount of scapegoating and victim-blaming.

It is this notion of 'lifestyle' that also unites the discourses of epidemiology and 'official' HIV/AIDS 'education' materials. Karpf (1988) has described the emergence of what she terms the 'look-after-yourself' model of health education in the late 1970s. From such a perspective 'illness is the result of harmful individual habits or a "lifestyle" undertaken voluntarily — eating the wrong foods, drinking too much, smoking, lack of exercise, and stress' (Karpf, 1988: 16). The 'look-after-yourself' approach to health education was intended to combat an overly medical view of health, for which it simply substitutes a highly voluntaristic picture of individuals 'taking charge' of their lives, and rejecting previous 'unhealthy' and irresponsible' lifestyles. As such, it has been widely instituted in many health education campaigns, although, as Karpf (1988: 17) points out, it assumes that individuals possess 'unqualified powers to shape their lives, with their future well-being their priority'. This also involves a virtual suppression of any consideration of the many powerful contingent circumstances that may inform decision-making. It is also a particularly inadequate approach in relation to questions of sexual behaviour, which comes to be seen as a simple arena of conscious choices, rather than as a complex arena of intense commercial and cultural pressures that compete to arouse and satisfy the workings of sexual fantasy. Finally, there is the added problem of creeping moralism that may inform distinctions between supposedly 'healthy' and 'unhealthy' sex, in a rhetoric that can easily slide into frank homophobia. It is especially important to reject spurious and highly misleading analogies between sexual behaviour and chemical addictions. These compound the double error of regarding smoking or alcoholism or narcotic drug use as purely personal, individual phenomena, while suggesting that any form of sexual activity outside the context of a full social and emotional relationship should also be regarded as shameful and damaging.[6] Such an approach is entirely incompatible with the aims and methods of effective safer sex education.

From the Individual to the Collective

The HIV epidemic also coincides historically with a quite separate crisis in the overall management and 'political economy' of sex and sexuality in the modern world. For example, state-directed HIV/AIDS 'education' campaigns have afforded an ideal opportunity for many governments to develop new strategies in their constant struggle to win popular consent to their larger political objectives in relation to population management and social policy. Not surprisingly, such strategies have stimulated widespread resistance, and it seems that levels of HIV/AIDS-related ignorance, prejudice and denial are highest in those countries such as Britain that have been bombarded with explicitly moralistic and directive kinds of AIDS 'education'. Hence the increased difficulties experienced by non-government AIDS service organizations that are obliged to face and deal with the direct consequences of campaigns which Patton has brilliantly characterized as: 'Too much, too late'.[7] These consequences include a steady escalation of the 'worried well' needing attention, and the drying up of funding for a 'problem' which it is erroneously believed has been resolved via government posters and television advertising.

This is why it is so vitally important to continue to emphasize that safer sex education should be concerned with developing individual and collective self-esteem in relation to *erotic* practice. For most official HIV/AIDS 'education' has only tended to reinforce negative perceptions of safer sex as a system of imposed constraints, that are only able to be complied with reluctantly, from motives of guilt and fear. It is unlikely that significant numbers of people will be able to sustain safer sex over time from such a perspective, which is also likely actively to discourage the adoption of safer sex on the part of the many others. Nor can mechanical behaviourist analyses explain the failure of such campaigns, save in terms of individual 'non-compliance', or so-called 'sexual addiction'. In the meantime, the delusion that HIV is only a risk from extraordinary sources that are external to the lives of decent, ordinary folk is casually reinforced.

It does not require a close psychoanalytic reading of government sponsored HIV/AIDS 'health education' materials to demonstrate their profound dread of an active, autonomous female sexuality, as exemplified in the 'Worrying Isn't it' campaign. Such fear on the part of many heterosexual men is evidently displaced and projected onto gay men, who are literally required to be 'feminized' in much public AIDS commentary. For effective HIV/AIDS education inevitably draws attention to the simple but clearly controversial fact that when everything is considered, *all* forms of consensual human sexual behaviour amount to much of a muchness. This is seemingly very disturbing to sexual identities that are massively stabilized by exaggerated notions of gender specificity, and the imagined 'otherness' of such supposedly unified categories as 'women' or 'homosexuals'. In this manner, possibly painful divisions in the self may be conveniently projected onto 'other people', and expressed as contempt. This process seems to be far more common among heterosexuals than lesbians or gay men. Indeed, the widespread phobic dread of AIDS that manifests itself daily in tabloid journalism and in the helpless compulsive HIV antibody testing of the 'worried well' is not unconnected to the fantasized perception that HIV infection implies a direct, if mediated, physical relationship with the bodies of gay men or people of colour, Dread of HIV infection thus speaks an excessive fear of transgressing profound social and psychic boundaries that evidently stabilize many aspects of heterosexual identity. That heterosexual identity may often *require* to be bolstered by the forces of unconscious homophobia and racism is a conjecture that deserves further enquiry. It may well be easier for some people to think of HIV in terms of miasmatic contagion, than to confront the actual modes of transmission that cannot be admitted to consciousness, for whatever reasons.

Notions of HIV antibody testing or quarantine as effective measures for the primary prevention are in this context only the most transparent re-inscription of those boundaries and categories forged by repression, that are experienced by many as indispensable to their most basic (if vulnerable) sense of self. Thus the struggle to achieve a psychic goal of masculinity or femininity may be rationalized and articulated in the readily available language of disease control. We should also recall that the available categories and identities of modern Western sexuality were originally constituted in a heavily medicalized discourse of sickness and health. Much of the imagery of AIDS was thus ready and waiting, and is by no means specific to the epidemic. When entire societies succumb to the excessive symptoms of sexual repression and anxiety, the consequences can be grim inded — as the history of HIV/AIDS-related legislation in such countries as Britain, Cuba, Sweden and the USA demonstrates with alarming clarity (Breum and Hendriks, 1988).

While such theoretical speculation may seem overly abstract to some, it is precisely *because* we face such a grim reality that we need to exercise all the intellectual adroitness of which we are capable. For Europeans like myself, who have helplessly watched the virtual decimation of an entire generation of fellow gay men, including many dear and much loved friends in cities throughout the United States, it is of the greatest importance to try to understand the continued denial of adequate funding and support for basic health care provision, health education, housing, anti-discrimination legislation and clinical trials of possible drugs for use in the treatment of HIV disease. It is our ethical and political responsibility to try our best, in the midst of a crisis that is frequently all but physically and emotionally overwhelming, to learn such lessons in order to be able to anticipate and counteract such tendencies in Europe, where the provision of socialized medicine and more enlightened social welfare policies have not prevented widespread discrimination against people living with HIV and AIDS, as well as their communities. As increasing numbers of gay men opt for the HIV antibody test as a means of access to good patient management, we can learn from the unexpected consequences of changing attitudes towards testing in the USA. For example, Helquist (1989: 30) has recently pointed out that 'organisations, like individuals, may also encounter conflicts . . . . Some AIDS activist groups have found that their seropositive members give top priority to AIDS treatment issues, while seronegative members want to emphasize prevention and policy concerns.'

In the present circumstances, we should emphasize that questions concerning safer sex education and treatment issues are not alternatives, but are strictly complementary, and of equal significance. Effective health education depends on the recognition that safer sex is an ongoing necessity for all gay men, regardless of our known or perceived HIV antibody status. At the same time, the need for ethically acceptable clinical trials for potential treatment drugs is equally an issue for *everyone* in the various communities affected by HIV disease. For nobody can know for sure if and when they might need them. And as Nick Partridge from the Terrence Higgins Trust has argued, there must be no question of our being any less supportive of people who may contract HIV in the future than we are of people living with HIV today.[8] In the meantime we need to sustain the development of the erotics of safer sex in the context of a morality that is founded on respect for diversity and choice, and which accords with Foucault's (1989: 330) rejection of any form of morality that seeks to be acceptable to everyone: 'in the sense that everyone would have to submit to it' — an aim that he identifies as 'catastophic'. It is precisely that aim which underpins so much official government sponsored HIV/AIDS 'education' around the world, a project that aspires to tether sexual identity ever more restrictively to the twin poles of 'the family' and the nation-state.

The erotics of safer sex remain the only effective means by which we can challenge and resist the literally deadly consequences of a stunting moralism that refuses to accept that *all* our consensual sexual needs are equally valid. This project is necessarily provisional, and closely contingent upon changing circumstances and available resources, including those of creative imagination. Safer sex constitutes both an erotics *and* an ethics; it has established a set of collective cultural practices that combine the affirmation of sexual desire in all its forms with an active, practical commitment to mutual care and responsibility. As the state and its many attendant institutions continue to look on, indifferent to our plight, we have enlarged our concept of gay identity that was forged in the tradition of gay pride, insisting that gay identity should *mean* safer sex. It is from this perspective that we now evaluate the dominant political and sexual rationalities of our times with a mixture of astonishment and horror. We are astonished by the relentless strategies of naked bio-medical policing that now passes for HIV/AIDS 'education' in so many parts of the world. We are horrified by the refusal of the state to accept its responsibilities to the complex population whose allegiance it claims.

As the epidemic worsens, we can only reasonably expect the gulf between these two models of HIV/AIDS prevention, and their respective research methods and priorities, to widen. The situation in Britain is very uneven. On the one hand, it is clear that younger people have a far more open-minded and generally sophisticated approach to questions of sex and sexuality than their parents and grandparents. On the other, it is equally apparent that older traditions — of moralism, of education, of party politics, of sexual and class identities — continue to dominate the field of cultural practice and cultural reproduction. Non-government AIDS service organizations are praised in public by government ministers, yet prevented from undertaking fully effective safer sex education in a period of ever-increasing state censorship. The government has also set its face against all forms of health education rooted in the hated concept of community development, while a leading spokesman for the Medical

Research Council, which supervises HIV/AIDS-related biochemical research, has publicly stated that he believes that treatment research raises a 'moral dilemma' since it might 'prolong the lives of people who would be infectious in the community' (Watney, 1989a: 18). The gulf between such 'pure science' researchers and the day-to-day lived experience of directly involved doctors and nurses faithfully duplicates the gulf between the rival models of health education that this chapter has considered. We cannot expect an easy or immediate resolution of these divisions, since HIV/AIDS education inevitably involves issues that are heavily loaded in political and ideological terms, from 'the family', national identity and gay rights to the complex realities of prostitution and injecting drug use in contemporary Britain. The attempted sexual counter-revolution that is such a central plank of British government policy means that effective HIV/AIDS education will continue to take place under the closest scrutiny of politicians and scandal-mongering journalists. The struggle between rival models of safer sex education meanwhile involves fundamental matters of life and death, and in the coming years it is likely to prove, for many, a fight to the death.

Notes

1 This is an extended version of a presentation given on 7 June 1989 as part of the 'Eroticism, Safer Sex and Behaviour Change' panel at the Fifth International Conference on AIDS, Montreal, Canada. It develops ideas originally presented in a paper, 'Theorising Rumour in Relation to Perceptions of Risk', at the Third Conference on Social Aspects of AIDS.
2 I am not aware of any such research in the UK. The current ESRC funded work of the Glasgow Media Group has no such specific aims.
3 The *Denver Principles* on the treatment and reporting of people living with AIDS date from 1983 and are reprinted in M. Callen (ed.) (1988) *Surviving and Thriving with AIDS: Collected Wisdom*, Vol. 2. (New York, People with AIDS Coalition). The forty-first World Health Assembly adopted a clear set of anti-discriminatory resolutions as WHA 41.24 in Geneva on 13 May 1988.
4 See the *British Medical Journal*, 297, 1197.
5 See 'Ins and Outs', *Time Out*, 977, 19.
6 See Ellen Herman's article 'Getting to Serendipity: Do Addiction Programs sap our Political Vitality?', in *Outlook*, Summer 1988, pp. 10–22.
7 Personal communication.
8 Personal communication.

References

AGGLETON, P., COXON, T. and WEATHERBURN, P. (1989) *Aids Health Promotion Activities Directed towards Gay and Bisexual Men in London (UK): A Briefing Document Prepared for the World Health Organisation Global Programme on AIDS*. Geneva, WHO/EPA.
ALTMAN, D., *et al.* (1989) *Which Homosexuality?* London, Gay Men's Press.
BRANDT, A. (1988) 'AIDS in Historical Perspective: Four Lessons from the History of Sexually Transmitted Diseases', *American Journal of Public Health*, 78, 4, p. 369–92.

BREUM, M, and HENDRIKS, A. (1988) *AIDS and Human Rights: An International Perspective*. Copenhagen, Akademisk Forlag.

CALLEN, M. (1983) *How to Have Sex in an Epidemic*, New York, News From The Front Publications.

CRIMP, D. (1988) 'How to Have Promiscuity in an Epidemic', in D. Crimp (ed.), *AIDS: Cultural Analysis, Cultural Activism*. Cambridge, Mass., Massachusetts Institute of Technology.

D'ERAMO, J. (1988) 'New Sex — Building a Gay Renaissance', *Mandate*, 14, 4, p. 72.

EVANS, A., *et al.* (1989) 'Trends in Sexual Behaviour and Risk Factors among Homosexual Men, 1984–87', *British Medical Journal*, 298, pp. 215–18.

FOUCAULT, M. (1980) *The History of Sexuality*, Vol. 1. New York, Vintage Books.

FOUCAULT, M, (1989) 'The Return of Morality', in S. Lotringer (ed.), *Foucault Live*. New York, Semiotext(e).

HELQUIST, M. (1989) 'The Helquist Report', *The Advocate*, 519, p. 30.

KARPF, A. (1988) *Doctoring the Media: The Reporting of Health and Medicine*. London, Routledge.

PATTON, C. (1985) *Sex and Germs: The Politics of AIDS*. Boston, Mass., South End Press.

SCHATZ, B. (1989) 'Coverage of Selected Drugs under State Medical Assistance (Medicaid) Programs in the USA'. Paper presented at the Fifth International Conference on AIDS, Montreal, Canada.

STALL, R. (1989) Implications of Relapse from Safer Sex', *Focus*, 4, 3, p. 3.

STIPP, H. and KERR, D. (1988) 'Determinants of Public Opinion about AIDS'. Paper presented at the annual meeting of the American Association for Public Opinion Research, Toronto, Canada.

WATNEY, (1987) *Policing Desire: Pornography, AIDS and the Media*. London, Comedia/Methuen.

WATNEY, S. (1989a) 'Introduction', in E. Carter and S. Watney (eds) *Taking Liberties: AIDS and Cultural Politics*. London, Serpent's Tail.

WATNEY, S. (1989b) ' A Common Tragedy: The Politics of AIDS', *Gay Times*, 130, pp. 42–5.

WATNEY, S. (1989c) 'Tasks in AIDS Research', *Gay Times*, 128, pp. 18–19.

Chapter 3

AIDS Invulnerability: Relationships, Sexual Behaviour and Attitudes among 16–19-Year-Olds

Dominic Abrams, Charles Abraham, Russell Spears and Deborah Marks

There are two pressing questions concerning young people and HIV: first, to what extent are young people at risk of HIV infection and, second, how can any existing risk be minimized? Both questions invite answers from many different perspectives of which the medical, socio-psychological and educational are perhaps most pertinent. In 1987 the Economic and Social Research Council (ESRC) funded a number of research projects designed to explore the social, attitudinal and behavioural aspects of the two questions. The Dundee project was the first to begin and was more modest in its aims than some of the others. Nevertheless, we hoped to clear some ground for future research and establish some of the key areas for investigation. In this chapter we describe the project and present some of its early findings, including important differences due to the sex and age of respondents. We conclude by drawing implications for health education policy and practice in relation to HIV infection.

Background

In 1986 little was known about young people's social and sexual behaviour in Britain. The lack of social scientific knowledge about young people had become a focus for theory and research in sociology, education and social psychology. In particular, the Economic and Social Research Council (ESRC) had just received final reports from projects under its Young People in Society initiative, and another (the '16–19 initiative') was under way. However, both of these initiatives, and other youth research (e.g. Hendry, 1983) tended to concentrate on political, economic and leisure activities. Thus, while much was being discovered about attitudes to new technology, about women workers in traditionally male occupations, about identity development, and political ideology, little if anything was being asked about another major area of change during adolescence, namely sexual behaviour. In this research context, with

AIDS becoming increasingly important as a public issue, it was clear that existing major research programmes had little to offer. First wave data from the 16–19 initiative longitudinal cohort study of 16–19-year-olds in Kirkcaldy, Fife, revealed that there were important sex and cohort differences in attitudes towards relationships, sex, homosexuality and sex roles (Abrams, 1987). Unfortunately, these issues had only been touched on using a few questionnaire items, and it was clear that a separate project would be required to explore AIDS-relevant issues more specifically. An important objective was to provide useful information which would increase the effectiveness of health educators and professionals in preventing future cases of HIV infection.

Context

Dundee seemed to be an important and interesting location in which to conduct research for a number of reasons. It is a small city of about 200,000 people set on the north bank of the Tay estuary in Scotland, north of Fife and Edinburgh, east of Perth and south of Aberdeen. Its major industries had undergone major decline during the past twenty years; the city had lost its carpet, jute, tyre and other factories. Recently, it failed to attract the Ford motor company to set up a new factory, and the city missed out on most of the North Sea oil development. It is known for having one of the highest proportions of working-class people in any city in Britain, and bears a high level of unemployment.

For many young people, post-school destinations are the Youth Training Scheme followed by casual or part-time work, or unemployment. The city is relatively isolated from other urban centres and its residents are not particularly geographically mobile. It is also physically divided by major inner-ring roads and through roads. Facing the estuary, at the west end are the prestigious buildings, large hotels, Dundee University and predominantly middle-class housing. Behind this are large council estates ('schemes') of which the most notorious are the high rise developments. These are starved of community resources and are noted areas of multiple deprivation. Prostitution and needle sharing among injecting drug users are supposedly commonplace in these schemes.

By 1986 it was already becoming clear that Dundee, along with Edinburgh, was experiencing a disproportionately high incidence of HIV infection. Edinburgh's arts festival and commerce make it a cosmopolitan city in which, unlike Dundee, a substantial proportion of HIV antibody positive people are gay men. Dundee is a conservative city in which homosexuality remains relatively covert. The majority of people identified as HIV antibody positive were injecting drug users, and that is still the case today (February 1989). Of 143 HIV antibody positive men and 60 HIV women, 117 and 43 (respectively) are heterosexual injecting drug users.

Theoretical Framework

Our research was theory driven. In general we aimed to relate a series of background variables including sex, age, class, locality and religion to intentions and actions regarding condoms, sexual behaviour and relationships, prejudice and AIDS-preventive behaviour. These considerations determined the content of the main survey questionnaires. At the outset we specified that four general theoretical perspectives seemed particularly relevant for exploring the social and cognitive processes mediating the relationship between background variables and intentions and actions. We assume that intentions and actions also feed back into the various social and cognitive processes.

First, social identity theory (Hogg and Abrams, 1988; Tajfel and Turner, 1979) provides a useful framework for understanding the intergroup dynamics of prejudice and social distance from social categories (for example, gay men, haemophiliacs, people with AIDS, etc.) as well as the motivational basis for these phenomena (Abrams and Hogg, 1988). The more recently developed self-categorization theory (Turner, 1985) outlines the cognitive consequences of social identity for perception of social norms. Second, we aimed to explore how far rational decision-making theories such as the theory of planned behaviour (Ajzen and Madden, 1986) and the health belief model (Becker, 1974; Rosenstock, 1974), which propose that intentions and behaviour can be predicted from various combinations of attitudes and values, could account for AIDS-preventive behaviour. Third, we drew upon theories of decision biases (notably prospect theory) to investigate the manner in which perceptions of the costs and benefits relative to the risks incurred, of various preventive actions, might be distorted according to the perspective of the perceiver (cf. Kahneman and Tversky, 1982). Finally, we referred to theories of social influence, including minority influence theory (Moscovici and Mugny, 1983) and referent informational influence (Hogg and Turner, 1987), reference group theory (Hyman and Singer, 1967) and Emlers's (1984) approach to reputation management. These seemed useful in considering both the *sources* and *modes* of influence. Sources include impersonal information, social categories and reference groups, and significant relationships of various kinds. Modes include informational and normative influence, social comparison and self-evaluation (see Abrams and Hogg, in press, for a review).

The Study

The project reported on here is a longitudinal cohort study of two groups of young people. The first involves a cohort of 16- and another of 18-year-olds in Dundee and Kirkcaldy, and the second is a cohort of first- and another of third-year undergraduate students at Dundee University and Dundee Institute of Technology. In addition, small samples of gay men and attenders at the Dundee and Perth Genito-Urinary Medicine clinics are being surveyed once only. The present chapter reports only on findings from the first wave for the cohorts of 16- and 18-year-olds. Respondents were sent a postal questionnaire, and a subsample was invited to participate in follow-up interviews. At the time of writing, the first wave of questionnaire and interview data are being analyzed, and a second wave questionnaire is being designed.

In February 1987, following negotiation with the Director of Education for Tayside, the rectors of all secondary schools in Dundee (and two comparison schools in Kirkcaldy) were asked whether they would be willing to release name and address lists of the pupils currently in their fifth year (S4) as well as those who had been on the list two years previously. Only three of the rectors refused (one on the basis that his school did not consider itself to be part of Dundee, another because he was anxious that parents might object, and a third because he did not have time owing to the teachers' pay dispute). Pilot research, which had started the previous October, culminated in a trial questionnaire being sent to 100 young people not included in the main survey. On the basis of the response distributions and extensive written comments from respondents, the questionnaire was reduced, revised and finalized in early April. In May we sent letters to all pupils on the list who were or would be over 16 years of age in April, saying we would later be sending them a confidential questionnaire and asking them to return a prepaid note to inform us if they did not wish to participate in the survey. Accounting for unobtainable addresses and refusals, we were left with an obtainable base of 1078 participants for the survey. Questionnaires were sent out at the end of May, and non-returns were followed up with a written and then a telephone reminder. The final response rate was 64 per cent (690), of whom 280 were young men, 410 were young women, 303 were from the older cohort and 387 were from the younger cohort.

Demographically the sample was very homogeneous: 95 per cent were of Scottish origin, 97.8 per cent were single, and 93.3 per cent lived in their parental home. Social class was measured using the Registrar General's classification according to father's occupation (a similar pattern is obtained when mother's occupation is included). The majority of respondents were from social classes C2, C1 and B (87.9 per cent). Of the 42.2 per cent claiming they were brought up according to a religion, 38.8 per cent were Protestant and 42.7 per cent were Catholic. The most popular national paper was *The Sun* (25.6 per cent), and the most popular local paper, the *Dundee Courier* (52.1 per cent). Both newspapers are sympathetic to the Conservative Party. However, of the 81.7 per cent who expressed a preference, 58 per cent supported the Labour Party, 19 per cent the SNP and only 10.7 per cent the Conservative Party.

Romantic and Sexual Involvement

The first task was to establish a profile of the romantic and sexual relationships experienced by respondents. Pilot research had established that a range of terms was used to describe various degrees of romantic involvement, but the the term 'going steady' was accepted as meaning having a medium- to long-term mutual emotional commitment. Since images of commitment and trust may be central to people's perception of prospective partners' likelihood of being HIV antibody positive, respondents were asked, using a free response format, how long a relationship had to last before it could be described as 'steady'. Interestingly, no clear consensus emerged. Respondents were as likely to suggest one month or less as six months or more (mean = 18.09 weeks, sd = 16.70 weeks, mode = 4 weeks). Moreover, there were no significant differences due to sex or cohort.

As can be seen in Table 1a, young women generally were more experienced in terms of romantic involvement. This is unsurprising in the light of previous research which has indicated that they tend to be a couple of years ahead of young men in forming romantic attachments (see Abrams, 1989, for a review). This has potentially a major impact on their social networks and leisure behaviour. However, for the present sample, the difference between the sexes was small, and was only significant on the measure of whether respondents had *ever* had a steady partner (Chi-square = 4.0, p < .05). What is clear is that respondents overwhelmingly did report having experienced romantic involvement, and roughly half of them described themselves as currently having a steady partner. Although the younger and older cohorts were equally likely to have had some romantic involvement in the past, the older cohort was much more likely to be involved currently (Chi-square = 29.1, p < .0001). This supported our prior assumption that the age span in this survey would be one in which fairly substantial increases in romantic involvement were taking place. Rather surprisingly, there was no significant sex difference in this pattern.

Another suprising finding in view of young women's greater interpersonal maturity was that young men were likely to have had more steady partners than young women (means = 2.25, 1.54; F = 11.30, p < .001). Specifically, although 26.9 per cent of young men had never had a steady partner and a further 49.6 per cent had had only one or two, men are more likely than women to have had four or more

Table 1a. Cell Percentages for Having 'Steady Partners' by Sex and Cohort

	Sex		Cohort	
	Male	Female	Younger	Older
Have partner now	45.0	50.6	39.2	60.3
Ever had partner	88.2	93.0	89.4	92.7

Table 1b. Percentage of Males and Females Indicating Different Numbers of Steady
Partners

	Steady partners			
	0	1–3	4–6	7+
Males	25.4	58.2	9.3	7.1
Females	28.0	63.1	5.5	1.3

partners (Chi-square (3df) = 21.98, p < .001). The percentage distributions in Table 1b illustrate this point.[1]

A similar pattern emerges on several other measures, such as a general index of romantic activity during the past year. This was based on responses to five items which asked whether the respondent had started going out with, 'gone steady' with, broken up with, gone out with different, and gone out with only one person. The response format was never, once, more than once in the last year. Thus the index reflects both the range and frequency of romantic activity. (Scoring on some items was reversed, and the summed score was divided by 3 to give scores on a scale from 1 (no involvement) to 5 (high involvement).) The alpha coefficient for this scale was 0.84. While older men were more active than younger men (means = 3.27, 3.09), the reverse was true for women (means = 3.10, 3.29) (F = 5.45, p < .05). More importantly, in terms of the frequency of new partners, on the item which asked whether the respondent had been 'going out with a steady partner but seeing others', young men were more likely to say 'once' or 'more than once' than were young women (Chi-square = 8.57, p < .05), as shown in Table 2.

Table 2. Sex Differences in Answers to the Question:
'In the last year have you ever been going out with a steady partner but seeing others'?

	Males	Females	Both
		(percentages)	
Never	82.0	89.7	86.7
Once	11.5	7.2	8.9
More than once	6.5	3.1	4.4

Evidence for the validity of the question concerning whether or not respondents currently had a steady partner is provided by answers to a question which asked for an estimate of the proportion of people of the respondent's own age that currently had steady partners. Young men perceived their peers as less likely to have a steady partner than did young women (47.3 per cent and 54.1 per cent respectively), and younger respondents perceived peers as less likely to have partners than did older respondents (49 per cent and 54 per cent respectively), (Fs = 18.61, 11.77; ps < .001). These differences in perceptions match the actual differences fairly closely.

Sexual Experience

Sexual experience was asked about separately because the pilot study revealed that a substantial proportion of respondents had romantic but not sexual relationships, and that when these were introduced in conjunction, the questions were intimidating to less experienced respondents. Indeed, some reported feeling mildly insulted by the presumption that having a partner implied engaging in sexual intercourse. Another lesson from the pilot research was that the term 'sex' covers a multitude of acts (cf. Coxon, 1987). It was important therefore both to define terms precisely and to ask about both penetrative and non-penetrative sex. At the first enquiry about sexual behaviour, the term 'have sex' was defined as meaning having penetrative sexual intercourse, as distinct from engaging in 'sex but not having intercourse'.

Men and older respondents reported having had substantially more sexual partners than women and younger respondents (F(sex) = 25.2, F(cohort) = 16.7, ps < .0001). The major shift appears to be between the younger and older men (F(sex x cohort) = 4.77, p < .05), as shown in Table 3. These cohort differences illustrate that the age groups span a period of considerably increased sexual activity. Moreover, 16.4 per cent of men and 22.9 per cent of women reported having had sex for the first time ever in the previous year, as did 21.1 per cent of the older and 19.4 per cent of the younger cohort. Men were more than twice as likely to have had sex several times during the past year (Chi-square = 104.23, p < .0001). Finally, respondents were asked whether they expected to have sex with someone in the next twelve months: 62 per cent of women and 73.0 per cent of men (Chi-square = 7.77, p < .01), and 77.2 per cent of older and 57.8 per cent of younger respondents (Chi-square = 25.77, p < .0001) expected to have sex. The responses to these items indicate quite clearly that approximately 20 per cent of each age group starts to engage in sexual intercourse in any one year. Presumably the rate of increase slows, but it could be reasonably be predicted that approximately 80–90 per cent of the older cohort will have had sexual intercourse by the time they reach 20.

Table 3. Cell Means for Number of Different Sexual Partners by Sex and Cohort

	Males	Females	Both
Older	4.64	1.69	2.90
Younger	1.96	0.83	1.28
Both	2.17	1.21	1.99

AIDS Information

The rapid increase in both romantic and sexual activity among 16–19-year-olds means that it is crucial to establish where young people find out about HIV and AIDS, and how likely they think their peers and themselves are to become infected. Respondents were asked whether they had ever been taught about a number of AIDS-relevant topics at school, and, if so, whether a specific lesson had ever been devoted to the topic. As can be seen in Table 4, AIDS came lowest, followed by relationships and drugs respectively. In the sense that other topics (sex, smoking and drinking) have a longer history of being taught in schools, this is not altogether surprising. Other data suggest that respondents do not *perceive* a link between education about sex and substance use on the one hand, and AIDS and relationships on the other. Moreover, it is worrying that only 7 per cent of the sample reported having received teaching on AIDS.

Table 4. *Percentage Reporting Having Ever Been Taught about, and Receiving Specific Lessons on Health and Sexual Behaviour Topics*

	Smoking	Sex	AIDS	Topic Drugs (percentages)	Drink	Relationships
Ever taught about in school?	89.6	87.6	27.0	61.0	70.6	48.3
(Of which) specific lesson?	67.1	86.7	27.9	59.5	61.8	47.6

A further set of questions asked to what extent (1 = very little, 5 = very much) each of a number of information sources would be attended to should the respondent wish to discover more about AIDS. Factor analysis of the responses revealed three orthogonal factors: *mass media* (television programmes, advertisements, radio programmes, newspaper advertisements and articles); *professionals* (GPs, nurses, social workers and teachers); and *significant others* (parents, partner, brothers and sisters, friends). These accounted for 37.7 per cent, 13.0 per cent and 9.8 per cent of the variance, and when items were combined to produce scales, these had alpha coefficients of .84, .81 and .72 respectively. Overall professionals were regarded as the most, and significant others as least, credible source of information. However, females were significantly more likely than males to attend to mass media and significant others (Fs = 11.87, 13.19, ps < .01 and < .001 respectively).

Having indicated the sources they regarded as most worthy of attention, respondents then had to tick the three sources of information from which they felt they had already learnt most about AIDS. TV programmes were cited most often, followed by leaflets, TV advertisements, magazine articles, GPs, parents and teachers respectively. Hence most information does *not* appear to be received from the most credible sources — clearly a problem when one takes into account research on source credibility effects (Chaiken and Stangor, 1987), which indicates that where people are not especially concerned or involved in an issue, a source credibility plays an important part in persuasion. This might imply that those who are least conscientious concerning HIV would respond most positively to messages from high credibility sources.

Precautions and Perceptions of Risk

Given the sex differences reported above, it was reassuring that 96.4 per cent of respondents agreed that 'males and females need to be equally careful to avoid catching the AIDS virus.' There were also no sex or cohort differences in the perceived seriousness of becoming HIV positive (see Table 5); only 22.8 per cent believed HIV seropositivity is unlikely to lead to AIDS and 72.3 per cent believed that most or all people with AIDS die.

Table 5. Perceptions of the Seriousness of HIV Infection

Item	1 None	2 Few	3 Some	4 About half	5 Most	6 Almost all	7 All	$\bar{x}$
				(percentages)				
How many people who get the AIDS virus develop AIDS?	0.3	5.1	17.4	26.9	29.3	15.0	6.1	4.49
How many people who get AIDS actually die of it?	0.7	4.5	10.3	12.3	18.3	22.6	31.4	5.36

The next issue is the vulnerability felt by respondents. This was approached in a number of ways. First, what situations posed a threat? Nine contexts were listed and respondents were asked how likely it was that a person could be infected in each (1 = not at all, 7 = extremely). Sharing needles and having sex were perceived as most risky, while going to the dentist, being in pubs, discos and public toilets, and sharing a glass or a cigarette were perceived as least risky. Unfortunately, both giving and receiving blood were perceived as moderately risky, indicating confusion in this area. These perceptions were stronger amongst the younger cohort (Fs = 4.24, 6.42; ps < .05). Young women regarded the dentist and having sex as riskier, but going to pubs and discos as less risky than did young men (Fs = 4.63, 13.69, 5.21; ps < .05, < .001, < .05 respectively).

Second, and as a more direct measure of social distance to people with HIV infection, respondents were asked whether they would engage in a series of acts with someone they liked who was HIV antibody positive. The majority would shake hands or swim with such a person (96.7 per cent, 88.6 per cent), and only a minority would use their toothbrush or razor (12.2 per cent, 10.3 per cent). However, there was no clear consensus about the two behaviours which entailed direct exchange of saliva, sharing an ice cream and kissing on the mouth (39.9 per cent, 43.4 per cent). This indicates a need for clarification in health education messages, and strong rejection of suggestions the HIV is transmitted easily through saliva (see Masters, Johnson and Kolodny, 1988, for an example of professionals' perpetuation of fallacious beliefs concerning AIDS).

Given respondents' perception that sex is risky and that their peers are generally sexually active, the question arises of how soon they expect HIV to be prevalent among people of their own age. Respondents were asked then to indicate how many people would be HIV antibody positive in one, five and ten years' time. The answers were startling. It was believed that roughly half of heterosexuals in their age group would be HIV positive in ten years' time. Taken together with the perception that HIV seropositivity culminates in death, this is an extremely pessimistic outlook, the psychological implications of which merit further investigation. A further finding was that of the 39.3 per cent of respondents who felt the sexes were not equally likely to acquire HIV infection, 86.4 per cent (33.9 per cent of total) believed that men were more at risk.

Before concluding that young people are anxious and despondent, it is salutary to note the manner in which these perceptions are related to respondents' personal lives. When asked when a cure might be found for HIV infection, 65.4 per cent thought it would be found within ten years. More important is the pattern of responses to the question, 'how likely are you to catch the AIDS virus' now and in five years' time. On a seven-point scale (1 = extremely unlikely, 7 = extremely likely), the modal response for both time periods was 1, and the means were 1.34 and 2.20; 82.5 per cent of respondents felt it was unlikely or extremely unlikely that they would be infected within the next five years. The implications of this are serious, since it means that despite perceiving their peers to be at risk, respondents exclude themselves from perceived vulnerability — they consider themselves to be 'AIDS invulnerable'.

Attitudinal Aspects of AIDS Beliefs

An obvious question is how 'AIDS invulnerability' fits in with other research which has identified large numbers of 'worried well' people. One way in which the two phenomena may be reconciled is through cognitive structures which credit the self with more responsibility and control over oneself than others have over themselves. Thus, while others are irresponsible and hence dangerous, the self is safe. Similar processes have been identified in the context of geographic mobility in terms of young people's understanding of economic influences on their lives (Abrams, 1988). To what extent is there any support for this invulnerability hypothesis from the present data?

First, 71 per cent of respondents say they would consider going for an 'AIDS test' if they felt worried about being HIV antibody positive. Second, as can be seen in Table 6, they are doubtful that they know all they need to about AIDS; they believe it best not to have sex too soon after starting to go out with someone, and it is then best to stick to one sexual partner. They do not particularly blame gay men, and are in strong agreement that getting AIDS would be 'one of the worst things that could happen' to them. On the other hand, and this is where the data give cause for concern, they are fairly convinced that none of their potential partners could be HIV antibody positive, and are uncertain or even disagree slightly that if they became HIV antibody positive it

Table 6. Cell Means for All Sex and Cohort Differences in Attitudes to Sex and AIDS

Item	Males	Females	F	Older	Younger	F	x̄
	(1 = strongly disagree, 5 = strongly agree)						
I know all I need to know about AIDS	2.56	2.48	1.08	2.53	2.50	0.10	2.51
Because of AIDS it is best to stick to one sexual partner	3.55	3.83	8.12**	3.61	2.41	6.97*	3.72
It is OK to have sex with someone once you have been going out with them for a few weeks	2.98	2.19	79.43****	2.61	2.41	5.67*	2.50
I do not think anyone I have had a sexual relationship with is likely to have the AIDS virus	3.52	3.43	1.44	3.56	3.38	5.57*	3.46
AIDS is one of the worst things that could happen to me	4.19	4.24	0.31	4.34	4.14	7.52**	4.23
If I did get the AIDS virus it would be because of my behaviour	3.01	2.63	18.40***	2.75	2.80	0.38	2.78
It is unfair to blame gay men for the spread of AIDS	3.26	3.67	20.61****	3.50	3.51	0.01	3.57

Notes: **** $p < .0001$
*** $p < .001$
** $p < .01$
* $p < .05$

would be a result of their own behaviour. Thus, on the one hand there is concern and caution, while on the other the sense of AIDS invulnerability.

These perceptions are not equally distributed across sex and cohort. Young men are less cautious sexually than young women, and more hostile to gay men (replicating findings from a cohort survey conducted in Kirkcaldy the previous year: Abrams, 1987). Older respondents are also less cautious, but are slightly more likely to agree that their partners will be HIV antibody positive.

Use of Condoms

Use of condoms during penetrative sex is possibly the most obvious form of preventive behaviour pertinent to young people, since the majority are actively engaging in sexual relationships. Early in the questionnaire, respondents were asked how effective condoms would be in preventing the transmission of HIV: 81.4 per cent believed that the use of a condom during sexual intercourse would prevent female to male transmission, and 88 per cent believed it would prevent male to female transmission. This consensus in beliefs about the efficacy of condom use, combined with fairly prevalent sexual caution, would logically seem to imply a positive attitude towards using condoms. However, there are countervailing forces including lack of familiarity, potential embarrassment and social reputation that need to be taken into account.

Respondents were generally familiar with what a condom is (97.5 per cent reported having seen one). However, there were large sex and cohort differences in usage. Young men were more likely than young women to have asked for a condom in a shop (36.2 per cent vs 10.75 per cent; Chi-square = 61.04, p < .0001), and were more likely to have used one during sex (46.3 per cent vs 36.4 per cent, Chi-square = 5.71, p < .05). Of greater importance is the evidence that condom use increases considerably between the ages of 16 and 18. Older respondents were approximately twice as likely as younger respondents to have asked for (31.3 per cent vs 12.66 per cent, Chi-square = 33.75, p < .0001) and used a condom (56 per cent vs 28.1 per cent, Chi-square = 49.84, p < .0001).

To assess the inhibitory effects of having to purchase comdoms, respondents were asked whether or not they would feel comfortable buying condoms in a range of different settings. As can be see in Table 7, both males and females felt fairly comfortable with the idea of buying condoms in a chemist, although young women overwhelmingly preferred a family planning clinic, and young men preferred a public toilet. Neither sex was particularly keen on purchasing condoms in health and beauty shops or supermarkets, and both placed record shops (e.g. attempts to sell 'Mates' condoms through the Virgin Record chain) at the bottom of the list. It seems, therefore, that impersonal and clinical settings are preferred for the purchase of condoms.

A further question asked from which sex respondents would prefer to purchase

Table 7. Percentage of Males and Females Who Said They Would Feel Comfortable Buying Condoms in Different Places

Location	Males	Females	χ^2
Supermarket	44.0	38.7	n.s.
Record Shop	37.0	22.9	14.51****
Family Planning Clinic	74.3	85.9	13.30***
Chemist	74.1	76.5	n.s.
Public toilet	83.1	68.9	16.19****
Health and beauty shop	41.5	42.8	n.s.

Notes: **** p<.0001
    *** p<.001

condoms. A very significant and extremely large sex difference emerged such that 65.9 per cent of males would prefer to buy from a man, and 94.1 per cent of females would prefer to buy from a woman (Chi-square = 248.4, p < .0001). From these data it appears that there are very strong social inhibitions surrounding both where and from whom condoms may be purchased and that these inhibitions are gender-specific.

Later in the questionnaire, respondents were asked to answer a number of Likert items concerning attitudes and intentions towards condom use. In the present chapter only three representative items from this part of the questionnaire are reported. In general there was a strong agreement that 'I would use a condom if I had sex with a new partner', although agreement was greater among females and younger respondents than among males and older respondents (Fs = 4.71; ps < .05). There was moderate agreement that 'I will carry condoms if I intend to have sex with someone new.' However, agreement was lower among females and younger respondents than among males and older respondents (Fs = 44.36 and 7.15; ps < .0001, < .01). Finally, while respondents were somewhat undecided about whether 'If I carried condoms people would think I wanted casual sex', females were more likely to agree than were males (F = 6.81, p < .01). The overall picture seems to be that young people are willing to purchase and use condoms, but that this is subject to certain social constraints. In particular, young women are less comfortable with the prospect of purchasing condoms in public settings, and will *only* feel comfortable buying condoms if served by a woman. Moreover, although young women are more willing to use condoms, they are less willing to carry them as this gives the impression of being promiscuous.

Sharing Knowledge, Views and Feelings about AIDS: Significant Others

At the end of the questionnaire, respondents were required to indicate on a three-point scale (Yes, Uncertain, No) answers to questions about people in each of four different relationships to themselves (parents, particular close friend of own sex, friends seen in a group, and partner). Factor analysis indicated that responses to these questions could be represented in two ways: some factors represented consensus across relationships regarding particular items; others represented correlations among items with respect to particular relations. In the present chapter it is only possible to report a few of the findings. Two items concerned whether respondents had ever discussed AIDS with each relationship, and whether they would talk to each if they were worried about AIDS (alpha coefficients for summed scores across relationships = .57 and .49 respectively). On a scale of 1 (applicable to all relationships) to 9 (applicable to no relationships), young men were highly significantly less likely to talk about AIDS (F = 37.2, p < .0001) even if worried (F = 14.34, p < .0001). Moreover, there was a slight but significant tendency for the sex differences to be larger in the younger cohort (Fs = 5.94, 4.0, ps < .05).

Three other items asked about the views held by the people in the four relationships. These questions were asked to gain an idea of the normative context for respondents' own attitudes (cf. Abrams and Hogg, in press). On the item, 'You should take care not to catch the AIDS virus' (alpha = .89), neither males nor females felt there was strong consensus. However, young women were significantly more likely to think others believed they should use a condom with a new partner (alpha = .67, F = 6.02, p < .05) and that they should say no to sex with a new partner (alpha = .71, F = 176.7, p < .0001). As discussed elsewhere (Abrams, Abraham and Spears, in preparation, a), when the impact of each relationship across items is assessed, there are marked differences both between sexes and for different kinds of relationships. Specifically, both males and females say they accept AIDS-relevant messages from a partner, but females are significantly more likely than males to accept messages from other relationships. This is particularly marked in the case of a close own-sex friend (F = 41.01, p < .0001), who for females has equal impact to a partner. For both young men and young women, the least influential relationship is friends seen in a group. The conclusion to be drawn from these findings is that the normative context provided by significant others is quite different for males and females. In particular, the former are resistant to AIDS-relevant messages from all sources other than a partner.

Reference Groups and the Wider Normative Context

The second form of normative context is that provided by perceptions of the behaviour and attitudes of reference groups. In line with social identity theory, it was predicted that gender-ingroup provides an extremely powerful normative framework for behaviour, and it is therefore important to establish what each gender perceives to be normative (Abrams, 1989; Abrams and Hogg, in press).

When asked to estimate the average number of sexual partners of a 20-year-old man and 20-year-old woman, a large difference is evident (means = 10.19, 7.94; modes = 10 and 5 respectively). There is also a sex difference in perceptions of the norms for women. Males believe that average number of partners is 9.82, whereas females believe it is 6.69 (F = 12.87, p < .01). Consistent with young men's perception of others as sexually more active, males also believe that people have sex more quickly after starting to go out together (Chi-square = 15.74, p < .01).

The moral overtones of 'changing partners regularly' are perceived as being different for men and women (cf. Spears, Abrams, Abraham and Marks, in submission). Specifically, although it suggests popularity with the opposite sex (for both men and women), it is significantly more likely to imply popularity with either sex for males than females. Moreover, young men are significantly more likely to perceive a sexually active woman as more popular with either sex than are young women. Frequent changes of partner are also significantly less likely to imply irresponsibility and low self-respect for males than females. Analysis of a composite score of moral character judgment (alpha = .88) revealed that younger respondents were more censorious than older respondents.

Finally, respondents were asked to what extent men and women would agree or disagree with certain items to which they themselves had responded earlier in the questionnaire. Most striking is the finding that females are perceived to hold more cautious attitudes and intentions than males and that female respondents perceive this difference to be much more marked than do male respondents (see Abrams, Abraham and Spears, in preparation, b).

Conclusion

The basic findings from this study are consistent with those of similar studies conducted elsewhere in the UK (e.g. Ford, 1988), and can be summarized as follows. The age span of 16–18 is a critical time in the onset and development of romantic and sexual relationships. Young people's response to AIDS appears to be mixed. On the one hand they are concerned (cf. Miller, 1987) about the presence and spread of the disease in the community at large, but on the other they have a strong sense of AIDS invulnerability, which seems to involve a perception that they have control over the risk at which they place themselves (cf. Widen, 1987). Males and older respondents in the present survey appear less concerned to take appropriate precautions, and are less sexually cautious than females and younger ones. The sex difference is partly attributable to the weaker ties that males have with significant others, and the belief that active sexuality is positively evaluated within their peer group.

A second important finding is the strong gender difference in orientations to condom purchase, possession and use. In particular, it appears much more difficult for young women to purchase and carry condoms even though they are more willing than young men actually to use them. This suggests that efforts to persuade young people to use condoms may not succeed unless they are targeted in gender-specific ways.

A third interesting finding is that although most information concerning HIV and AIDS is gained from the mass media (cf. MacDermott, Hawkins, Moore and Cittadinose, 1987), this is not an especially credible source. It would seem that guidance and information from professionals may provide a more fruitful avenue of AIDS education, perhaps in combination with structured peer tutoring. It does not appear from the present data that mass media messages or informal discussion among groups of friends will on their own have as much impact as intended. Given the lack of specific education received by respondents concerning HIV, it would seem that an obvious avenue for health education development might be classroom-based workshops led by high credibility professionals (such as GPs). The use of high credibility sources increases the likelihood that messages will be accepted as accurate and unbiased. Combining this with peer discussion may consolidate this effect by heightening interest, involvement and the acquisition of further information.[3]

Notes

1   All Chi-square statistics are based on raw data, not percentages. Where data are reported from multi-item sections of the questionnaire, all significant differences are supported by significant multivariate Fs for that section. Unless stated otherwise, all Fs have approximately 1660 degrees of freedom, with slight variations due to missing data.
2   For reasons of economy of space, only a sample of the findings is presented here. Further information is available on request.
3   The research in this chapter was supported by an ESRC grant (XA44 250001), entitled 'Young People's AIDS-Relevant Preventive Cognitions in Dundee and Kirkaldy awarded to Abrams and Abraham in 1987. We wish to thank Paschal Sheeran and Teresa O'Neill, who work with us on the project.

References

ABRAMS, D. (1987) 'Attitudes to Sexual Behaviour and Homosexuality in the 16–19 Initiative First Wave Data'. Working paper, University of Dundee.

ABRAMS, D. (1988) 'Self-denial as an Aspect of Group Identification'. Paper presented at the Australian Bicentennial Meeting of Social Psychologists, Leura, 23–25 August.

ABRAMS, D. (1989) 'Differential Association: Social Developments in Gender Identity and Intergroup Relations during Adolescence', in S. M. SKEVINGTON and D. BAKER (eds), *The Social Identity of Women*. London, Sage.

ABRAMS, D. and HOGG, M. A. (1988) 'Comments on Motivational Status of Self-esteem in Social Identity and Intergroup Discrimination', *European Journal of Social Psychology*, 18, pp. 317–34.

ABRAMS, D. and HOGG, M. A. (in press) 'Social Identification, Self-categorisation and Social Influence', in W. STROEBE and M. HEWSTONE (eds), *Review of European Social Psychology*, Vol 1. London, Wiley.

ABRAMS, D., ABRAHAM, S. C. S. and SPEARS, R. (in preparation, a). 'The Role of Significant Others in Consolidating Attitudes and Behaviour with Regard to AIDS'.

ABRAMS, D., ABRAHAM, S. C. S. and SPEARS, R. (in preparation, b) 'Reference Group Norms and Social Identity: The Relevance of Social Consensus to AIDS-related Attitudes and Behaviour'.

AJZEN, I. and MADDEN, T. (1986) 'Prediction of Goal-directed Behaviour: Attitudes, Intentions and Perceived Behavioural Control'. *Journal of Experimental Social Psychology*, 22, pp. 453–74.

BECKER, M. H. (1974) 'The Health Belief Model and Sick Role Behaviour', *Health Education Monographs*, 2, p. 409.

CHAIKEN, S. and STANGOR, C. (1987) 'Attitudes and Attitude Change', *Annual Review of Psychology*, 38, pp. 575–630.

COXON, T. (1987) 'Something Sensational: The Sexual Diary as a Tool for Mapping Detailed Sexual Behaviour', *The Sociological Review* 35, pp. 353–67.

EMLER, N. P. (1984) 'Differential Involvement in Delinquency: Toward an Interpretation in Terms of Reputation Management', in B. A. MAHER and W. B. MAHER (eds), *Progress in Experimental Personality Research*, Vol. 13. New York, Academic Press.

FORD, N. (1988) 'A Survey of AIDS Awareness and Sexual Behaviour and Attitudes of Young People in Bristol'. University of Exeter, Institute of Population Studies.

HENDRY, L. B. (1983) *Growing Up and Going Out: Adolescents and Leisure*. Aberdeen, Aberdeen University Press.

HOGG, M. A. and ABRAMS, D. (1988) *Social Identifications: A Social Psychology of Group Processes and Intergroup Relations*. London, Routledge.

HOGG, M. A. and TURNER, J. C. (1987) 'Social Identity and Conformity: A Theory of Referent Information Influence', in W. DOISE and S. MOSCOVICI (eds), *Current Issues in European Social Psychology*. Vol. 2. Cambridge, Cambridge University Press.

HYMAN, H. H. and SINGER, J. L. (1967) *Readings in Reference Group Theory and Research*. New York, Free Press.

KAHNEMAN, D. and TVERSKY, A. (1982) 'The Psychology of Preferences', *Scientific American*, 246, pp. 160–73.

MACDERMOTT, R. J., HAWKINS, M., MOORE, J. and CITTADINOSE, S. (1987) 'AIDS Awareness and Information Sources among Selected University Students', *Journal of American College Health*, 35 pp. 222–6.

MARKS, D. ABRAHAM, S. C. S., ABRAMS, D. and SPEARS, R. (in submission) 'AIDS and Health Education Policy for Young People'. University of Dundee.

MASTERS, W. H., JOHNSON, V. E. and KOLODNY, R. C. (1988) *Crisis: Heterosexual Behaviour in the Age of AIDS*, New York, Grove Press.

MILLER, D. (1987) *Living with AIDS and HIV*. Basingstoke, Macmillan Education.

MOSCOVICI, S. and MUGNY, G. (1983) 'Minority Influence', in P. B. PAULUS (ed.), *Basic Group Processes*. New York, Springer-Verlag.

ROSENSTOCK, I. M. (1974) 'The Health Belief Model and Preventive Health Behaviour', *Health Education Monographs*, 2, pp. 354–86.

SPEARS, R., ABRAMS, D., ABRAHAM, S. C. S. and MARKS, D. (in submission) 'Social Judgements of Sex and Blame in the Context of AIDS: Gender and Linguistic Frame'.

TAJFEL, H. and TURNER, J. C. (1979) 'An Integrative Theory of Intergroup Conflict', in W. G. AUSTIN and S. WORCHEL (eds), *The Social Psychology of Intergroup Relations*. Monterey, Calif., Brooks-Cole.

TURNER, J. C. (1985) 'Social Categorization and the Self-concept: A Social-Cognitive Theory of Group Behaviour', in E. J. LAWLER (ed.), *Advances in Group Processes Theory and Research*, Vol. 2. Greenwich, Conn., JAI Press.

WIDEN, H. A. (1987) 'The Risk of AIDS and the Defense Disavowal Dilemmas for the College Psychotherapist', *Journal of American College Health*, 35, pp. 268–73.

Chapter 4

Blame and Young People's Moral Judgments about AIDS

Stephen Clift, David Stears, Sandra Legg, Amina Memon and Lorna Ryan

This chapter reports some of the findings from the first phase of the HIV/AIDS Education and Young People Project based in Canterbury, England (Clift *et al.*, 1989). As part of this project, information has been collected from a large sample of young people concerning their understandings of HIV infection and AIDS, their beliefs about the seriousness of AIDS, their beliefs about infection risks and personal vulnerability to infection, and their attitudes towards a variety of AIDS-related issues. The present chapter is concerned with aspects of young people's moral constructions of AIDS. It focuses in particular on their attributions regarding HIV infection and the feelings which follow from these.

The issues discussed in this paper are well illustrated by two examples taken from the written accounts we have collected. Here, for example, are the comments of a 15-year-old boy, which express a highly blaming and unsympathetic attitude towards a particular individual with AIDS.

> ... I watched a QED program on the subject of 'AIDS' — a young lady had the disease. Virtually the first thing the narrator said was, 'caught the disease after a casual one night affair with a man she hardly knew in Hollywood. She certainly did not know he was bisexual — and certainly did not know he had 'AIDS'. I have no sympathy for her because if she is going to conduct herself in this appalling manner — i.e. having sex outside of marriage with someone she hardly knew — knowing the risks (maybe not 'AIDS' but other appalling STDs) then, quite frankly, she deserves whatever comes her way as a result. She was from a good home and there was really no excuse. Just imagine if everyone had one sexual partner and there was no homosexuality — would there be a problem? I think 'AIDS' is doing some good — it is making people sit up and think about the way

53

they conduct themselves sexually. The sooner people's moral values go up, the sooner AIDS will disappear, and surveys such as this with questions asking 14–15 years olds 'have they ever had sex' will not be necessary. We don't want lessons on how to avoid 'AIDS' by using condoms etc., teach a few moral values — the results may be surprising ... (Male, 15)

This can be contrasted with the following account from a 16-year-old girl, who, in contrast to the boy above, completely rejects the notion of victim-blaming within the context of AIDS.

... Recently in school we had a discussion on AIDS. One particular boy put his ideas about the disease across by saying gays, drug-users etc. who have AIDS are to blame for their having contracted the disease. He also said that everyone who has AIDS and doesn't wear a condom are to blame and he has no sympathy for them. Naturally, this annoyed me immensely, not only was his 'accusations' not true, but they were also totally pathetic. It seems to me he has been watching too many 'durex' adverts and not enough good advisory documentaries. It is sad to think that people blame AIDS sufferers in this way. Even if the person was 100% healthy and through one night didn't wear a condom, this person doesn't deserve to die of AIDS. People should be better educated with such matters instead of having pathetic, ignorant ideas ... (Female, 16)

Background to the Canterbury Project

Social and psychological research concerned with investigating the knowledge, beliefs and attitudes of different groups regarding HIV infection and AIDS is accumulating rapidly (Clift and Stears, 1988; Warwick *et al.*, 1988a, 1988b; DHSS, 1987; Abrams *et al.*, 1989; Currie, 1989; McQueen and McGlew, 1989; see Memon, 1989, for a recent review). Central concerns of such research have been to establish what individuals know about AIDS and the attitudes they hold (Reid, 1988; Searle, 1987) and to assess the extent to which these have changed as a result of public information campaigns or more local educational interventions (DHSS, 1987; Clift and Stears, 1988; Clifford *et al.*, 1988; Hill and Mayon-White, 1987). Research has also investigated the extent to which individuals engage in risky practices (Ford and Bowie, 1988; McKeganey and Barnard, 1989; Coxon, 1988) and begun to explore the relationships between cognitive and attitudinal factors and the likelihood that an individual will engage in behaviours which involve a risk of infection (Fitzpatrick *et al.*, 1989).

The techniques most commonly used to collect information are self-completion questionnaires and structured interviews. Only rarely, as in the work of Warwick *et al.* (1988a, 1988b) and Hastings and Scott (1988), has use been made of semi-structured interviews and group discussions to investigate people's understanding and attitudes. Despite the widespread use of questionnaire techniques, however, relatively little attention has been given to identifying the principal dimensions involved in lay constructions of AIDS and in developing instruments to assess these. Reliable and valid instruments are needed to explore the factors which mediate reactions to people with HIV infection and AIDS and which affect the likelihood of individuals engaging in risk reduction strategies.

The present research arose directly out of an earlier study concerned with undergraduate students' beliefs and attitudes regarding AIDS and the changes apparent over a six-month period (Clift and Stears, 1988, 1989). The results of this research offered an initial and tentative mapping of the principal dimensions of young people's responses to AIDS. Starting from a questionnaire composed of fifty-six items, thirteen distinct clusters of items were identified by Elementary Linkage Analysis (McQuitty, 1957) and a number of these were combined to form two scales: the first concerned with 'worry' over contact with people infected with HIV; the second concerned a variety of 'moral' issues associated with AIDS. These scales were significantly correlated and were found to be related to such factors as political identification and religious belief. One of the concerns of the present project was to build on the findings of this earlier study and to extend the research to a younger and more representative sample of young people. More specifically, the intentions of the project were as follows. First, it aimed to collect data on the understandings, beliefs, attitudes and behaviours of young people aged 14–18 living in the south-east of England. Second, it aimed to identify the principal cognitive, attitudinal and behavioural factors underlying such data. Third, it was concerned to examine sex and year group differences on these variables, and explore the relationships between them. Finally, it was hoped that the study would provide a basis for the systematic construction of more sensitive instruments for use in a later phase of the project.

In common with much of the research conducted so far on individuals' beliefs and attitudes, our earlier work with undergraduate students was based entirely on the use of questionnaires for data collection and the work reported here has also relied heavily on this approach. We have begun to shift, however, towards the collection of more qualitative data which can be interpreted within the framework provided by the analysis of information from questionnaires.

Sample and Procedure

The sample consisted of 1080 fourth, fifth and sixth formers drawn from four secondary schools. Two of the schools were in Canterbury, one in Hove and one in South London. The sample included 573 boys and 507 girls; 472 fourth year, 375 fifth year and 233 sixth year pupils. All pupils completed a six-part questionnaire on different aspects of AIDS. Part 1 consisted of items concerned with worry over contact with infected individuals, the seriousness of AIDS, perceived vulnerability and moral and social attitudes. Parts 2 and 3 were concerned with risk assessments and knowledge of AIDS. Part 4 asked for information of sexual and drug taking behaviour and attitudes towards sexual experience and condom use. Part 5 requested information on such matters as religious beliefs, church membership and ethnic group identification. Finally Part 6 asked respondents to write an account of their own views on any aspect of HIV infection and AIDS.

Analysis and Results

This chapter reports on the findings from part 1 of the questionnaire and relates these results to the written accounts given in part 6. As part 1 was constructed to assess four issues — concern over contact, seriousness, vulnerability and moral/social attitudes — it was anticipated that the items concerned with these issues would emerge as distinct clusters on analysis. The correlation matrix for these items was subject to a principal axis factor analysis, and five factors with eigen values greater than one were rotated to the oblimin criterion. Table 1 reports the factor pattern with loadings > 0.25 given (for this analysis the sample size is reduced to 990 due to the listwise deletion of cases having one or more missing value). As expected, worry over contact, vulnerability and seriousness emerged as separate factors. For the moral and social items, two factors emerged which can be labelled 'morality' and 'blame'. Table 2 reports the correlations between factors. It is clear from this table that 'morality', 'blame' and 'contact' are positively intercorrelated: young people who are moralistic and blaming in their outlook are more likely to express reluctance over being in contact with infected individuals. This finding replicates the previous finding reported by Clift and Stears (1988, 1989) that 'worry' over contact is associated with a moralistic perspective on AIDS.

Factor scores were calculated for each of the five factors by the regression method (Norusis, 1988), and Table 3 reports the results of a two-way analysis of variance for each factor, with sex and year group as independent variables. As the factor scores are standardized, each has a mean of zero and a standard deviation of one. Significant sex and/or year group differences emerged for all factors. It is clear that substantial sex and year group differences emerged for the 'blame' factor, with males and the younger age groups being more blaming than females and the older age groups. The remainder of this chapter focuses on the blame factor, and illustrates the variation in young people's views on AIDS it represents.

Table 1. *Oblimin Factor Pattern for Twenty-three Items in Part 1 of the Questionnaire*
(N = 990)

			Factors			
	1	2	3	4	5	C
I would eat a meal made by a person with AIDS	-78					57
I would be happy to share a cup with a person who has AIDS	-78					57
I would not be happy about a person with AIDS staying the night in my house	63					51
I would not be happy to kiss a person who has HIV	56					35
I would be worried about becoming infected with HIV if someone is my class had the virus	53					30
I am very unlikely to become infected with HIV in future		66				47
I am worried about becoming infected with HIV in future		-53				30
Some of my friends could become infected with HIV in the future		-37				24
I know enough to avoid becoming infected with HIV in the future		34				14
The number of people with AIDS in this country will always be small		26	-25			14
If a person with AIDS is treated, they can get better and lead a normal life again			-55			32
There is no cure for AIDS			54			29
If a person develops AIDS, they are certain to die			42			25
AIDS is something only gay men and drug users need to worry about			-30			20
To help stop the spread of HIV, sex education in schools should stress the need for ' no sex before marriage'				53		28
AIDS is a big problem in Britain because standards of sexual behaviour are low in our society				52		26
AIDS is a warning from God that levels of sexual behaviour in society are too low				48		33
If people lived normal and responsible lives, problems like AIDS would never arise				45		42
Gay men are to blame for bringing HIV into this country					51	42
Children born with HIV deserve treatment more than drug users who become infected with HIV by sharing needles					45	31
I don't feel sorry for people who become infected with HIV through having sex					40	32
Because of AIDS, sex between men should be against the law					38	42
AIDS is a very painful disease						09

Table 2. Correlations between the Five Oblimin Factors
(N = 990)

	Contact	Vulnerability	Seriousness	Morality	Blame
Contact	—				
Vulnerability	03	—			
Seriousness	01	− 07	—		
Morality	35[b]	14[b]	08	—	
Blame	37[b]	24[b]	− 10[a]	32[b]	—

Notes: a p<0.01
     b p<0.001 (two-tailed)

Table 3. Means on Five Factor Scores for Year and Sex Groups and Results of ANOVA
(N = 990)

Factor		Year groups 4	5	6	Total	F_{sex}	F_{year}	$F_{sex \times year}$
1 Contact	M	− .22	.07	.02	− .07	5.524[a]	6.140[c]	1.102
	F	− .00	.09	.19	.08			
	M + F	− .12	.08	.10	− .00			
2 Vulnerability	M	− .11	− .07	− .24	− .13	27.342[d]	4.491[b]	0.090
	F	.15	.21	− .02	.14			
	M + F	.01	.07	− .14	.00			
3 Seriousness	M	.13	− .05	.03	.05	3.795[a]	2.966[a]	0.802
	F	− .00	− .07	− .12	− .05			
	M + F	.07	− .06	− .04	− .00			
4 Morality	M	− .12	.00	.24	.00	0.012	7.974[d]	1.048
	F	− .04	− .03	.13	− .00			
	M + F	− .08	− .01	.18	− .00			
5 Blame	M	− .32	− .06	.05	− .15	38.016[d]	15.469[d]	0.649
	F	.34	.17	.37	.16			
	M + F	− .15	.06	.20	.00			

Notes: a p<0.05
     b p<0.01
     c p<0.005
     d p<0.001

The Blame Factor

The blame factor is defined by four issues: the attribution of collective blame to gay men, the advocacy of legal restrictions on homosexual behaviour, a lack of sympathy for people who become infected with HIV through sexual activity, and the judgment that certain groups are more deserving of treatment than others. Young people scoring in the bottom and top 20 per cent of the blame factor (N = 197 and 198 respectively) were identified, and their written accounts in part 6 of the questionnaire compared. The accounts of young people who are highly blaming are discussed first, followed by the contrasting views of young people who are highly non-blaming.

The High Blame Group

In a small number of cases within the highly blaming group, the written accounts expressed an extremely punitive orientation towards 'people with AIDS'. Such people, it is suggested, should be killed, mutilated or removed from society.

> . . . I think people with AIDS should all be put on an island to end their years, so people are then more safer from these queers, sex maniacs and drug users . . . . (Male, 16)

> . . . They should kill people with AIDS or even better put them away somewhere with themselves . . . . (Male, 15)

> . . . The people who have AIDS should be shot or have 'I HAVE AIDS' stamped on their foreheads. They are a bunch of toss pots and they are FAGGOTS!! . . . . (Male, 15)

As these examples suggest, homophobia is a significant theme in the accounts offered by the members of the high blame group, and anti-gay prejudice is often expressed with extreme virulence. In some cases, gay men are considered directly responsible for the development of the AIDS epidemic, and as a result gay men collectively are seen as deserving extreme forms of punishment. In some cases, young people express a desire to administer punishment personally. More typically, however, the view is that homosexuality should be banned. Coupled with these attitudes are views of homosexuality as 'unnatural', 'immoral', 'sick', 'hateful' and 'disgusting'.

> . . . The gay bastards spread AIDS and if I catch them I'll cut there dicks off and kick the shit out of them . . . . (Male, 14)

> . . . I think all gays should be shot. I hate gays they are sick bastards . . . . (Male, 15)

> . . . I think that AIDS was started when queers started to become big as it has only started recently. I think that people who have become afflicted with AIDS from have sex with the same sex deserve it . . . . (Male, 16)

> . . . My views on AIDS are that there should not be gays. If there weren't in the first place AIDS would never had started. People should take it much more seriously and be incouraged to NOT sleep around . . . . (Male, 14)

> . . . I also feel that homosexuality should be made illegal because as well as being a cause of AIDS its immoral and totally disgusting . . . . (Male, 17)

In what is perhaps the most vicious account to emerge from the entire sample, it is bisexual men who are singled out as the particular object of loathing.

> . . . I feel that the problem of AIDS is really down to bisexual males. I feel that without these people AIDS would have been confined to the gay population which, as the Chief Superintendent of the Greater Manchester police said 'are wallowing in a hell of their own making'. I have no sympathy with gays whatever their problem or bisexuals who are the real murdering culprits for introducing the disease into the innocent heterosexual world who are now paying for their filthy behaviour . . . . (Male, 18)

Gay men are most commonly the object of such bigotry and abuse, but other groups — bisexuals, drug users, prostitutes, lesbians, people who are 'promiscuous' and 'foreigners' are all inveighed against in this way. All the accounts quoted above, in which gay men are the sole focus of attack, come from boys. The following group of extracts comes from girls; it is interesting to observe that in these blame and responsibility with regard to infection are attributed more widely.

> . . . I think there should be a law against gays and lesbians because they are not natural and if it wasn't for them then we would have the cure. Also the foreigners should be kept in their own country because they are spreading the disease . . . . (Female, 15)

> . . . Prostitutes should be arrested for their irresponsible behaviour towards other members of the human race . . . . (Female, 14)

> . . . Homosexual behaviour should be stopped. Drug addicts should be locked up, with the drug slowly taken away . . . . (Female, 15)

> . . . Gays should be banned because they are the starters and it is their fault if they get it, bi-sexual people are thoughtless as they pass it on to normal people. There should be more warnings about babies catching it from their infected mothers . . . . (Female, 15)

The Blame-Sympathy Equation

The examples given so far have involved some form of collective blaming with respect to the origins and spread of AIDS (rarely are HIV infection and AIDS distinguished in these accounts), coupled with advocacy of social controls or sanctions directed at particular categories of people. Not surprisingly, the two groups mentioned most often are gay men and drug users. Equally common among young people low on the blame factor are statements in which certain types of individuals are considered responsible for their infection, whereas others are seen as 'innocent victims'. In the former case, infection is often attributed to actions over which the individual has control, and in the latter, to events outside the individual's control. Where some control is perceived to exist, the action involved may be described as 'stupid', 'wilful', 'reckless' or in some sense 'wrong'. Expressions of sympathy or the lack of it are often linked to this fundamental distinction concerned with control and responsibility.

> ... I feel sorry for some people who catch AIDS by accident, but I don't feel sorry at all for gays or pimps or drug dealers.... (Female, 15)

> ... The people I feel sorry for are the haemophiliacs who can transmit AIDS through a blood transplant and also people who's husband or wife have AIDS and then transmit it to their partner. The junkies who inject AIDS feel sorry for themselves but it's their own fault.... (Female, 15)

> ... Certain people allow themselves to be infected with the disease through stupidity i.e. drug addicts, gays, prostitutes, etc. and from them the disease spreads through normal sexual intercourse, blood transfusions, etc.... (Male, 16)

> ... If drug takers catch AIDS then it is their fault, but when babys are born with the virus they should have the drugs first and more attention should be paid to them.... (Male, 14)

One particular expression of the blame and sympathy equation is the view that some people deserve treatment and others do not. Sometimes this distinction is drawn very dramatically, and the view is held that some people should receive no treatment at all and simply be left to suffer and die. In other cases, the issue is who should receive priority in treatment and the first call on scarce resources. A related issue is the view that certain people who develop AIDS deserve to suffer.

> ... I believe that a strict screening procedure is necessary for blood used for transfusion therefore reducing the chance of AIDS being caught by haemophiliacs. Secondly, those who have contacted AIDS through drug abuse, sleeping around or homosexual activity ought to be left to rot because they have caught what they deserve and we should be helping the haemophiliacs and the babies born with AIDS.... (Male, 18)

> ... I think that most of the blame should be put on the careless people like drug takers and adults that have more than one partner. Babies that are born with AIDS are the innocent ones and should be the only one treated. Cures for the disease are being developed just to be used on people that made trouble for themselves.... (Male, 15)

The Low Blame Group

The examples quoted in the last section come from young people who score below the twentieth percentile on the blame factor. For those at the opposite end of the dimension, the idea that certain groups can be blamed for the origin and spread of AIDS is totally unacceptable, as is any form of prejudice, discrimination or oppression of people with HIV infection or AIDS. These views are generally associated with a rejection of homophobic attitudes and prejudice against drug users.

> . . . I think AIDS is a very serious problem and what annoys me most is that a lot people especially young blame it on homosexuals, which is not fair, because diseases start all different ways and nobody's to blame . . . . (Female, 16)

> . . . I don't think people should blame gays as I think this is really prejudiced. People should be aware of homosexuality but it shouldn't be taught to very young people, though I don't think it has anything to do with AIDS now although more gay people might have been infected in the past . . . . (Female, 15)

Other accounts are more explicit and lengthy and begin to explore in more detail the issues surrounding the collective blame position and some of its implications. In some cases, young people suggest that AIDS is being used as an excuse by individuals, certain sections of the media and the government to abuse and further oppress minority groups, particularly gay men. This construction of events is generally tied in with commentary on the nature and origins of homophobic attitudes. For others, blaming is seen as unhelpful, irrelevant and positively harmful, both to people with AIDS and to the lives of individuals and groups associated with AIDS. The argument put forward is that trying to find someone or some group to blame can do nothing to help confront the reality of AIDS; the important thing is to deal effectively with the problem. The next example ties together many of these issues, and is particularly interesting for its reference both to blame and to the issue of social distancing. The account expresses very well the relationship between 'anxiety' over contact and 'blame' which emerges from the factor analysis reported in Tables 1 and 2.

> . . . I think that no community, gay or otherwise, should be blamed for the AIDS virus. A lot of people use AIDS as an excuse to persecute a certain group of people or religion, which is wrong. The media have not helped much in telling people the correct facts about AIDS. Many people have become paranoid about it to the extent that they won't shake hands or use the same cutlery in a restaurant as everyone else does. . . . A lot of young people hate gays, mostly because they have been told that they are to blame for the deaths of people with AIDS. I have heard my cousins of four and

seven years old call people 'fucking gay' and 'yuk, you've got AIDS! . . . .'
(Female, 15)

In other accounts, the blaming perspective is criticized both for its harmful consequences and for its irrelevance. What is needed, it is argued, is positive, constructive action in finding a cure, in supporting people with AIDS and in ensuring that people are properly educated. Again, it is interesting to see in the following account the way in which the issue of 'blame' is linked with rejection and social distancing.

> . . . I also feel that the AIDS problem is being blamed very much on homosexuals and that a growing resentment towards them is developing in our society. This causes great problems as homosexuals feel ashamed and so may not feel that they want to accept help available to them. AIDS sufferers are also vulnerable to attack from others, due to a growing 'hysteria' towards the virus. These sufferers should be allowed to work for as long as they are physically able and NHS funded hospices should be set up to allow them to die comfortably and with as much self-respect as possible. If you have AIDS, then this information should be kept strictly confidential, e.g. you shouldn't have to be screened if entering another country. (Female, 18)

Breaking the Blame-Sympathy Link

Among those young people who are highly non-blaming according to their blame factor score, there are some who express concern and sympathy only for certain categories of people with HIV or AIDS. The more blatantly prejudicial accounts are rare, however, and a variety of 'transitional' forms is more common. In some accounts, for example, different cases of infection are construed in terms of control but the implication to differential sympathy is rejected — e.g. 'this person only has himself to blame but I still feel sorry for him.' In other cases, sympathy is felt for groups which have 'brought AIDS upon themselves' but to a lesser degree than for those infected through 'no fault of their own'. Another transitional form involves a shift from distinctions made at the level of group categorization to distinctions made directly with reference to knowledge and control, e.g. 'I feel sorry for people infected eight years ago, but people infected now only have themselves to blame' or 'I don't feel sorry for people who know the risks and yet engage in risky activities.' Related to this is the emergence in some accounts of 'the person who knowingly infects others' or 'the person who knowingly has sex with an infected person' as a particular focus of the 'blame-sympathy' issue. In the latter case, for example, the individual is perceived to carry the blame for their own infection if they do not take proper precautions. Perhaps because the specific issue of control is more salient for some of these young people, we also find some of the rare examples of non-blaming attributions towards drug users among members of this group.

> . . . I feel sorry for people who are infected with the AIDS virus, unless they have had unprotected sex with a number of different partners, or have shared a needle to inject drugs. I do not feel that it is gay people who have brought AIDS to Britain and I am not against people who have the AIDS virus. I feel that some people are really ignorant and selfish, if they know they have the AIDS virus and yet they have unprotected sex with their partners . . . . (Female, 14)

> . . . People who know they are having a sexual relationship with an HIV carrier should wear a condom. If he doesn't I have no sympathy. If a baby gets it or someone who doesn't know their partner has got HIV get it then I feel sorry for them . . . . (Male, 15)

> . . . I feel that the majority of people who have HIV could have avoided it by taking more interest in their own future and well being and modifying their habits accordingly. This being the case though people with HIV deserve normal humane compassion and care providing they make every effort to stop themselves infecting others . . . . (Male, 18)

> . . . I feel differently about various people who have caught HIV. If they are haemophiliacs then I feel really sorry for them and also people who have sex with one partner but that partner is infected. Regarding drug takers and homosexuals I still feel sorry for them, but to a lesser degree . . . . (Male, 17)

> . . . I feel sorry for people who have contracted AIDS or HIV especially if they got it 8 years ago. Now that we know so much about AIDS there is no excuse really to get AIDS, but I wouldn't condemn those who have . . . . (Female, 16)

Beyond those occupying transitional positions, a larger number of young people among the non-blaming group express unconditional sympathy for anyone infected with HIV or with AIDS. These young people are well aware of the serious nature of AIDS and the suffering it involves. For them, all people in this position should be cared for and the circumstances of minority groups should not be made worse by having to cope with prejudicial attitudes, social ostracism, discriminatory practices and oppression. The view is often expressed that people with AIDS should be treated as 'normal' or like 'anyone else' who has an illness and that treatment in separate hospitals or wards is not a good idea. These young people often express an interest in knowing more about the personal circumstances of people with AIDS and a desire to give them practical help. Some suggest that if they knew someone with AIDS they would go out of their way to befriend them, and some see people with AIDS as providing positive examples of people meeting a life-threatening illness with fortitude and courage.

> . . . I feel sorry for anyone who has AIDS and I think everyone should help in the best way they can and not treat anyone who has AIDS as outcasts . . . . (Female, 14)

> . . . I think that people who get AIDS should be treated whoever they are (drug users, gays, prostitutes, etc.) and no preference should be given . . . . (Female, 14)

> . . . I can only feel very sorry for people who are infected and more should be done to help them . . . . (Male, 17)

> . . . People who are infected with the AIDS virus should not be treated as social outcasts but helped medically and supported by their community. They should not be treated as though they have done something but should be treated, as far as possible, as though they have done nothing wrong . . . . (Male, 16)

> . . . Those who have AIDS should be well looked after as I believe they have a lot to give society about how to endure the pain and how to avoid the virus in the first place . . . . (Male, 18)

Among the non-blaming group, young people often describe how they would like to behave towards someone infected with HIV or with AIDS and how they would want to be treated if they became infected. These young people express no anxiety about becoming infected through social contact and voice a wish to counteract the prejudice and discrimination they feel infected people will experience in society.

> . . . If I knew someone who was infected by HIV, I would not be terrified of them or cut myself off from them. I would try to care for them (though not in a patronising way). I would carry on as normal and try to help them through the prejudice that they would undoubtedly receive . . . . (Male, 16)

> . . . I feel that when someone becomes infected you should treat them exactly the same as anyone else, many people get teased because they have the disease, this is wrong. If I knew someone with the disease I would treat them exactly the same, I would not be afraid of going near them, or sharing a cup or plate with them . . . . (Female, 15)

Personal Experience of AIDS

While some young people imagine what it would be like to know someone with AIDS, a number of young people in our sample were able to write from experience of knowing a person infected with HIV or with AIDS. Significantly, all of these accounts are provided by young people who reject all forms of blaming and are highly sympathetic towards the circumstances of people with HIV or AIDS. Almost all of these accounts raise highly significant issues concerned with the personal and social dimensions of AIDS.

> . . . At my last school there was a boy in my brother's year who was haemophiliac and had contracted HIV. He was treated just the same as other people but the school did have rules if he cut himself and the boy would let anybody except the school nurse [sic] who would wear rubber gloves touch his blood. Nobody treated him any different . . . . (Male, 17)

> . . . I myself have a relation, a haemophiliac child of 15, who has the virus, but at present is only a 'carrier'. However I am sure you can imagine how we felt when we found out. Yet despite our help, fellow children reacted badly at his school and as a result he had to move to another school. It is still very difficult to explain to other people that they are at no risk from him. They are all so scared. I think, however, that whatever is done to tell people about AIDS nothing will quell this enormous fear that it has struck into many people until a cure is found. I do think that more could be done to inform people how to look after people with AIDS who have not yet needed to be admitted into hospitals, as it seems that so far nothing has been said about this . . . . (Female, 18)

A further five young people described direct contact with friends or acquaintances with HIV or AIDS. Two are quoted here and the second provides an eloquent summing up of many of the themes which characterize the non-blaming position in relation to AIDS.

> . . . I actually know someone with HIV and my friendship with him has not changed. I know there is no way I can contract the virus off of him just by sharing his company. He needs friends just like all the other sufferers do. Ignorant people who joke about AIDS and make snide comments make me want to be sick! . . . . (Female, 17)

> . . . I would be happy to be friends of an AIDS carrier. They need a lot of help and I would be willing to give it. My friend has AIDS and it doesn't bother me at all. AIDS sufferers are not aliens. Many of them don't consciously do things to get AIDS. You can't blame people for it. Society is to blame. There ought to be a much more responsible attitude to AIDS. Hostels and hospital should be set up for people who suffer from AIDS. They need as much help as possible to rebuild their lives. Its not fair that people with AIDS should be outcast. Society won't accept them so they have no one to turn to . . . . (Female, 15)

Discussion

In comparing the accounts written by the most blaming and least blaming groups of young people in our sample, a number of significant themes emerged. In part, these themes correspond to the issues which serve to define the blame factor, but the material available from part 6 of the questionnaire allows us to go considerably beyond the sparse and lifeless dimension defined by factor analysis.

Among the most blaming, we find a tendency to blame groups such as gay men and drug users for the epidemic and advocacy of collective punishment and social and legal controls directed at entire social groups. Gay men are a particular target of abuse, and homophobic sentiments are commonly expressed, although many other stigmatized and marginalized groups are the target of prejudice. The 'innocence versus guilt' construct is commonly employed by highly blaming young people, and this is reflected in the frequent linkage between judgments of blame and a lack of sympathy. Significant here is the perception of personal control or lack of it over the activity which led to infection. Finally, we find some people regarding AIDS as a deserved condition and making the judgment that certain groups are less deserving of care and treatment than others.

Among the least blaming group, in contrast, we find a clear rejection of collective blaming and condemnation of any form of prejudice, discrimination or oppression against social groups associated with AIDS. Judgments about control over the source of infection are still important, but these are more often 'individualized' in character and the implication to feelings of sympathy or lack of it is considerably weakened and even rejected. More common, however, are expressions of unconditional positive regard toward infected people and an active concern to befriend and support people with AIDS. Finally, we find cases among the least blaming group of young people who have personal experience of relatives, friends or acquaintances who are infected with HIV or who have AIDS.

These findings raise a wide variety of significant questions of a theoretical, empirical and practical nature. How, for example, do differences in the tendency to blame relate to other aspects of young people's understanding, beliefs and attitudes regarding AIDS? How also do they relate to potentially relevant social and psychological factors such as socio-economic status, political and religious affiliations, ethnicity and so on? What theoretical perspectives can help us to go beyond the descriptive exercise of documenting variation and its correlates? What are the social and educational implications of the differences found?

In attempting to address some of these issues, it should be said at the outset that while the focus of this research is on young people aged between 14 and 18, the variations described are clearly not specific to this age group. The positions identified undoubtedly could be found in any broad cross-section of the adult population and we found little in the accounts collected which could be characterized as specifically 'childlike' or 'youthlike'. Nevertheless, the evidence does suggest that developmental considerations may be important in understanding the ways in which young people make sense of different aspects of AIDS. In the area of values, attributions and feelings, we can begin to see how judgments about AIDS may reflect general levels of cognitive and moral development. It is not difficult, for instance, to see some parallels between the various positions distinguished along the blame dimension and the broad distinctions drawn by Kohlberg (1976) between pre-conventional, conventional and post-conventional levels of moral judgment. Although Kohlberg's work has been subject to trenchant criticism (e.g. Phillips and Nicolayev, 1978), there may be some value in looking at individual constructions of AIDS from this perspective, particularly as re-formulated from a feminist viewpoint in the recent work of Gilligan (1977).

The suggestion that a cognitive-developmental perspective may be of value in understanding variations of the blame factor should not, however, be taken to imply that these differences arise independently of cultural and interpersonal influences. The basic Piagetian epistemology underlying Kohlberg's work is one of interactive constructionism which views individuals as actively engaged in making sense of the material, social and symbolic environments around them. The positions we have documented reflect to some undetermined degree the influence of cultural representations transmitted through the family, peer group, education and media, and it remains to explore more fully the complex relationships of culture, social context and individual constructions of AIDS.

One significant result from our present study, which is relevant to the last point, is the finding that constructions focused on 'blame' are 'gendered' to a substantial degree. While it is true that some girls are blaming, and that rather more boys are compassionate, the trend emerges very clearly that tolerance and concern are most prevalent among young women, whereas bigotry, punitiveness and lack of sympathy are more common among young men. These differences are likely to reflect more general processes of differential gender socialization which construct 'masculinity' and 'femininity' in the context of family, peer group, community and school. One consequence of this linkage could be that boys may resist adopting more tolerant and sympathetic attitudes in relation to AIDS as this would carry the implication of becoming less 'masculine'.

The suggestion that variation on the blame factor may reflect more general social-psychological processes highlights a further point that such variation is not specific to AIDS, and would undoubtedly emerge in relation to other health issues and many contentious social problems. Eiser *et al.* (in press) have recently shown, for instance, that young people's views of AIDS are very similar to their perceptions of lung cancer and very different from their views on asthma and diabetes. The issue of 'blame' emerged as a significant factor in these discriminations. Young people's moral constructions of AIDS should, therefore, be set within the context of their beliefs and attitudes concerning health and illness and within the yet broader framework of theory and research on attitudinal structure. It is likely, for instance, that young people who are highly blaming with respect to AIDS will also hold relatively traditional and punitive attitudes on a wide variety of issues (women's rights, immigration, unemployment etc.) which combine to define a general factor of 'conservatism' in social attitudes (Wilson, 1973).

A further theoretical perspective which has clear relevance to understanding individual positions on the blame factor is attribution theory (Weiner, 1985). The written accounts suggest that judgments of personal control over the events which lead to infection are of central importance in the process of attributing blame and in structuring the feelings experienced for infected individuals. Attribution theory identifies 'locus', 'stability' and 'controlability' as major dimensions of causal attribution, and links causal attributions with differential cognitive, emotional and behavioural consequences (Weiner, 1988). Progress in understanding the dynamics and consequences of blaming in relation to AIDS may be achieved by exploring the applications of attribution theory to this issue.

Finally, significant educational issues are raised by the findings reported here. It is likely that in any class of fourth, fifth or sixth formers, the entire spectrum of opinion documented in this article around the issue of blame will be represented. Among the questions this raises are the following. Should education in HIV infection and AIDS concern itself with the issue of blame and the wide variety of issues which surround it? Are schools and other environments addressing these issues in their provision of HIV/AIDS education? If they are, how are they doing so — what resources are used and what methodologies are employed? Finally, what are the effects of teaching about HIV and AIDS on young people's moral constructions, their attributions and their feelings for infected people? All of these questions regarding education on HIV/AIDS are being addressed within the second phase of the HIV/AIDS Education and Young People Project based in Canterbury, and it is hoped that the research currently underway will provide answers of practical significance to teachers and young people alike.

Acknowledgments

Thanks are due to the South East Thames Regional Health Authority and the AIDS Education and Research Trust (AVERT) for their financial support, and to the teachers and pupils who participated in this study.

Stephen Clift et al.

References

ABRAMS, D., ABRAHAM, C., SPEARS, R. and MARKS, D. (1989) 'AIDS Invulnerability: Relationships, Sexual Behaviour and Attitudes among 16–19-Year Olds', Chapter 3 in this volume.

CLIFFORD, B., MESSENGER-DAVIES, M., PHILLIPS, K., PITTS, M. and WHITE, D. (1988) 'How Teenagers Respond to a Video: Learning AIDS', *Times Educational Supplement*, 24 September, p. 134.

CLIFT, S.M. and STEARS, D.F. (1988) 'Beliefs and Attitudes Regarding AIDS among British College Students: A Preliminary Study of Change between November 1986 and May 1987, *Health Eductation Research*, 3, 1, pp. 75–88.

CLIFT, S. and STEARS, D. (1989) 'Undergraduates' Beliefs and Attitudes about AIDS', in P. AGGLETON, G. HART and P. DAVIES (eds), *AIDS: Social Representations, Social Practices*, Lewes, Falmer Press.

CLIFT, S.M., STEARS, D.F.A. LEGG, S., MEMON, A. and RYAN, L. (1989) *Report on Phase One of the HIV/AIDS Education and Young People Project*. Canterbury, HIV/AIDS Education Research Unit, Christ Church College.

COXON, T. (1988) 'The Numbers Game: Gay Lifestyles, Epidemiology of AIDS and Social Science', in P. AGGLETON and H. HOMANS (eds) *Social Aspects of AIDS*, Lewes, Falmer Press.

CURRIE, C. (1989) 'Young People in Independent Schools, Sexual Behaviour and AIDS', Chapter 5 in this volume.

DHSS (1987) *AIDS: Monitoring Responses to the Public Education Campaign February 1986 to February 1987*. London, HMSO.

EISER, C., EISER, J.R. and LANG, J. (in press) 'How Adolescents Compare AIDS with Other Diseases: Implications for Prevention', *Journal of Pediatric Psychology*.

FITZPATRICK, R., MCCLEAN, J., BOULTON, M., HART, G. and DAWSON, J. (1989) 'Variation in Sexual Behaviour in Gay Men', Chapter 8 in this volume.

FORD, N. and BOWIE, M. (1988) 'Sexually Related Behaviour and AIDS Education', *Education and Health*, October, pp. 86–91.

GILLIGAN, C. (1977) 'In a Different Voice: Women's Conceptions of Self and Morality', *Harvard Educational Review*, 47, 4, pp. 482–517.

HASTINGS, G.B. and SCOTT, A.C. (1988) 'The Development of AIDS Education Material for Adolescents', *Journal of the Institute of Health Education*, 26, 4, pp. 164–71.

HILL, A. and MAYON-WHITE, T. (1987) 'A Telephone Survey to Evaluate an AIDS Leaflet', *Health Education Journal*, 46, 3, pp 127–9.

KOHLBERG, L. (1976) 'Moral Stages and Moralization: The Cognitive-Developmental Approach', in T. LICKONA (ed.), *Moral Development and Behavior*. New York, Holt.

MCKEGANEY, N. and BARNARD, M. (1989) 'Drug Injectors' Risk for HIV', Chapter 10 in this volume.

MCQUEEN, D. and MCGLEW, T. (1989) 'A Survey of Undergraduate Opinion of AIDS'. Paper presented at the Third Social Aspects Conference, South Bank Polytechnic, 11 February 1989.

MCQUITTY, L.L. (1957) 'Elementary Linkage Analysis for Isolating Orthogonal and Oblique Types and Typal Relevances', *Educational and Psychological Measurement*, 17, pp. 207–29.

MEMON, A. (1989) 'Young People's Understanding, Beliefs and Attitudes Regarding AIDS: A Review of Research'. HIV/AIDS Education Research Unit, Christ Church College, Canterbury (submitted for publication).

NORUSIS, M.J. (1988) *SPSS/PC+ Advanced Statistics V2.0*, Chicago, Ill., SPSS Inc.

PHILLIPS, D.C. and NICOLAYEV, J. (1978) 'Kohlbergian Moral Development: A Progressing or Degenerating Research Program?' *Educational Theory*, 28, 4, pp. 286–301.

REID, D.A. (1988) 'Knowledge of School Children about the Acquired Immune Deficiency Syndrome', *Journal of the Royal College of General Practitioners*, 38, pp. 509–10.

SEARLE, E.S. (1987) 'Knowledge, Attitudes and Behaviour of Health Professionals in Relation to AIDS', *Lancet*, 3 January, p. 26.

WARWICK, I., AGGLETON, P. and HOMANS, H. (1988a) 'Young People's Health Beliefs and AIDS', in P. AGGLETON and H. HOMANS (eds), *Social Aspects of AIDS*, Lewes, Falmer Press.

WARWICK, I., AGGLETON, P. and HOMANS, H. (1988b) 'Constructing Commonsense: Young People's Beliefs about AIDS', *Sociology of Health and Illness*, 10, 3, pp. 213–33.
WEINER, B. (1985) *An Attributional Theory of Motivation and Emotion*, New York, Springer Verlag.
WEINER, B. (1988) 'Attribution Theory and Attributional Therapy: Some Theoretical Observations and Suggestions', *British Journal of Clinical Psychology*, 27, pp. 93–104.
WILSON, G.D. (1973) (ed.) *The Psychology of Conservatism*. London, Academic Press.

Chapter 5

Young People in Independent Schools, Sexual Behaviour and AIDS

Candace Currie

This chapter reports on findings from a study in which the sexual behaviour of young people is viewed from a lifestyle perspective and, in particular, is seen as a dimension of health-related behaviour. A lifestyle approach involves examining the social and environmental contexts within which health behaviours are performed (Aaro, Wold, Kannas and Rimpela, 1986). It means incorporating into the study design the measurement of factors such as the family and school environment, which may not directly influence health but are nevertheless important in understanding how lifestyles and their component health-related behaviours develop and change. Using this approach, the sexual behaviour of young people can be examined not in isolation but in relation to other lifestyle factors including smoking, drinking, exercise and eating habits, relationships with parents and attitudes towards school.

By considering the relationship between sexual behaviour and other patterns of health behaviour, one can determine whether engaging in sexual relations at a young age is associated with a lifestyle which incorporates potentially health enhancing behaviours such as regular physical activity, or with potentially health damaging activities such as smoking and alcohol abuse. Findings from the second World Health Organization (WHO) Health Behaviour among Schoolchildren Survey show that the association between sexual behaviour and other lifestyle factors may be important in relation to the design of programmes which aim to promote health in this age group (WHO, 1988). This chapter explores the idea that the promotion of healthy and responsible people may also be approached from a lifestyle perspective.

The study described here is a pilot for a component of a major survey to be conducted in Scotland and fourteen other European countries which are collaborating in an ongoing cross-national study of young people's health behaviour for the World Health Organization. The main study has a longitudinal design with cross-sectional surveys being repeated at three-year intervals and is now in its third survey year, the first and second being 1983 and 1986 (Aaro *et al.*, 1986; Currie, McQueen and Tyrrell, 1987). The third survey will be carried out in Scotland at the end of 1989; it is the first to include an optional component on young people's sexual behaviour and AIDS, which countries may choose to include if they wish. The reason for the inclusion of this topic is that the international research group felt the need to respond to the growing threat of AIDS to young people. However, it was agreed that it would be inappropriate to view sex as merely an AIDS-related behaviour and to frame questions in that light. Instead, it was decided to explore young people's behaviour in the context of their lifestyles as a whole and as part of an overall process of social, emotional and physical maturation. Through this route, it might be possible to identify where AIDS fits into the picture of a developing sexuality.

The Study

The pilot study reported on here was conducted in December 1988 and involved a sample of 300 young people in school, aged approximately 11, 13 and 15 years of age. Pupils were drawn from four independent schools in Edinburgh, since agreement to use the questionnaire was given readily by the headteachers of these schools. It is intended that the main survey to be carried out at the end of 1989 will sample from both state and independent schools from all regions of Scotland. Of the four schools in the study, two were co-educational, and two were single sex: one a boys' school, the other a girls' school. A previous survey showed that the majority of pupils attending these schools are from social classes I and II as classified by father's occupation (Currie *et al.*, 1987).

Only the 15-year-olds in the sample were asked questions relating to sexual behaviour. Of the sample of 115 15-year-olds, sixty-five were young men and fifty were young women. The survey employed a self-completion questionnaire given out in the classroom by the researcher. The teacher was not present. Confidentiality and anonymity were assured, and after completing the questionnaire, respondents were asked, if they had time, to put any comments on the questionnaire on the back of the last page.

Most of the questions relating to sexual behaviour in the pilot were selected and adapted from a study of young people's sexuality conducted in Finland (Kontula and Rimpela, 1986). This was an in-depth study of sexual knowledge, attitudes and behaviour and, as such, employed a great many more questions on sexuality than it is feasible to include in this survey, which has a much broader scope.

The questions relating to sexual behaviour were constructed as follows: 'Have you ever experienced the following things? Write down the age you were the first time.' Then the following items of behaviour were listed: kissing on the mouth, light petting (above waist), heavy petting (below waist), and sexual intercourse. The meaning of the term 'sexual intercourse' was not defined. The terms 'sexually active' and 'sexually experienced', as used interchangeably in this chapter, are defined as having experienced any of the above behaviours. It should be noted that the questions referring to these behaviours did not specify whether they were performed with persons of the same or the opposite sex. There were no questions about sexual behaviour performed alone — solo masturbation, for example.

Questions regarding the experiences of being in love, and having a steady relationship were worded as follows: 'Have you ever been really in love with a boy or girl whom you know?', 'Have you had a steady relationship with a girl friend or boy friend?', 'Do you have a steady girl- or boyfriend at present, if yes, how long have you been going steady?' As before, none of these questions specifically referred to partners of the same or opposite sex.

Sexual Behaviour

By the age of 15, significantly more young women (82 per cent) than young men (61 per cent) reported that they have experienced kissing on the mouth ($x^2 = 4.4$, df = 1, p < 0.05). However, with regard to other behaviours, gender differences were not significant. Thus 68 per cent of young women and 50 per cent of young men reported having experienced light petting; 48 per cent and 32 per cent respectively reported that they had experienced heavy petting; and 10 per cent and 12 per cent respectively said they had had sexual intercourse.

Among young women, age at the onset of periods is correlated with age of first sexual behaviours. Pearson product-moment correlation coefficients are calculated between age at menarche and age when various sexual behaviours are first experienced using minimum pairwise deletion of missing cases. Values for r and their significance levels are as follows: light petting r = .44 (p < 0.01); heavy petting r = .41 (p < 0.01); sexual intercourse r = .56 (p < 0.001).

In addition to studying the physical aspects of sexual development, it was considered important to examine the emotional aspects. In response to questions concerned with the experience of being in love and having steady relationships, around half of the 15-year-olds surveyed said that they had been in love at least once, and around half reported that they have had a steady relationship. Current steady relationships ranged from one week to almost two years in their duration.

Sources of Information about Sexual Matters

In response to an open-ended question, 'Where do you get most of your information about sexual matters?', the main sources mentioned were parents, friends, books or the mass media, and school, with some young people giving several sources. Young women and young men differed in their preferred sources of information: 40 per cent of young women compared to 10 per cent of young men mentioned parents; 60 per cent and 36 per cent respectively mentioned friends; 48 per cent and 52 per cent said books or mass media; and 18 per cent and 28 per cent respectively reported that they got most information from school.

So whereas young women most commonly cited their friends as sources of information on sexual matters, young men most often mentioned books, other literature and television, the second most commonly cited category among young women. Although friends were the second most likely common source of information for young men, they were still much less likely to mention this source than were young women. Parents were the third most popular source for young women who were four times more likely to use their parents than young men for whom this is the least commonly reported source. Young men are more likely than young women to mention school, and for young men this source is preferred to parents. In summary, young women were more likely than young men to acquire information through discussion with others, whereas young men seemed to prefer using more private ways that do not necessitate talking about sex. Another gender difference is that young women were more likely to use a variety of sources of information.

Communication about Sex with Parents and Friends

The young people involved in this study were asked how often they had discussed various topics relating to sexuality with their parents. The following figures give the percentages of young women and young men respectively who reported having discussed each topic at least once with their parents: contraceptives, 65 per cent and 32 per cent; relationships with girl- or boyfriend, 88 per cent and 54 per cent; becoming pregnant/getting a girl pregnant, 72 per cent and 25 per cent; menstruation (periods), 98 per cent and 14 per cent; the disease AIDS, 88 per cent and 56 per cent; other sexually transmitted diseases, e.g. herpes, gonorrhoea, 47 per cent and 16 per cent.

In agreement with the question on sources of information, young women were markedly more likely than young men to discuss all these sex-related topics with their parents. Compared to other sexual issues, AIDS came high on the agenda for discussion between parents and respondents. Nevertheless, around half of the young men had never discussed AIDS with their parents. This finding contrasts with young women where almost all have discussed the subject. Furthermore, discussions about AIDS, as with the other topics, were more frequent between young women and their parents than between young men and their parents. Hence, whereas around 30 per cent of the former reported having discussed AIDS many times, fewer than 10 per cent of the latter did this.

Respondents were also asked whether they had discussed the above topics seriously with their friends. If one presents the results in the same way, young women and young men respectively reported having discussed the following topics at least once with friends: contraceptives: 89 per cent and 48 per cent; relationships with girl- or boyfriend, 98 per cent and 70 per cent; becoming pregnant/getting a girl pregnant, 93 per cent and 52 per cent; menstruation (periods), 94 per cent and 23 per cent; the disease AIDS, 90 per cent and 67 per cent; other sexually transmitted diseases, e.g. herpes, gonorrhoea, 67 per cent and 27 per cent.

Again in agreement with the open-ended question on sources of information, these data show clearly that young women were more likely than young men to have talked to their friends about sex, the topic of AIDS being no exception. Moreover, on all subjects, including AIDS, both young women and young men were more likely to have talked with friends than parents.

If one puts responses from these two sets of questions together, one obtains percentages of respondents who have discussed the topics with neither parents nor friends and perhaps with no one else either, since only rarely were other people, such as sisters or brothers, mentioned as sources of information on sex. Data on young women and young men respectively give the following percentages for each topic: contraceptives, 6 per cent and 46 per cent; relationships with a girl- or boyfriend, 2 per cent and 27 per cent; becoming pregnant/getting a girl pregnant, 6 per cent and 44 per cent; the disease AIDS, 4 per cent and 25 per cent; other sexually transmitted diseases, e.g. herpes, gonorrhoea, 27 per cent and 68 per cent.

The findings show that a large proportion of young men talked neither to parents nor to friends about these sexual matters. Most importantly, one-quarter of 15-year-old young men may not have discussed AIDS with anyone. Young women were far more likely to have discussed these sexual issues with either friends or parents and often both.

Communication about Sex and Sexual Experience

On the relationship between sexual behaviour and frequency of talking about sexual matters with parents and friends, there were some broad differences between young women and young men, and between young people who only have experience of kissing and light petting and those who have engaged in heavy petting and sexual intercourse.

Table 1 presents Pearson product-moment correlations, calculated as described above, and shows that among the young men interviewed, those who are sexually experienced are likely to have discussed sexual matters more frequently than those who are not, but there are differences between them depending on the extent of sexual experience. Young men who had experienced kissing and light petting are likely to have discussed sexual matters more often, with both their parents and their friends, than young men who have not engaged in these activities. However, although young men who have practised heavy petting and sexual intercourse were more likely to discuss sex frequently with friends than their relatively inexperienced peers, this did not hold for discussion with parents.

Table 1. Correlations between Sexual Behaviour and Communications about Sex

Young men (N = 47)	Kissing	Light petting	Heavy petting	Sexual intercourse
Discuss with parents				
Contraceptives	.33**	.34**	.18	.23
Relationships	.60***	.50***	.26	.10
Pregnancy	.46***	.32**	.24	.40**
AIDS	.35**	.32**	.12	.05
Other STD	.24	.30	.26	.34*

Young men (N = 47)	Kissing	Light petting	Heavy petting	Sexual intercourse
Discuss with friends				
Contraceptives	.65***	.68***	.52***	.37**
Relationships	.58***	.58***	.37**	.22
Pregnancy	.64***	.67***	.53**	.40**
AIDS	.48***	.50***	.30	.25
Other STD	.40***	.41***	.46***	.43***

Young women (N = 36)	Kissing	Light petting	Heavy petting	Sexual intercourse
Discuss with friends				
Contraceptives	.41**	.14	.13	.17
Relationships	.42**	.32	.08	.16
Pregnancy	.66***	.45***	.29	.17
AIDS	.28	.16	.07	.09
Other STD	.41**	.33	.18	.26

Notes: * p < 0.05
** p < 0.01
*** p < 0.001

No such associations are found for young women between sexual behaviour and frequency of talking about sex with parents. Thus those who are sexually active were not more likely to discuss sex frequently with parents. Furthermore, although young women who have engaged in kissing and light petting were more likely to discuss some sexual matters with their friends than their peers who are not yet sexually active, this did not apply to young women who had engaged in heavy petting and sexual intercourse (Table 1); here young women and young men differ.

It should be remembered that the study used a small sample and the numbers of young people who reported engaging in heavy petting and sexual intercourse were even smaller. Bearing this in mind, and that the main survey will be repeated with a much larger sample (around 1000 15-year-olds) from a range of social backgrounds, it might nevertheless be hypothesized that engaging in sexual activities does not lead to increased discussion about sex with parents — indeed, the reverse may be true. For young men, sexual experience and discussing sex with friends are clearly associated. For young women, this appears to be true when sexual behaviour includes kissing and light petting, but if they are involved in heavy petting or sexual intercourse, then they may be less inclined to discuss sex with their friends.

Sexual Behaviour and Lifestyle

The associations between five measures of health-related behaviour — frequency of smoking, drinking alcohol, getting drunk, dieting and taking regular hard physical exercise — and measures of sexual experience — whether or not respondents have engaged in kissing, light or heavy petting and sexual intercourse — were explored. Table 2 gives correlation coefficients calculated as above. The data show that young women and young men who have begun to engage in sexual activities are more likely to be daily smokers, and when they drink to do so to excess, than their peers who have not begun to be sexually active. So the subgroup of young people who are engaging in sex also tend to engage in other behaviours with potential health risks.

Table 2. Correlations between Sexual Behaviours and Other Health Behaviours

Young women	Smoking N = 41	Drinking N = 41	Drunkenness N = 41	Dieting N = 42	Exercise N = 42
Kissing	.27	.06	.29	.20	.28
Light petting	.39**	.08	.38**	.20	.19
Heavy petting	.46***	.29	.50***	−.07	.05
Sexual intercourse	.56***	.50***	.81***	.16	−.27
Young men	Smoking N = 43	Drinking N = 43	Drunkenness N = 43	Dieting N = 49	Exercise N = 49
Kissing	.29	.24	.43***	.04	.28
Light petting	.35**	.29	.56***	−.20	.21
Heavy petting	.39**	.32*	.56***	−.13	.12
Sexual intercourse	.18	.54***	.53***	−.08	−.03

Notes: *p <0.05
**p <0.01
***p <0.001

The other dimensions of lifestyles considered are related to family life and school life. In relation to family life, there are two questions which provide measures of the quality of parent-child communication. The first one asks respondents how easy it is for them to talk to their parents about things that really bother them, and the other asks whether they feel foolish when they talk to their parents. In Table 3 correlations between these measures and the measures of frequency with which respondents discussed sexual matters with their parents are presented.

Table 3. Correlations between Measures of Parent-Child Communication

Young women (N = 39)	Ease of talking to mother	Ease of talking to father	Feel foolish when talking to parents
Discuss with parents			
Contraceptives	.40**	.32*	−.32*
Relationships	.59***	.52***	−.39**
Pregnancy	.52***	.51***	−.37**
AIDS	.54***	.29	−.18
Other STD	.44***	.22	−.30*

Correlations between Sexual Experience and School Variables

Young men (N = 50)	Liking for school	Good opinion of performance
Kissing	−.18	−.43***
Light petting	−.32**	−.35**
Heavy petting	−.46***	−.50***
Sexual intercourse	−.37**	−.43***

Notes: *p < 0.05
**p < 0.01
***p < 0.001

The correlations in Table 3 show that, among young women, discussions about sexual matters were more likely to occur in families where daughters find it easy to talk to their parents about their problems and do not feel foolish for doing so. For young men, there were no associations between the two sets of variables, suggesting that discussions about sex are less dependent on there being an easy relationship between sons and parents.

In relation to school life, young people were asked to rate how much they liked or disliked school, and they were asked to rate their teacher's opinion of their performance in class. As shown in Table 3, among young men, a negative attitude towards school and own performance at school were associated with being sexually active at 15 or earlier; these associations were not found among young women.

Discussion

Around half of the young women and one-third of the young men have engaged in heavy petting and around 10 per cent report having had sexual intercourse. The sample was, however, drawn from schools where most children come from professional families, and so it might be questioned how good an estimate it provides of the prevalence of sexual experience in the teenage population in Scotland. Earlier studies of young people's sexuality conducted in England found no difference between social class groups and sexual experience among young women (Schofield, 1965; Farrell, 1978). Farrell's study, but not Schofield's, found that young men from working-class backgrounds become sexually experienced at a younger age than did middle-class young men. So estimates of the prevalence of sexual behaviours from this pilot may be low for young men but more accurate for young women.

Data from this small pilot study indicate that in Scotland there may have been up to a ten fold increase in percentage of young women who have had first intercourse by age 15 since 1982 (Bone, 1985), but such a pattern would have to be confirmed with the larger survey. Furthermore, comparing the Scottish figures with those from England and Wales in 1974, Bone found that Scottish young women are less likely than those in the rest of Britain to have penetrative intercourse in their teens. Thus in 1982, and by the age of 16, 6 per cent of Scottish young women had had penetrative intercourse, whereas the figure was 12 per cent in England and Wales in 1974, some eight years earlier (Farrell, 1978). Exact figures are not important here; it is sufficient that in Scotland a small but significant percentage of young people engage in heterosexual penetrative sex by the age of 15 and some members of this subgroup may therefore potentially be at risk of HIV.

Sources of Information on Sexual Matters

Young men in the sample rely to a greater extent on literature and the media for information on sex than on friends or parents and, although they may get adequate factual information from these sources, they may be missing out on more personal advice regarding the development of their own sexual behaviour. This may be especially important in relation to AIDS where not just facts but a safe code of behaviour need to be learned. For example, young people embarking on their sexual careers need to learn how to protect themselves from the risk of contracting HIV, but this risk should be seen in perspective and within the broader context of developing responsible sexual behaviour.

A quarter of young men were found to discuss AIDS with neither their parents nor friends. Young women used books and the media as much as young men, but used friends and parents much more than their male counterparts. Young women also used a greater variety of sources and specifically made greater use of close personal sources of information. Because of the range of sources of information that young women used to find out about sex, when it comes to gathering information on AIDS they may be better placed than young men. Indeed, it was found that a mere 4 per cent of the former have discussed AIDS with neither parents nor friends.

Allen's (1987) study of education in sex and personal relationships, which surveyed 200 young people and their parents sampled from three cities in England, found that different sources of information are used for different reasons. Friends and mothers are used because of familiarity and lack of embarrassment; however, young people are aware of the limitations of friends their own age in terms of getting reliable factual information. When asked where they thought they would get the most accurate information about sex and contraception, young women were most likely to say their mother whereas young men chose their teacher or their doctor. Only a small percentage of young women or young men cited their friends. However, although young men think of doctors and teachers as reliable sources, few would actually turn to these people, claiming that they would feel too awkward. Allen found that children preferred their friends because even with all their unreliability they were still considered the most understanding and trustworthy. After mothers, friends were the most likely people to be turned to with questions on sex, contraception or relationships.

In the study described here, school as a source of information was cited least by young women; young men were almost three times as likely to mention school, but nonetheless a mere 28 per cent do so. This suggests that either schools are not providing much information or that pupils find the information unhelpful. Schools potentially have a very important role in sex education, and in Allen's (1987) study are considered by both parents and young people themselves to be the most important source of information and education about sex and contraception. These pilot data suggest that schools do not always fulfil these roles or only do so for a minority of pupils.

As with education about contraception, AIDS education for young people needs to address the whole subject of sexuality and should be placed within the context of age-specific lifestyles as a whole. It has been suggested that in school and elsewhere sexual behaviour should not be discussed simply in the context of disease. Young people need to be taught decision-making skills that can enable them to protect themselves and their health, and sex needs also to be seen in a positive light (Tandy and Bax, 1988). Many young people in Allen's study felt that school should teach not only about sex and contraception but also about the development of personal relationships. AIDS education perhaps needs to be integrated into such a curriculum and not treated as an isolated subject.

Talking to Parents about Sex

Results show that respondents who were more sexually experienced were no more likely to have discussed sex with their parents than those who were inexperienced. Put another way, discussion about sex is not associated with early coitus. This may be reassuring to those who believe that teaching young people about sex will encourage them to experiment, but also suggests that parent-child communication about sex has little impact on sexual behaviour.

There has been and continues to be much debate as to the influence of parent-child communication about sexual matters on young people's sexual behaviour. Most recent discussion has centred on the question of whether open communication about sex and contraception between parents and their teenage children has any effect on contraceptive behaviour (Knox and McGlew, 1986). Studies fall into two broad categories. On the one hand, there are those such as Farrell (1978), Fox and Inazu (1980) and Bury (1984) which suggest that the evidence is convincing that parent-child (and particularly mother-daughter) communication may have a variety of 'positive' outcomes including the postponement of sexual activity, or, in those who are already sexually active, the practice of more effective birth control. The processes by which these effects are brought about are, however, not well understood.

More recent research, which examines in detail the exact nature of mother-daughter communication from each side of the relationship, as well as the effects of this communication on the young person's behaviour, has, however, failed to substantiate the 'unproven assumptions' previously made on the basis of indirect evidence (Knox and McGlew, 1986). Thus Newcomer and Udry (1984, 1985) have found that neither parental attitudes towards premarital sex, nor parent-child communication about sex and contraception, appear to affect young people's subsequent contraceptive behaviour. Cvetkovich and Grote (1983) suggest that responsible contraceptive behaviour is more to do with maturity and the young person's acceptance of her/his own sexuality than with communication with parents about sex. Most young people find that these discussions are limited due to parents' inability to think of their children as sexually capable people.

The controversy continues as to the significance of parent-child communication, but what is clear from many studies is that parents and their offspring often find discussing sexual matters difficult and embarrassing, and that both consider that school is, at least potentially, the most important source of information (Allen, 1987). Kendall and Coleman (1988) suggest that the inability on the part of adults in general, and not just parents, to accept young people's sexuality is the cause for the poor management in our society of the sexuality of the young. This poor management means that there is no commitment to an educational policy which provides the framework for teaching young people about all aspects of sex in the context of wider personal relationships. It also means that rarely is there an existing framework within which the subject of AIDS can be sensitively dealt with.

Discussing Sex with Friends

Respondents discussed sex more with their friends than with their parents. However, whereas for young men sexual experience increases the likelihood that they have talked about sex with their friends, the same is not true for young women. Again, this finding is open to several interpretations. One is that young women talk to such an extent to their friends that no differences appear between those who are sexually inexperienced or experienced. The other is that once they have started having sex, young women are rather less inclined to discuss their personal lives, perhaps due to ambivalence about their own behaviour. Whereas for young men, among their peers, it is socially acceptable and even desirable to gain sexual experience and the reputation that goes with it, it is still the case for young women that reputation is something to be guarded. The defence of reputation may be crucial to young women's social standing, certainly around the age of 15 or so (Lees, 1986). Being sexually active may be something that young women prefer to keep to themselves. Friends are probably not a source of reliable advice on practical matters (Allen, 1987), but could perhaps, if they felt less ambivalent about their own behaviour, provide emotional support. Since young women are growing up within such a confusing moral and emotional climate, it is little wonder that forward thinking and decision-making regarding their sexual behaviour may elude them. AIDS brings with it yet another fear regarding the possible outcome of sexual encounters, and if education about AIDS is not integrated into broad-based programmes on sexual relationships, it may become just another factor contributing to conflict with which young people and perhaps especially young women, view their emerging sexuality.

A Lifestyle Approach to Understanding Young People's Sexuality

Using the lifestyle perspective, one observes that young women and young men who embark on sexual activity at a young age are at 15 more likely to smoke and consume alcohol, at least at this stage in their lives. For young men, disaffection from school is also associated with early sexual activity. Girls who find their parents difficult to talk to about their problems also communicate less with their parents about sexual matters.

The lifestyle approach to studying young people's sexual behaviour allows the consideration of whether sexual behaviour in this age group appears to be a largely negative or positive health behaviour. Early sexual activity, as we have seen, is associated with behaviours such as smoking and alcohol use, which are often considered to be forms of risk-taking and potentially health compromising, especially if continued into adulthood. A previous study of 15-year-olds using a sample of 1500 young people in Scotland found that smoking and drunkenness were correlated with poorer self-rated health (Currie and McQueen, in press). The evidence suggests that sexual behaviour has some of the features of risky behaviour and negative health behaviour.

Health risk-taking has been claimed to have multiple developmental functions for young adults. It has been proposed tht only through risk-taking can they cope with the developmental demands of learning to deal with intoxicants such as tobacco and alcohol (Franzkowiak, 1987). The same argument could be applied to sexual risk-taking. However, the risks can be reduced so that as few young people as possible have to face the long-term consequences of unplanned pregnancy or HIV infection.

The way in which adults view young people's sexuality may have an important role in shaping adolescent perceptions of their own sexual behaviour (Kendall and Coleman, 1988). In particular, the way in which sex educators, be they parents or teachers, deal with the subject may influence how young people feel and act, and may have increased the negative aspects of sex in young people's minds. A recent Finnish survey has shown that fear is a major component of young people's feelings about sex (Rimpela, 1989). For the sexually active young person with a negative view of their own behaviour, conflict can arise, and this may lead to greater risk-taking. For example, if a young woman is brought up to believe that premarital sex is wrong, she may not intend to have intercourse until it actually happens. Planning ahead and taking responsibility for contraception could mean accepting that she is sexual and that she may have intercourse (Bury, 1984). By avoiding considering contraception, it may be possible to maintain a sexually inactive self-image whereby the occurrence of sex is perceived as an exception (Gross and Bellew-Smith, 1983). If denial of emerging sexuality led to avoidance of sexual encounters, then young people in this ambivalent state would avoid the risks of unprotected sex. However, it seems clear that this group may be in particular need of guidance regarding responsible sexual behaviour. This has serious implications for AIDS prevention in young people, and presents a challenge to adults involved in education in personal and sexual relationships. It is within this spirit that Kendall and Coleman (1988) suggest that adults must acknowledge the fundamental importance of young people's sexuality and, having done so, must take on the responsibility for creating national policies related to the provision of confidential contraceptive advice and availability, and school sex education set within the context of education about personal relationships.

It is proposed that the lifestyle approach to studying young people's sexual behaviour and AIDS can be valuable from the point of view of designing appropriate educational programmes. In particular, it suggests a more holistic style of sex education and AIDS education, one which takes lifestyles as a whole into account. This study found that those embarking on sexual activity at a young age tend to have certain characteristics: they are engaging in what are considered by adults (but perhaps not teenagers themselves) to be risky behaviours, they may have problems relating to parents and they may be alienated from school. To reach this subgroup, there is the need to take their overall lifestyle into account.

Finally, possible limitations of the sample should be considered. The sample cannot in any sense be said to represent 15-year-olds in Scotland as a whole. Although in Edinburgh 20 per cent of 15-year-olds attend independent schools (Currie *et al.*, 1987), this is not typical of Scotland overall, where the most children attend state schools. Moreover, there is a different social class structure in the two types of school, with the sample here consisting of children from predominantly professional families. Health-related behaviours such as smoking and drinking have been found to differ according to class among young people and, independent of social class, differences in behaviour of pupils attending the two types of school have been observed (Currie and McQueen, in press). It may be that sexual behaviour also varies according to these factors. Nevertheless, one might speculate that the differences are likely to be of degree rather than in terms of interrelations between sexual behaviour and other health behaviours. Such issues can only be resolved when the main study has been undertaken.

References

AARO, L. M. WOLD, B., KANNAS, L. and RIMPELA, M. (1986) 'Health Behaviour in Schoolchildren: a WHO Cross-national Study', *Health Promotion*, 1, pp. 17–33.

ALLEN, I. (1987) *Education in Sex and Personal Relationships*. London, Frances Pinter.

BONE, M. (1985) *Family Planning in Scotland in 1982*. OPCS Social Surveys Division, London, HMSO.

BURY, J. (1984) *Teenage Pregnancy*. London, Birth Control Trust.

CURRIE, C., and McQUEEN, D. V. (in press) 'Difference in Patterns of Drinking and Smoking in 15 Year Old Scottish Schoolchildren', *Drogalkohol* (in German). Also (in English) Working Paper No. 31, Research Unit in Health and Behavioural Change, University of Edinburgh.

CURRIE, C., and McQUEEN, D.V. and TYRRELL, H. (1987) 'First Report of the RUHBC/SHEG/WHO Survey of the Health Behaviour of Scottish Schoolchildren (Lothian Region) Aged 11, 13 and 15 Years', Working Paper, Research Unit in Health and Behavioural Change, University of Edinburgh.

CVETKOVICH and GROTE (1983) 'Adolescent Development and Teenage Fertility', in BYRNE, D. and FISHER, W. A. (eds) *Adolescents, Sex and Contraception*, London, Lawrence Erlbaum Associates.

FARRELL, C. (1978) *My Mother Said: The Way Young People Learn about Sex and Birth Control*. London, Routledge and Kegan Paul.

FOX, G. L. and INAZU, J. (1980) 'Patterns and Outcomes of Mother-Daughter Communication about Sexuality', *Journal of Social Issues*, 36, 1, pp. 7–29.

FRANZKOWIAK, P. (1987) 'Risk-taking and Adolescent Development: The Functions of Smoking and Alcohol Consumption and Its Consequences for Prevention', *Health Promotion*, 2, 1, pp. 51–61.

GROSS, A. E. and BELLEW-SMITH, M. (1983) 'A Social Psychological Approach to Reducing Pregnancy Risk in Adolescence', in D. BYRNE and W. A. FISHER (eds), *Adolescents, Sex and Contraception*. London, Lawrence Erlbaum Associates.

KENDALL, K. and COLEMAN, J. (1988) 'Adolescent Sexual Behaviour: The Challenge for Adults', *Child and Society*, 2, pp. 165–77.

KNOX, H. and McGLEW, T. (1986) 'Mother-Daughter Communication: Birth Control and Unplanned Teenage Pregnancy; A Review'. Report commissioned by the Scottish Health Education Group.

KONTULA, O. and RIMPELA, M. (1986) 'Maturation, Human Relations and Sexuality in Schoolchildren (The Kiss-Study)'. Protocol from Department of Public Health, University of Public Health, Finland.

LEES, S. (1986) *Losing Out*, London, Hutchinson.

NEWCOMER, S. F. and UDRY, R. J. (1984) 'Mothers' Influence on the Sexual Behaviour of Their Teenage Children', *Journal of Marriage and the Family*, 46, pp. 477–85.

NEWCOMER, S. F. and UDRY, J. R. (1985) 'Parent-Child Communication and Adolescent Sexual Behaviour', *Family Planning Perspectives*, 17, 4, pp. 169–74.

RIMPELA, M. (1989) 'The Finnish Experience of Monitoring Health Behaviour: Implications for Health Promotion'. Paper presented at WHO:HBSC study meeting: current status and future plans. Report from Research Unit in Health and Behavioural Change, University of Edinburgh.

SCHOFIELD, M. (1965) *The Sexual Behaviour of Young People*. London, Longman.

TANDY, A. and BAX, M. (1987) 'AIDS: Health Education in Schools: The Role of the Community Child Health Services', *Child and Society*, 2, pp. 148–57.

WHO (1988) *Health for All Young People in Europe: Results from a Cross-National Survey of Health Behaviour among Schoolchildren*. Copenhagen, WHO.

Chapter 6

'Adolescents', Young People and AIDS Research

Ian Warwick and Peter Aggleton

In this chapter we will examine some of the taken for granted assumptions that inform emerging research agendas concerning young people and AIDS. Our interest in this field has been stimulated by recent conversations with psychologists and other social researchers, as well as by our recent reading of a number of research papers which view quite uncritically the relationship between biological maturation and young people's social development. These papers, and the discourse which surrounds them, most usually seek to identify in 'adolescents' (as young people in these studies are invariably called) certain qualities which are likely to render the person concerned particularly vulnerable to HIV infection and AIDS. These qualities often include emotional instability, a propensity to sexual experimentation, risk-taking, alcohol abuse and an involvement with illicit drugs. These attributes are often assumed to inhere quite unproblematically in all 'adolescents', but more especially in street youth, working-class youth, college students and young people from minority ethnic communities.

We will begin by identifying the origins of ideas like these. In so doing, particular attention will be focused on varieties of psychological explanation that seek to individualize and pathologize youth as a stage of life to be passed through en route to a mature and stable adulthood. Next we will discuss briefly the systems of disciplinary provision that have been rendered legitimate by ideologies that construct substantial numbers of young people as 'adolescents'. Specifically, we will examine the contribution that psychology has made in identifying a range of 'therapeutic' interventions that can be used to facilitate the smooth transition from a refractory 'adolescence' to a stable adulthood. Finally, we will explore some of the ways in which representations of youth as deficient, irresponsible or developmentally immature inhere in the research agendas to which many social scientists working in the field of HIV and AIDS currently subscribe. Notions such as these, we will argue, present an overly homogeneous view of young people and do violence to the socially differentiated nature of youth. Moreover, they are likely to lead to ill-conceived and poorly planned health education/promotion interventions, if indeed this is their aim. Just as seriously, they deflect attention from adults' own beliefs and practices to focus this instead upon those of young people.

Representations of 'Adolescence'

Current media representations of youth attempt to fit young people into a tripartite system of newsworthiness. Within this, the young person becomes either gifted, deprived or depraved (Muncie, 1988). Positive images of youth are most often associated with being a sporting star and being an entertainer in television and/or mainstream popular music. A propensity to victimization or an involvement in criminal activities most often characterizes deprived youth, with depravity being linked to gang or mob membership in the case of boys, or to sexual non-conformity in the case of girls (Falchikov, 1986).

However, it would be a mistake to restrict our attention solely to media representations. Since the late nineteenth century, social researchers too have played a key role in constructing young people as inherently deviant. For psychologists in particular, the concept of 'adolescence' has had a long history. Stanley Hall's (1905) original textbook on the subject, entitled *Adolescence: Its Psychology and Its Relations to Physiology, Anthropology, Sociology, Sex, Crime, Religion and Education*, laid the conceptual foundations for subsequent theorizing, as well as for much of what currently counts as 'common sense'. Hall argued that in the transition from children to adults people mimic the phylogeny of the human race. With growing maturity, we leave behind our animalistic childhood to embrace adolescent savagery en route to civilized adulthood. ' . . . The adolescent is neo-atavistic, and in him the later acquisitions of the race slowly became prepotent. Development is less gradual and more salutary, suggestive of some ancient period of storm and stress when old moorings were broken and a higher level attained . . . ' (Hall in Musgrove, 1964: 56).

In Hall's eyes, and in the eyes of many thereafter, the intervening years between childhood and adulthood were marked by a period of storm and stress. Even as society urges adolescents on towards greater maturity, other forces threaten to pull them back to a primitive state of stone-age animalism. Through analogies such as these, and through the institutional practices of a newly developing psychology, 'adolescence' became associated, if not synonymous, with the potential for deviance and pathology. The problem thereafter became one of ensuring that the adolescent was kept properly in the realm of psychological rather than medical expertise (Rose, 1985).

Although Hall's psycho-biological and determinist approach viewed the cause of 'adolescence' as essentially biological, Cyril Burt recast this. In 1925, fresh from his own deliberations on the 'feeble minded', the architect of psycho-eugenics turned his attention to the 'young delinquent' (Burt cited in Rose, 1985). Burt believed that the cause of delinquency lay in a misdirected general emotionality, a problem caused by faulty upbringing and, in particular, by interaction with an unstable mother. The site of correction was to be either the home, the family or the special treatment centre. By asserting that the psychologist had a role to play, not only in the assessment and identification of the delinquent, but in treatment via the re-direction of wayward impulses, psycho-eugenics laid the foundations for a new clinical space, concerned with, and directed towards, troublesome young people (Rose, 1985).

Foundations for the elaboration of this space, along with others of psychological import, had been laid some years earlier by academics in universities intent on refining their newly emerging status (Ben-David and Collins, 1966). As a consequence of these activities, the newly conceptualized young person was imbued with a range of distinctively mental qualities which set him (or her) apart from those who were older or younger. By this move, psychology claimed from bio-medicine the right to speak for young people, constructing 'adolescence' as a stage of life, a transition to be passed through on the road to adulthood. The qualities attributed to this period vary in detail from account to account, but most emphasize young people's desire to experiment (especially with drugs and in sexual relationships), their inability to see situations from other people's point of view (especially those of adults), their need to risk-take and to test boundaries (especially those to do with parental or teacherly authority), and their concern to live for the moment rather than the future.

All these features individualize, pathologize and homogenize 'adolescence'. By ignoring material inequalities between adults and young people, between young women and young men, between middle-class young people and working-class young people, between black youth and white youth, and between those who are able-bodied and those who are disabled; and by turning a blind eye to the creative, innovative and resistant aspects of youth subcultures (see, for example, Hall and Jefferson, 1976; Hebdige, 1979; McRobbie and Nava, 1984; and McRobbie, 1989), psychology has succeeded in constructing young people en masse as potentially irresponsible, immature and, above all, in need of adult tutelage, supervision, guidance and control.

The consequences of a mode of analysis which constructs young people as irresponsibly hedonistic, developmentally immature or deficiently skill-less can be seen clearly in mid-twentieth century analyses of juvenile 'delinquencies' and 'immoralities'. These came quickly to be understood as attributes of social and psychological growth in adolescence and only indirectly the result of economic and political conditions (Gillis, 1977). Ideas such as these were later popularized and widely disseminated through textbooks for parents and in guides for the trainee teacher or prospective youth worker (see, for example, The Home and School Committee of the English New Education Fellowship, 1954; Klein, 1963). Books with titles such as *The Adolescent in Your Family* (US Department of Health, Education and Welfare, 1955) and *Your Teenage Children* (Gibberd, 1964) advocated expert intervention when the strain on adults proved too much. The cover of the latter, for example, suggested that most parents would be 'glad of guidance from anyone who claims to be an expert on the *special* difficulties that *inevitably* arise at this stage' (emphasis added).

During the 1960s and 1970s, and coincident with growing student unrest in colleges and universities in Europe and North America, young people were singled out as being especially prone to rebellion. This could occasionally lead to generational conflict on a grand scale, as some, finding it difficult to 'separate from dependent or affectionate childhood ties', exhibited 'an exaggerated sense of independence to convince themselves and others that they can stand on their own feet' (Group for the Advancement of Psychiatry, 1966: 27). Moreover, young people's search for independence and their desire to question aspects of the status quo could cause particular difficulties in their encounters with adults. In their dealings with students, for example, college staff were advised to expect rapid transitions from civilized and adult 'consultations across the table' to cunning, dangerous and overgrown childish tantrums (Gunn, 1970: 45).

In this situation, themes that had remained dormant since the early twentieth century gained new importance. Qualitatively, 'adolescents' remained much the same as they had always been, the problem now lay in managing the tensions that could arise in their relationships with the adult world. The challenge for teachers, parents, youth workers and physicians lay in how best to intervene so as to manage this wayward stage of life; the growth of counselling, guidance and allied practices, whose task it is to normalize the waywardness of youth, is perhaps best seen in this light.

Ideas like these have captured the imaginations of many older people, shaping the ways in which they think, talk and write about those younger than themselves. As a result, they have become the 'common sense' that informs everyday understandings of young people and youth. Unfortunately, many social researchers too have cast their critical faculties aside, accepting as truth what are in reality little more than twentieth century theories about 'adolescence'. As Clarke (cited in Muncie, 1988: 9) has put it, 'the link between (all modern) representations of youth is the underlying assumption of the *different* and *deviant* nature of youth.'

Young People and AIDS

In this section, we will examine contemporary research agendas around young people and AIDS to assess the extent to which they have been captured by the ideologies of 'adolescence' described above. In order to do this, we will review some of the studies on young people and AIDS carried out since 1986. A broadly chronological approach will be adopted, although within this we will aim to identify key thematic concerns within and between different investigations.

The Unknowledgeable Adolescent

In an early paper, DiClemente, Zorn and Temoshok (1986) surveyed the knowledge, attitudes and beliefs about AIDS of 1326 'adolescents' in San Francisco. Students enrolled in family life education classes were presented with a checklist of ready-made statements about AIDS. They were required to indicate whether the statements were 'True' or 'False', or whether they did not know. The authors were concerned to find out whether students living near, what they called, a 'high density AIDS epicenter' — San Francisco in this case — possessed greater knowledge than students living elsewhere. They contrasted their findings with those from an earlier paper by Price *et al.* (1985) which had suggested that high school students were neither informed nor concerned about AIDS. They concluded that geographic proximity to an AIDS 'epicenter' was indeed relevant to how much students knew about the syndrome, with San Franciscan students showing higher levels of knowledge and greater concern than their counterparts elsewhere.

In a later edition of the journal in which DiClemente *et al.*'s paper was originally published, Wiesman and colleagues (1987) take exception to these conclusions, arguing that differences in knowledge between the two groups of young people are in fact artefacts of the measurement procedures adopted — a claim the original authors subsequently reject (DiClemente *et al.*, 1987). However, completely unrecognized in this debate are certain key assumptions about young people and their beliefs. Data collection procedures which consist of lists of 'True' or 'False' statements must, by their nature, construct those who are assessed by them as *cognitively deficient* in some respects. Furthermore, by suggesting that there are clear-cut answers to questions such as 'Having sex with someone who has AIDS is one way of getting it' or 'I am less likely than most people to get AIDS', schedules such as those employed by DiClemente *et al.* do violence to the available bio-medical knowledge (which distinguishes clearly between a virus and a syndrome, and which suggests that only certain kinds of sexual activity pose the risk of infection), as well as to the complex processes involved in risk perception. These issues are not examined by researchers who seem intent on demonstrating young people's deficiencies in the belief that 'knowledge about high-risk behaviours associated with AIDS virus infection [sic] could help limit the spread of disease in [the adolescent] population' (DiClemente *et al.* 1986: 1443).

The High Risk Adolescent

The notion of the 'high risk adolescent', whereby *all* young people are characterized as equally at risk for HIV, makes one of its many appearances in Strunin and Hingson's (1987) report on a telephone survey conducted among 860 young people in

Massachusetts. Their paper begins with the uncompromising statement that 'adolescents are as a group at high risk for exposure to acquired immunodeficiency syndrome (AIDS)' (Strunin and Hingson, 1987: 825). We must presume that by talking so loosely of exposure to AIDS they in fact mean exposure to HIV. The authors continue by pointing out, quite correctly on this occasion, that at the time of their study, reported cases of AIDS among 20–29-year-olds were increasing. But on what grounds are we to accept that people in their mid-20s are 'adolescents'? Potential difficulties such as this are quickly glossed over by the not entirely accurate suggestion that there can be a 'latency period' of between one and four years before AIDS develops, and by the quite unsubstantiated assertion that 'given adolescents' drug use and sexual behaviours, that group is at risk for AIDS' (Strunin and Hingson, 1987: 825). Via rhetorical devices such as these, readers are seduced into accepting a priori the waywardness of youth, even when data in the same paper fail to substantiate such a proposition. Strunin and Hingson, for example, found that 45 per cent of the young people they spoke to had not had 'sexual intercourse'! Of those who had, the 20 per cent who had changed their behaviour now made use of what the authors characterize as 'truly effective precautions' such as 'avoiding sex' or 'using a condom' (Strunin and Hingson, 1987: 827). From findings such as these, it is clearly less than fair to characterize young people en masse as a 'high risk group'.

The Overdetermined Adolescent

Yet another way in which young people have been constructed in relations to AIDS can be found in studies such as the extensive *Canada Youth and AIDS Study* (King *et al.*, 1989). Heralded as one of the most important investigations of its kind, this involved an investigation into the knowledge, attitudes and behaviour of over 38,000 young people in Canada. Yet the picture which emerges is one of young people whose behaviour is barely under control, this being determined either by their biology and the bodily changes that accompany puberty, or by peer group pressures. In the rationale for the *Canada Youth and AIDS Study*, we are warned:

> Many social scientists see the years between adolescence and young adulthood as a period of considerable stress. Associated with the emotional and physical changes that accompany puberty, there is pressure to conform to peer values, and a need to establish some clearer direction at a time of great uncertainty. (King *et al.*, 1989: 1)

These statements invite us to embrace wholesale a conception of 'adolescence' in which complex desires, motivations and actions, arising in specific material contexts, and in classed, aged, gendered, cultured and sexually differentiated subjects, are to be reduced to a refractory biological base. Thankfully, however, biology is not entirely destiny, in this respect at least. Outside influences too have a role to play, but all too often these create further problems. Thus we read that ' . . . adolescents face pressures to use drugs, especially alcohol, that impair their judgment and ability to make decisions at a time when they are beginning to be sexually active. This combination tends to lead to unplanned sex without precaution' (King *et al.*, 1989: 5).

Claims such as these, which are usually made for entire groups of young people with little or no substantiating evidence, constitute the 'common sense' around which many current research protocols are constructed. To give a further example, and one which rehearses almost verbatim these same arguments, Eiser, Eiser and Lang (forthcoming) preface their recent study of 'younger adolescents' with the claim that late adolescence is a stage of 'great vulnerability to AIDS and HIV infection, given the tendency to engage in frequent sexual activity and to experiment with illegal drugs.' Quite what the evidence is to suggest that the respondents in this particular study were likely to display these same behaviours later in life (their survey was a study of young students in secondary schools in south-west England) remains unspecified. Such is the power of these claims, they need no justification. It is as though by invocation young people *are* this way, and when they are not, we need have no doubt that their real interests, motivations and behaviours will be largely ignored by studies which seem more intent on bolstering conventional fictions than in enquiring into the variety of ways in which young people respond to HIV and AIDS.

The Tragic Adolescent

Yet another variation can be found in Wishon's (1988) alarmingly poetic yet singular view of young people's concerns. Preceding a quote from Wordsworth's poem, 'We Are Seven', the reader is informed that 'most victims of AIDS die; and especially among the young, when they die, they die despairing — lamenting the future they've been denied, shattering in convulsive fashion the heartfelt myth of the young, that they are invincible (Wishon, 1988: 213). In Wishon's mind, AIDS does indeed equal death. But not only this, a terrible death, and one that is all the more tragic because young people are involved. From accounts such as these, it would appear that young people really are innocent. Not for them, the hazards of low paid, dangerous and monotonous employment, not for them inadequate and appalling housing conditions, not for them physical and emotional abuse that so many experience on the grounds of their sexuality, race or gender, and not for them the realities of disease, illness and death. He continues, 'dying from AIDS is distinctly unpeaceful, and we are constant witness to hundreds of young among the dying who perish "before the flower of their creativity has enjoyed even brief bloom"' (Wishon, 1988: 219).

But for some there is a grim inevitability. Young gay men, young injecting drug users and young women having sexual relationships with a person with HIV infection or AIDS face en masse the bleakest of futures. Wishon explains, 'in most cases, AIDS is a death sentence steadfastly awaiting the . . . youth who are at greatest risk of becoming victims — . . . adolescent homosexuals and intravenous drug abusers, adolescent female partners of patients with AIDS or carriers . . . (Wishon, 1988: 218). Quite why 'female partners' should be singled out in this way is explicable only in terms of a logic which constructs some groups (here 'adolescent homosexuals' and 'intravenous drug abusers') as culpable and others as more undeserving. According to this frame of reference, young gay men and injecting drug users can *never* acquire HIV 'innocently' — only those who became infected as a result of heterosexual contact with them can lay claim to such a status. It is important to recognize that representations such as these are not 'truths' but social constructions, no less typical than they are vilificatory and patronizing. Of course, not all young gay men and young injecting drug users are at risk in quite the way Wishon would have us believe — some may have taken on safer sex and safer injecting practices quite a while ago, and others may never have been at risk in the first place. Even if some young people are more vulnerable to infection, this may have more to do with the ways in which they are systematically denied access to information about risk reduction, and the freedom and resources to act upon this knowledge, than to their status as 'victims', be they 'innocent' or otherwise.

The Irresponsible Later Adolescent

One particular kind of young person singled out for special concern in recent social research on HIV and AIDS is the college or university student. Given the wealth of studies that have now been carried out, one suspects that this focus has been as much motivated by researchers' easy access to undergraduates as by a desire to support college students in their responses to HIV. In conducting research in planning AIDS health promotion on campus, it is rare to find lecturers and teaching staff as objects of concern. Not for them, it seems, the peer pressure to engage in sexual activity. Nor do tutorial staff exercise poor judgment in their choice of sexual partners. Still less, do they experience the temptation to experiment with recreational drugs; instead it is the college student who has the monopoly on such wayward emotionality, and it is students who have difficulty with their sexuality, students who believe that AIDS is of no relevance to them, and students who must be the focus of professional intervention.

Thus Richard Keeling, Director of Virginia University's student health service, is able to say, without pausing for a moment to consider his peers' beliefs about AIDS (or their sexual practices for that matter), that a sense of invulnerability, *augmented* by peer pressure, *and* a desire for immediate gratification, *and* a willingness to experiment, *and* a high number of sexual partners, places college students particularly at risk (cited in Biemiller, 1987: 32; emphasis added). In another report, this same health service director acknowledges the need to consider others, both on and off campus. But while Keeling views the barely controlled sexual appetites of students as a cause of concern, he also wishes to protect them from what he describes as 'the spread of AIDS from the big cities'. 'Students', he reminds us, 'are *commonly* experimental; those in college may act out differing elements of their sexuality, exercise poor judgment in their selection of sexual partners, and be introduced to recreational drugs' (Keeling, 1986: 25). As a final warning he suggests ominously that 'they may not confine their sexual exploration to dealings with other students: they may interact with an institution's employees or the community as well. AIDS is no longer just a disease of the big cities; it has gradually moved out of the metropolitan areas' (Keeling, 1986: 25).

Concerns similar to these are voiced in McDermott and colleagues' (1987: 223) study of AIDS knowledge among 'select university students'. Working from the assumption that 'students have both relatively high levels of sexual activity and the potential for multiple sexual partners' (who does not have this *potential*, one wonders), they developed a twenty-statement inventory which was administered to 500 students in a large university in mid-western USA. Two questions on the twenty-item inventory focused on sexual behaviour. Students were invited to mark each item 'True' or 'False'. The first statement read, 'One way of decreasing the chance of getting AIDS is to avoid casual sex.' The second read, 'A person who engages in indiscriminate sexual behaviour increases the risk of contracting AIDS.' For the first question, 78.9 per cent got it 'right', and for the second, 68.3 per cent — percentages which McDermott and colleagues find less than reassuring. 'It is alarming', they say, 'that so many persons in a sexually active group fail to associate casual sex or indiscriminate sexual behaviour with disease risk' (McDermott *et al.*, 1987: 224). We should, of course, be alarmed for quite different reasons.

First, these researchers seem unable (or unwilling) to distinguish between a cause (HIV) and an effect (AIDS) in the statements they ask students to respond to, collapsing the two together via phrases such as 'getting AIDS' and 'contracting AIDS'. Second, not a shred of evidence is offered for the claim that young people as a whole are more sexually active than, say, people in their late 20s and early 30s, still less does it seem necessary to demonstrate that the particular young people surveyed in this study were so. Third, deeply ambiguous and highly value laden phrases such as 'casual sex' and 'indiscriminate sexual behaviour' are strewn around the inventory without the least attempt at clarification. Finally, safer sex is here equated with the avoidance of 'casual sex' and careful selection in the choice of sexual partners — a woefully inadequate approach to take, given understanding of the ways in which HIV is and is not transmitted.

Ian Warwick and Peter Aggleton

Varieties of Adolescent, Varieties of Risk

Imagery such as that discussed above is even more evident in Ford's (1988) recent survey of AIDS awareness and sexual behaviour among young people in Bristol. Beginning from the claim that 'in terms of general attitudes to life a more permissive attitude is . . . positively related to hedonism', he examines the relationship between 'sexual behaviour, sexual philosophy, AIDS awareness and other aspects of lifestyle' (Ford, 1988: 38). Using cluster analysis, Ford is able to identify a tripartite typology of young people's sexual philosophies which, he claims, may have broad summary implications for AIDS education. Young people, he claims, can adopt a 'traditional-restrictive', a 'liberal-romantic' or a 'radical-recreational' approach in their sexual relationships. The first of these categories describes those who are 'virgins', young people who believe strictly in 'no sex before marriage'. The second group restricts sex to steady relationships, and the third condones sex with multiple partners outside a primary sexual relationship. To Ford, the last group is the most worrying, being predominantly hedonistic and having the highest percentage of fathers in manual occupations. Such middle-class concern about young working-class people's recreational involvements is, of course, far from new (see, for example, Pearson, 1983).

Ford's analysis is replete with moral judgments and questionable conceptions of safer sex. He insists, for example, that 'monogamy is recommended as the safest means of avoiding the AIDS virus' (Ford, 1988: 26), and suggests that safer sex involves 'the limitation of an individual's sexual activity to within an exclusive, monogamous relationship, and the use of a condom as a prophylactic' (Ford, 1988: 2). This emphasis on condoms reveals as much about dominant beliefs in the inevitability of bodily penetration in authentic sexual encounters as it does about young women's and young men's own preferences and behaviours. As a result, it becomes as unproblematic to enquire into young people's sexual behaviours as it is to construct a typology of sexual philosophies. For example, Ford is keen to find out about what he terms the 'precautionary actions' that 'virgins' and 'non-virgins' might take, and asks young people whether they intend to 'insist on the use of a condom, find out about their partner's past sexual experience and ask the partner to have a blood test to check for the AIDS virus' (Ford, 1988: 27).

In this half sentence, Ford conjures up a number of popular illusions. First, the question shows little awareness of the factors which make it difficult, if not impossible, for many women to 'insist' that their male partners use a condom when having penetrative sex (cf. Holland et al., 1989). Second, it fails to recognize that knowing your sexual partner is not a reliable form of safer sex. As is becoming clear from the *Women, Risk and AIDS Project*, 'knowing' can be an extremely poor guide to risk assessment, since it relies to heavily on stereotypical, and possibly invalid, information. Indeed, some of the young people interviewed in connection with this project were not at all concerned about HIV infection *because* they felt confident that so long as they restricted their sexual partners to people living on the same housing estate, and whose sexual histories they knew about, there could be no risk of infection (Ramazanoglu, 1989). Finally there is no recognition here of the limitations of testing as a means of risk reduction (see Patton's chapter elsewhere in this volume, Chapter 1). In this account, safer sex becomes reduced to a set of individual, and often quite impractical and unrealistic, actions that it is supposed *others* should take.

Implications

We have reviewed the studies cited above for two main reasons. First, we are concerned that popular myths about youth and 'adolescence' are in the process of being uncritically reproduced within contemporary social research on HIV and AIDS. Second, we are alarmed when social researchers seriously propose that investigations such as those reviewed can be used as the starting point for AIDS health education/promotion involving young people.

As we have argued, much contemporary research accepts a priori and without question the view that young people as a group are unknowledgable, irresponsible in their relationships with others, immature and easily led. In our opinion, such representations are singularly unhelpful in making sense of the socially differentiated nature of young people's experience in relation to HIV and AIDS. In future work, it will be vital to enquire into the different ways in which young women and young men, young heterosexuals and young lesbians and young gay men, young middle-class people and young working-class people, young blacks and young whites, the young disabled and the young able-bodied have responded to AIDS. This research should begin to map out the heterogeneity of beliefs, understandings and knowledge that informs the behaviour of specific groups of young people in different contexts.

Major problems also arise when well meaning adults, who may themselves be less adequately versed in issues to do with HIV and AIDS, rush in with checklists of items gleaned from medical reports or newspaper columns. Ill-defined concepts, medically misleading terminology and prejudiced language can be found in numerous inventories that have supposedly been designed to assess young people's knowledge and beliefs about HIV and AIDS. Thus there is endless talk about the 'AIDS virus' the 'AIDS test', 'getting AIDS', 'catching AIDS' and 'avoiding AIDS' in interview and questionnaire schedules — terminology which is likely to tell us more about researchers' own confusions about the difference between a virus and a syndrome than about anything young people believe.

Profoundly ambiguous terms, such as 'deep kissing', 'light petting', 'sexual intercourse' and 'steady partner', abound in many research instruments. Similarly, the often used phrase 'have sex' can hold a multitude of meanings. It can refer variously to oral sex, vaginal sex, anal sex, masturbation, or any combination of these. It can describe an act involving one person, two women, two men, or a woman and a man. It can describe circumstances in which one or both partners experience an orgasm, or a situation in which neither does. It can describe events in which there was an exchange of semen and/or cervical and vaginal secretions, or ones in which steps were taken to ensure that this did not occur. Bearing this in mind, what does it really mean to ask a young person (or an adult for that matter), 'Did you use a condom when you last had sex?' In contexts such as these, surely we are entitled to ask, Is this the best that publicly funded social researchers can come up with?

Then there is the issue of prejudiced language to contend with. To what extent should researchers include items which are blatantly moralistic, racist, sexist, anti-lesbian and anti-gay in the questionnaires and interview schedules they develop, and to what extent should we assume that predominantly white, middle-class heterosexual social scientists are able to recognize when statements do indeed have these qualities? Judging from most of the research instruments we have seen, there is grave cause for concern here.

But it is when social researchers claim that their investigations into young people's beliefs can lay the foundations for future AIDS health education and health promotion that we should perhaps be most sceptical. For a start, effective AIDS health education/promotion is about much more than the provision of bio-medical information. It is about the interface between this knowledge and lay beliefs; it is about attitudes, emotions and feelings; it is about perceptions of risk in specific situations; it is about the social empowerment of groups; and it is about the elimination of structures which systematically deny young people access to the resources they need (Homans and Aggleton, 1988; Aggleton, 1989). Were question-naires and interview schedules to include items relating to this wider range of issues, and were the social researchers who administer them better networked with their colleagues working as health educators and health promoters, there would be grounds for more optimism.

If future social enquiry into young people and HIV/AIDS is to inform health education and health promotion initiatives, it needs to do several things. First, it should be less concerned with advocating certain moral positions than at present — be these to do with the nature of young people, with sexual behaviour or with injecting drug use. Given that we live in a world in which there is not one but a multitude of moral stances — some defined by religious systems of belief, others not — efforts to privilege one moral code above all others are unlikely to be successful, even in the short term. Given also the diversity of human sexual identities and desires, health education and health promotion which speak only to a restricted range of safer sexual behaviours are likely to be ill-conceived.

Second, social research of this kind must begin to examine the diversity of young people's experiences, enquiring into the interplay between bio-medical knowledge and lay beliefs for individuals who are socially differentiated from one another, at least on the grounds of class, gender, ethnicity, sexuality. Given the rich legacy of women's experience and feminist scholarship, there is no reason at all to suppose that young women's experience and needs in relation to HIV and AIDS will be the same as young men's. Likewise, there is no reason to suppose either that the interests of young black people in urban areas will match those of young whites in rural settings. These different starting points should be the subject of future social research so that AIDS health education and health promotion can be made more relevant and more socially empowering for the range of social groupings that exist today.

Finally, the beliefs and understandings of adults need to be the subject of closer scrutiny. Many adults remain unfortunately wedded to generalized notions of young people reminiscent of early twentieth century thought. Questioning such ideas could usefully throw some light on the uses to which such notions are being put in contemporary research on young people and HIV/AIDS. Are they, for example, important in establishing and maintaining particular ideas about young people's sexuality? How do findings from research then become part of age-related regulatory ideologies? How best can key policy-makers, for example, begin to challenge popular prejudices against young people? Similar sorts of questions raise important issues for researchers' own understandings of HIV infection and AIDS, as well as the health education and health promotion strategies which they recommend be adopted with young people.

It has been our intention in this chapter to present a critical reading of the rapidly growing research literature relating to young people and HIV/AIDS. We have become increasingly alarmed about the ways in which young people are frequently represented in relation to issues to do with HIV infection and AIDS. Our alarm, and occasional anger, at what we have read will, we hope, be felt by others who also wish to challenge dominant ideologies in and around AIDS research which appear to have more to do with shoring up popular prejudices about young people than examining their unequal status in a differentiated society.

References

AGGLETON, P. (1989) 'Evaluating Health Education about AIDS', in P. AGGLETON, G. HART and P. DAVIES. (eds), *AIDS: Social Representations, Social Practices*. Lewes, Falmer Press.

BEN-DAVID, J. and COLLINS, R. (1966) 'Social Factors in the Origins of a New Science: The Case of Psychology', *American Sociological Review*, 31, 4, pp. 451–65.

BIEMILLER, L. (1987) 'Colleges Could Play Crucial Role in Halting Spread of AIDS Epidemic, Public Health Officials Say', *Chronicle of Higher Education*, 33, 22, pp. 1–32.

DiCLEMENTE, R.J., ZORN, J. and TEMOSHOK, L. (1986) 'Adolescents and AIDS: A Survey of Knowledge, Attitudes and Beliefs about AIDS in San Francisco', *American Journal of Public Health*, 76, 12, pp. 1443–5.

DiCLEMENTE, R.J., ZORN, J. and TEMOSHOK, L. (1987) 'Response by DiClemente *et al.*', *American Journal of Public Health*. 77, 7, pp. 876–7.

EISER, C., EISER, R.J. and LANG, J. (forthcoming) 'How Adolescents Compare AIDS with Other Diseases: Implications for Prevention', *Journal of Pediatric Psychology*.

FALCHIKOV, N. (1986) 'Images of Adolescence', *Journal of Adolescence*, 9, pp. 167–80.

FORD, N. (1988) *A Survey of the AIDS Awareness and Sexual Behaviour and Attitudes of Young People in Bristol*. Exeter, University of Exeter, Institute of Population Studies.

GIBBERD, K. (ed.) (1964) *Your Teenage Children: How You Can Help Them*. London, Macdonald.

GILLIS, J. R. (1977) *Youth and History: Tradition and Change in European Age Relations: 1770 to the Present*. New York, Academic Press.

GROUP FOR THE ADVANCEMENT OF PSYCHIATRY, COMMITTEE ON THE COLLEGE STUDENT (1966) *Sex and the College Student*. New York, Atheneum.

GUNN, A. (1970) *The Privileged Adolescent: An Outline of the Physical and Mental Problems of the Student Society*. Lancaster, Medical and Technical Publishing Co.

HALL, G. S. (1905) *Adolescence: Its Psychology and Its Relations to Physiology, Anthropology, Sociology, Sex, Crime, Religion and Education*. New York, Appleton.

HALL, S. and JEFFERSON, T. (1976) *Resistance through Rituals*. London, Hutchinson.

HEBDIGE, D. (1979) *Subculture: The Meaning of Style*. London, Methuen.

HOLLAND, J., RAMAZANOGLU, C. and SCOTT, S. (1989) 'Managing Risk and Experiencing Danger: Tensions between Government AIDS Education Policy and Young Women's Sexuality'. Paper presented at the British Sociological Conference: Sociology in Action. Plymouth Polytechnic, 21–23 March.

HOMANS, H. and AGGLETON, P. (1988) 'Health Education, HIV Infection and AIDS', in P. AGGLETON and H. HOMANS (eds), *Social Aspects of AIDS*. Lewes, Falmer Press.

KEELING, R. P. (1986) 'AIDS on Campus: What You Should Know', *AGB Reports*, 63, 2, pp. 24–8.

KING, A. J. C., BEAZLEY, R. P., WARREN, W. K., HANKINS, C. A., ROBERTSON, A. S. and RADFORD, J. L. (1989) *Canada AIDS and Youth Study*. Ottawa, Center for AIDS Health Protection Branch, Health and Welfare Canada.

KLEIN, J. (1963) *Human Behaviour and Personal Relationships*. Leicester, National Association of Youth Clubs.

MCDERMOTT, R. J., HAWKINS, M. J., MOORE, J. R. and CITTADINO, S. K. (1987) 'AIDS Awareness and Information Sources among Selected University Students', *Journal of American College Health*, 35, 5, pp. 222–6.

MCROBBIE, A. (1989) (ed.) *Zoot Suits and Secondhand Dresses*. Basingstoke, Macmillan.

MCROBBIE, A. and NAVA, M. (eds) (1984) *Gender and Generation*. Basingstoke, Macmillan.

MUNCIE, J. (1988) 'Depraved or Deprived: The Problem of Adolescence', in *Open University (D211) Social Problems and Social Welfare. Block 1*. Milton Keynes, The Open University Press.

MUSGROVE, F. (1964) *Youth and the Social Order*. London, Routledge.

PEARSON, G. (1983) *Hooligan: A History of Respectable Fears*. Houndmills, Basingstoke, Macmillan Education.

PRICE, J. H., DESMOND, S. and KUKULKA, G. (1985) 'High School Students' Perceptions and Misperceptions of AIDS', *Journal of School Health*, 55, pp. 107–9.

RAMAZANOGLU, C. (1989) Findings reported at MRC AIDS Behavioural Research Forum, London, 17 May 1989.

ROSE, N. (1985) *The Psychological Complex: Psychology, Politics and Society in England 1869–1939*. London, Routledge and Kegan Paul.

STRUNIN, L. and HINGSON, P. (1987) 'Acquired Immunodeficiency Syndrome and Adolescents: Knowledge, Beliefs, Attitudes, and Behaviours', *Pediatrics*, 79, 5, pp. 825–8.

THE HOME AND SCHOOL COMMITTEE OF THE ENGLISH NEW EDUCATION FELLOWSHIP (1954) *Advances in the Understanding of the Adolescent*. Sheffield, Home and School Council.

UNITED STATES DEPARTMENT OF HEALTH, EDUCATION AND WELFARE, CHILDREN'S BUREAU (1955) *The Adolescent in Your Family*. Rev. ed. Washington, US Department of Health.

WIESMAN, J. M., NATALE, J. A., LIN, J. C., GARRET, A. T., FITZGERALD, P. J., DAVIS, K. E., LEVIN, L. S. and HELGERSON, S. D. (1987) 'Adolescents' Knowledge of AIDS near AIDS Epicenter', *American Journal of Public Health*, 77, 7, p. 876.

WISHON, P. M. (1988) 'Children and Youth with AIDS', *International Journal of Adolescence and Youth*, 1, pp. 213–27.

Chapter 7

On Male Homosexual Prostitution and HIV

Peter Davies and Paul Simpson

In 1536 the Imperial Diet of the Holy Roman Empire — the European Parliament of its day — met to consider, among other things, the threat posed to the contemporary social order by a virulent and life threatening sexually transmitted disease, syphilis. They met against a background of a Europe facing an unprecedented ideological split. Religious schism was exacerbating petty rivalries among many of the principalities nominally in thrall to the Empire, and there was open or barely suppressed conflict among many of them. Economic tension, due to the entrepreneurial aggression of the Italian states and the incipient inflation due to the influx of precious metals from the new world, also threatened an order that dated back politically to Charlemagne and ideologically to the first Roman hegemony. The response of the Diet to the threat posed by syphilis (see Jacquart and Thomasset, 1988) was to issue an edict prohibiting 'all concubines or other extra-marital sex relations such as prostitution' (Bullough and Bullough, 1987: 152).

In our own century, whether as a response to syphilis (see Brandt, 1985) or to HIV, the impulse to re-assert monogamy as a bulwark against epidemic disease remains intact. The historical accident that AIDS was first recognized among gay identified men focused interest on one group, that of male homosexual prostitutes, about which little was or is known. This interest was first articulated around the role of such men as a 'bridge' between existing 'high risk groups', particularly the 'gay community' and injecting drug users, and the 'general population', which for the purposes of this formulation consists solely of heterosexual and almost monogamous couples.

The fallacy of conflating *social* categories with *physical* processes has been well rehearsed, as has the pernicious pertinacity of the notion of a 'general population' beleaguered by pools of infection. Male prostitutes remain, however, because of the nature of their work, perhaps uniquely at risk from HIV transmission. In order that those risks may be reduced, an understanding of male homosexual prostitution both as an individual negotiation and as a social formation is urgently needed.

However, the first thing that strikes the researcher is the extreme paucity of published material on male homosexual prostitution. This is, no doubt, partly due to the fact that the practice is marginal to two phenomena that are themselves peripheral to academic interest: prostitution and homosexuality. But, more than that, it is the potential of male homosexual prostitution to contradict current orthodoxies that guarantees its academic invisibility. These contradictions are fundamental. Because it involves a contract between two men, male homosexual prostitution confounds those who regard (female) prostitution as a simple rehearsal of gender inequality. Because, in some cases, the punter (or client) pays for the orgasm of the prostitute, it challenges those who would reduce prostitution to a form of consumer capitalism: mere payment for pleasure; and because it exists at all in the era of gay liberation, it embarrasses those who extol the revolutionary egalitarianism of the gay community.

Rediscovering the Male Prostitute

Classical Greece and Rome

There is, to our knowledge, no definitive or even comprehensive survey of the history of male homosexual prostitution (but see Benjamin and Masters, 1964). Rather, it is the subject of passing allusion in works dedicated to the rediscovery of the homosexual in history, the occasional essay and as footnotes to the study of the female variant. What follows collects and digests some of these sources but makes no claim either to exhaustive or to original research. We argue that the historical material on male homosexual prostitution, though sparse, nevertheless allows the tentative conclusion that the phenomenon was common in many previous ages and is trans-historical, at least in the loose sense that the institutional forms appear to be remarkably consistent over time. These forms and the types of prostitute that emerge are the first theme of this section. The second theme, which notes the economic and particularly patriarchal power relations that underpin male homosexual prostitution, is not fully developed in this chapter since the discussion is both wider and more complex than exigencies of space and considerations of continuity allow us to include.

Foucault (1985) uses Aeschines' tract *Against Timarchus* and Demosthenes' *Erotic Essay* to point out that in classical Greece it was not permissible for a man who had been a prostitute to hold public office. Aeschines charges Timarchus with having been a prostitute and thus ineligible for office. The arguments adduced allow the meaning and implications of the category 'prostitute' in classical Greece to be outlined. Timarchus is said to qualify for the epithet because of his number of partners, his indiscriminateness and his acceptance of payment for services. But these are deemed insufficient to label him a prostitute and thus ineligible for office since he is neither registered as a prostitute nor has he lived in a brothel.

This confusion points to the difficulty of labelling a person (then or now) as a prostitute simply on the basis of the exchange of cash or goods. The classical Greeks maintained an ambivalent attitude towards homosexual love and sex. It was thought to be neither natural nor unnatural but 'para physin', outside nature. In this society, such criteria (number of partners, indiscriminateness and acceptance of gifts) would render an altogether unacceptable number of men ineligible for office. Hence, official forms of registration and restriction evolved.

The essential problem, as Foucault points out, is:

> ... the difficulty caused ... by the juxtaposition of an ethos of male superiority and a conception of all sexual intercourse in terms of the schema of penetration and male domination. The consequence of this was [in classical Greece], on the one hand that the 'active' and dominant role was always assigned positive values but on the other hand it was necessary to attribute to one of the partners in the sexual act the passive, dominated and inferior position .... (Foucault, 1985: 220)

Here is highlighted the essential paradox of male homosexual prostitution, the essential incompatibility between a masculine (as in dominant, active, insertive) self-image and the implicit inferiority of accepting money for sexual favours. Foucault goes on to say that, while this kind of relationship presented little problem when it involved a woman or a slave, who were 'naturally' inferior, the case was altered when it involved a free-born man. Thus, he argues, any boy involved in a sexual relationship with a man was involved in a paradox that Foucault calls the 'antinomy of the boy'. While the man could legitimately and honourably love, desire and enjoy a boy, the boy 'could not and must not identify with that role' (*ibid.*: 221). Since he would grow up to inhabit the dominant role, he could not afford to be or to have been the passive, inferior object of desire. The prostitute, Foucault suggests, is the man who enjoys, relishes and accepts the inferior role. Thus, Timarchus's real crime was that he ' ... placed himself and showed himself to everyone in the inferior and humiliating position of a pleasure object for others; he wanted this role ... he profited from it ... ' (Foucault, 1985: 219). This leads us to the intriguing speculation that the true precursor in classical Greece of the modern gay man is not the ubiquitous lover of boys, but the prostitute: not Phaedrus but Timarchus.

A similar pattern to that noted in classical Greece (i.e. widespread homosexual love and sex but a disdain for male homosexual prostitution) appears to have been the norm in the case of Rome, though in this case the documentary evidence is more abundant. The appearance of male homosexual prostitution is linked by Verstraete (1980) to the emergence of a slave-owning economy: some slaves being kept, he argues, for their sexual services. He points to the poet Martial who, found in flagrante delicto with a boy by his wife, excuses himself by pointing out that the boy is a slave and not a Roman citizen. From this, Verstraete argues that 'a homosexual relationship between citizens would have scandalized the most tolerant circles of Roman society' (Verstraete, 1980: 228). Boswell disagrees with this analysis and suggests that the stigma attached not to citizens who engaged in homosexual acts *per se* but to those who became prostitutes

> ... due to the fact that (1) prostitution represented the bottom level of a profession already viewed with disdain by well-born Romans (i.e. commerce) and (2) anyone, citizen or slave could avail himelf of the services of a prostitute. The prospect of a Roman citizen servicing a slave sexually and for money was to invite contempt and disgust . . . . (Boswell, 1980: 77)

Nevertheless, Boswell does claim to detect 'a strong bias against passive sexual behaviour on the part of a citizen' (*ibid.*: 74). This disapproval hardened in the later Empire with the adoption by the Emperors of Christianity and its radical views on the body (see Brown, 1988) and in 390 AD male prostitutes in Rome were publicly burned.

It is with the Romans that we are first able to identify distinct types of male homosexual prostitute. The Romans, for example, distinguished between *exoleti*, who were sexually insertive, and *catamiti*, who were receptive in homosexual intercourse (Boswell, 1980: 79). But more interestingly, there appear to have been types distinguished by their areas of trade.

> ... In addition to male brothels, male prostitutes frequented alleyways or the arches of buildings where female prostitutes also plied their trade. Many public places in Rome were pickup points for male and female prostitutes and male prostitutes frequented the public baths to meet customers . . . . (Boswell, 1980: 77–8)

On an intriguingly modern note, he adds: ' . . . Colors and styles of clothing appear to have been used as symbols for availability as prostitutes and for the role preferred . . . ' (Boswell, 1980: 778).

It is difficult not to see in these three types — those in the brothels, the street walkers and frequenters of the public baths — the spiritual ancestors of those who work today in astoundingly similar milieux in European and North American cities, although reason and historical sensitivity revolt against it.

The Middle Ages

Reference to male homosexual prostitution re-appears in the verse of the tolerant eleventh century, and male brothels, according to one anonymous poem, existed in Chartres, Orleans, Sens and Paris, with the intriguing suggestion that they employed only those with large genitals. This discrimination, Boswell suggests, leads one to suspect that such establishments were not uncommon. Such liberalism was to disappear in the comprehensive moral backlash of the thirteenth century, at which time male homosexual prostitution, along with homosexuality in general, was denounced as symptomatic of Muslim decadence and degeneracy (Boswell, 1980).

The twin themes of economic power and of different types re-appear, merged, in the late middle ages. Male servants, whose main duty is the sexual gratification of their masters, are recorded in sixteenth century London (Bray, 1982). Bray also records that male brothels were denounced by writers in 1598 and 1649, and that the theatre appears to have been provided with male prostitutes, though whether these were in demand by patrons or richer and older actors is unclear. Similarly, court records note the existence of male brothels in London in 1720 (Weeks, 1977).

The Nineteenth Century

In the nineteenth century prostitution of all types flourished behind the facade of a prim and repressive morality, but whereas women prostitutes tended to be a distinct lumpen-class, male prostitution appears a more casual affair. There were brothels but also more casual prostitution. In the brothels of 1840, the going rate for a boy was £10 (Bray, 1982: 37), and in 1889 a major scandal erupted over boy prostitution in a Cleveland Street brothel (Weeks, 1977), with a hint of royal involvement in the person of Prince Albert Victor, son of the Prince of Wales.

Weeks (1977) also comments on the casual, situational prostitution of the Guards regiments, encouraged by low pay and poor conditions of service. The rewards of prostitution were substantially greater than those of more orthodox employment and many working-class youths found their way into this lucrative trade. He further comments on the attractions these horny-handed sons of toil held for the Victorian middle-class man.

> ... [T]here is a strong element of sexual colonialism in the avidity with which the upper middle class male approached his 'trade'. According to Sir Edmund Backhouse, Oscar Wilde preferred working-class youths because 'their passion was all body and no soul'. But there was also a yearning to escape the stifling middle-class norms. E. M. Forster wanted 'to love a strong young man of the lower classes and be loved by him and even hurt by him'. Edward Carpenter proclaimed his love for the poor and uneducated: 'The thick-thighed, hot, coarse-fleshed young bricklayer with the strip around his waist.... (Weeks, 1977: 40–1)

The Twentieth Century

In the twentieth century Kinsey, Pomeroy and Martin (1948: 596) state that 'homosexual prostitutes are, in large cities not far inferior in number to the females who are engaged in heterosexual prostitution' and, ever the biologist, Kinsey even examines in detail the problems involved in managing multiple erections and orgasms as a male prostitute (Kinsey *et al.*, 1948: 216). Pomeroy (1972), in his memoir of Kinsey, reports on Kinsey's travels in Italy in 1955 where he noted that the Spanish Steps, the Colosseum and the houseboats on the Tiber were major areas of male homosexual prostitution.

Cory and LeRoy (1963) provide a racy account of the hustling scene in an American city in the early 1960s and, at the same time, in this country Hauser (1962), in a book that is remarkably wide-ranging for its time, distinguished five types of male homosexual prostitute. These are: the 'young volunteer', a 'young boy often of very tender age, who has been misled into this form of activity'; the 'call-boy', an older, more intelligent, often employed man who hustled on the telephone; the ' "cottage" type', whom Hauser reviles as 'the lowest type of prostitute' and who is defined by his area of work (the cottage); the 'club and pub prostitute', also labelled from his place of work; and the 'roller', whose inclusion among prostitutes is surely problematic, in that he earns money through threat or use of physical violence on men he has lured with promises of sex.

In Britain in the late 1960s and early 1970s the decriminalization of certain tightly defined male homosexual activities and the import from the United States of gay liberation changed the terms of the debate about homosexuality. In the euphoria of gay liberation, it was easy to believe that, with great visibility, a form of legality and the consequent greater availability of homosexual sex, the demand for the services of the homosexual prostitute would soon dry up. Harris reports one of his hustlers as opining that ' . . . since the Wolfenden proposals became law . . . you have to approach people . . . hunt for prey. Before that they came up to you. Now you have to hustle . . . ' (Harris, 1973: 65). Fifteen years later, the euphoria evaporated, this turns out to have been a vain hope. The hope of a new order dissipated as business realized that the new gay community was a source of profit and commercialism permeated the gay scene. West (1977: 221) claims that 'homosexual brothels of any kind have been largely eliminated.' Instead of withering away, the availability of homosexual prostitutes increased as advertising in the gay press was capable of reaching a wider clientele and demand remained high despite the replacement of the pre-1967 imperatives of secrecy and anonymity with norms of promiscuity and athleticism.

Evidence of the contemporary incidence of male homosexual prostitution is sparse and limited to the United States. Bell and Weinberg (1978), in their massive survey of gay lifestyles in the USA, suggest that there are two types of prostitute: the straight hustler (see below) and the gay hustlers, who were 'in the life' for whatever the market could bear. They report that one-quarter of their white homosexual respondents had been paid for sex at least once (Bell and Weinberg, 1978: 85–93 and 311). This suggests a substantial group of (admittedly casual) prostitutes. However, without finer detail in the reporting of their figures, it is impossible to distinguish between those who have been paid once only and those for whom it forms a substantial part of their sexual activity. Moreover, they report that 28 per cent of their white respondents had paid for sex at least once, though only 1 per cent said that this was for more than half of their partners.

This latter finding is broadly confirmed by Jay and Young (1977) who report that 76 per cent of the respondents in their large study of gay men in the USA had never paid for sex. Exactly the same proportion had never been paid for sex. The same authors are aware of the diversity of ways in which the prostitutes meet their clients: '...on well-known streets and corners or other pick-up spots such as bus stations, through ads in gay or ''underground'' newspapers through massage or escort services, as part of an organised call-boy service, even by advertising on bulletin boards in gay neighbourhoods...' (Jay and Young, 1977: 259).

There is an intriguing congruence that emerges between the institutional forms of prostitution across the ages. While it can never be clear whether these forms are indicative of different types of prostitute or merely represent different opportunities for the trading of sexual favours, it does appear that, over time, three broad 'types' recur. There are those who ply their trade on the streets and in well known locales, those who are attached to brothels and those who are servants and slaves. We do not intend a crude ahistoricism but merely point a curious congruence over time and between cultures. All the more interesting, therefore, is the way that this continuity has been submerged in contemporary descriptive literature, to which we now turn.

The Myth of the Male Prostitute

A casual perusal of the extant literature which purports to describe male homosexual prostitution presents the reader with two compelling stereotypes: that of the straight hustler, and that of the teenage runaway prostitute. These two portraits, often merged into a single, sorry account, dominate contemporary sociological descriptions and fuel popular and journalistic stereotypes. A compelling, if implicit, part of the tale is the theme of seduction. According to this paradigm, male homosexual prostitutes are heterosexuals who are seduced by older, predatory homosexuals and this seduction is achieved by economic force majeure. The account is thus a compelling portrait of innocence betrayed, outraged and defiled. Yet to take this portrait to represent a complete picture of male homosexual prostitution is to mistake exemplification by synecdoche. The mistake is the result of a selective inattention by researchers and unwarranted generalization from idiographic accounts by readers and does not necessarily reflect the actual preponderance of such prostitutes in the real world.

Rarely can the study of a social phenomenon be so dominated by a single piece of work as is this subject by Reiss's (1961) article, 'The Social Integration of Queers and Peers'. Based on interviews with '18.6 per cent of . . . 1008 boys between the ages of 12 and 17' (Reiss, 1961: 436; incidentally, the quoted percentage suggests 187.49 interviews), the article provides a vivid and thoughtful description of the world of the straight hustler. Reiss's work draws on earlier work by Butts (1947) who introduced the notion of the young heterosexual man engaging in male homosexual prostitution in order to make a living. Butts noted that the boys he interviewed liked to talk with girls 'to assure themselves that they aren't queer' (Butts, 1947: 674). Few admitted taking pleasure from homosexual activity; most said they found it repulsive and that the fees they charged varied with the service required. Reiss's contribution is a description of the group norms that governed the interaction between the 'peers', the prostitutes, and the derided 'queers', their clients.

Clearly, Reiss is describing here once again the 'antinomy of the boy'. Like the eromenos in classical Greece, the straight hustler is caught in a contradiction. Engaging regularly in despised homosexual acts and moreover in the economically inferior role of a prostitute, he nevertheless wishes to retain a dominant, heterosexual, masculine self-image. In Reiss's formulation, this contradiction is neutralized in the prevailing norms of the peer group, which emphasize the financial rewards of the trade and enjoin disavowal of any pleasure in the act. Most importantly, however, a heterosexual self-image is reinforced by restricting the hustler to the insertor role in oral intercourse.

Reiss's portrait resonates with the second strand of the literature, that of moral indignation. The themes of seduction, of innocence betrayed and of economic necessity leading to the denial and subversion of a boy's natural sexuality are prominent in Harris's (1973) account of male homosexual prostitution in London and reach their apogee in Lloyd's (1979) piece of tabloid sensationalism masquerading as serious investigation.

Harris begins his account of the Dilly Boys with a portrait of 'Jimmy', who, by the prominence of the account, is clearly intended to serve as exemplar of the type. Jimmy arrives in London at the age of 16, having left his parental home following an 'unhappy series of incidents' (p. 12). Alone in the city, he finds himself, by chance, in Piccadilly, where he is approached and befriended by an older man who offers accommodation, which Jimmy accepts. There, Jimmy refuses the sexual advances of his host (p. 14). At this point, Harris indulges in an excess of piety, quoting Jimmy's observation on his hustling peers: 'Such nice boys doing things like that'; and reporting Jimmy's avowed heterosexuality (p. 15). Incidentally, this utterance is a wonderful example of the poverty of the written word. One longs to hear the tone and inflection of the comment, which could easily, completely and relevantly alter its meaning. On his second day in the capital, Jimmy is picked up in an amusement arcade and, this time, in return for accommodation, he does not 'resist the sexual advances made to him' (p. 17). As the limitations of his options become apparent, Jimmy makes 'a conscious choice out of drift and deviance' (p. 19) and becomes a full-time male homosexual prostitute until he is arrested two weeks later and returned to his parents (p. 20).

There are two specific criticisms of this piece of work, which illustrate the problems implicit in this type of investigative research and which underline how dubious it is to generalize from it. Jimmy's drift into prostitution, as recounted by Harris, seems to happen very easily: the stages appear almost contrived. This impression may, of course, be a misapprehension due to the nature and style of the prose, but two points continue to niggle. The first concerns Harris's statement that Jimmy 'happened to be present' when he, Harris, was talking about his research on Jimmy's second day in London (p. 15). It is difficult to believe that this is entirely happenstance or that it had no effect on Jimmy's future career. The ethics of ethnographic research is a subject beyond the scope of the present essay but it would be interesting, to say the least, to hear the exact content of that conversation.

Second, we are told that, despite Jimmy's protestations of heterosexuality, he receives a letter from a friend (having left home abruptly and written only one letter without an address to his parents, how, one asks, did he receive a letter in return?) which enquires: 'what's the score with the gay scene in London?' Harris himself comments at this point, 'it is not common for this description of homosexuals to be used outside the homosexual scene' (p. 15). Quite so. One *is* bound to wonder whether Jimmy's innocence is assumed for the benefit, and to enlist the sympathy, of the researcher.

Consider, by contrast, Seabrook's (1976: 174) account in his admittedly impressionistic set of portraits and descriptions of erotic locations, in which 'Mike', an 18-year-old dilly boy, says 'they [his peers] might tell you they don't [enjoy homosexual sex] but they're fucking liars' and later, asked if he 'likes girls', he replies: 'Yeh, course I do, . . . [grins] Not for sex though . . . A lot of the boys make out all they want is some nice chick who's gonna love them and all that.'

This contradictory evidence prefigures two general points about the way in which research of this sort is construed. First, it is simply not possible to choose between these two accounts, to give valid reasons for preferring Mike's account to that of Jimmy. Idiographic research of this sort does not address itself to questions of incidence, representativeness and falsification. Rather, it attempts a description of a certain geographically and temporally defined phenomenon. To prefer one account to another involves a decision about the quality of the research that is invidious and often made *ad hominem*.

Neither Reiss nor Harrris nor any of the researchers who have provided descriptions of similar forms of street prostitution makes any claim that their particular group contains all those who might be termed male homosexual prostitutes. Yet the stereotype has come to dominate the literature and this domination is taken to indicate the universality and uniqueness of the type it describes. For example, Hoffman's (1979) article entitled 'The Male Prostitute', in one of the more reputable readers on gay sexuality and lifestyles, consists of a digest of Reiss, a case history of a straight prostitute and a single paragraph that allows that 'there are, of course, many hustlers who admit to being gay' (Hoffman, 1979: 281).

Similarly, there is simply no evidence to substantiate West's claim in his supposedly authoritative discussion of homosexuality that '... most full-time hustlers are youths or young men in the age range 16–25, drop-outs from respectable society, disorganised in their habits, conspicuously work-shy, living from hand to mouth' (West, 1968: 222). Nobody knows how many full-time hustlers there are and nobody, certainly, has elicited from them enough information to substantiate the claim that West makes. We repeat: this assumption that the part is representative of the whole is unfounded and based on unwarranted extrapolation from the particular to the general.

Mention of West leads us to consider the second of our general points: the easy assumption of moral outrage that characterizes so many accounts of this subject. This may be explicit, as in Lloyd's (1979) farrago, but more objectionable is the moral baggage that weighs down supposedly scholarly accounts. Of these authors, West is perhaps a paradigm. West's (1968) treatment of the whole question of homosexuality is vitiated by his assumption of pathology and his reliance on mainstream psychiatric paradigms and clinic samples. His approach is always patronizing, often offensive and sometimes downright misleading. To take one example almost at random from his discussion of prostitution, he quotes often and approvingly from research by a Danish police officer, Jersild (1956):

> ... In Jersild's research (which, incidentally, shows how the realistic and practical approach of the policeman can be combined with a humane attitude) he found that young male prostitutes very often came from those emotionally and socially impoverished family backgrounds which are the well-known breeding grounds of delinquency in boys and immorality in girls. There was a very high incidence of broken homes, police records, reform school committees, excessive drinking, educational backwardness, unemployment and work-shyness. He found that many of the boys [had been] apparently stimulated further in this direction [i.e. towards prostitution] by their experience of the joys of a parasitic existence and of the ease with which money could be got by bullying and robbing perverts.... (West, 1968: 129).

The disapproving tone, the offensive vocabulary and the wilful ignorance of the reality of poverty of this (and many other) passages would not be out of place in a popular newspaper. From such a distinguished academic, the standard of argument and insight is simply indefensible. Indeed, it is difficult to believe that such work can be taken seriously especially when, in his later work (West, 1977), which claims to re-assess the conclusions of the earlier, he includes statements of such stunning banality as: ' . . . Male hustling differs in important respects from ordinary [sic] prostitution, both because the traders are men and also because the relationships are homosexual' (West, 1977: 221).

But West is simply mirroring a widespread distaste and fear. Scandals over male prostitutes are a recurring feature of our society's attempts to reinforce the ideology of the family. Female prostitution is seen as a crime against society and an indictment of financial inequalities. Male homosexual prostitution is all that and a crime against nature too. According to a recent, and supposedly authoritative, review of the law on sex and sexuality,

> . . . Whereas the predominant concern about heterosexual molestation of girls is that they may find the experience off-putting and thereby become anxious, frigid or even lesbian [sic], the concern for boys involved homosexually with older men is that they may find the experience attractive and be seduced into homosexuality . . . . (Howard League, 1985: 27).

Are we really supposed to take seriously the contention that molestation frightens girls and attracts boys? Such a crude, if convenient, aetiology that ascribes adult homosexuality in both sexes to male seduction reveals an ignorance of the complexity of sexuality and of the indigenous experience of lesbians and gay men that would be ludicrous were it not of such moment.

In London Today

Despite the dominance of the stereotypical male prostitute in the literature, even a casual perusal of the 'Services Offered' columns in the gay press suggests the existence of other types plying their trade in different ways and using different titles. In a recent issue of the popular *Gay Times*, for example, there are some eighty-six advertisements, collected under headings 'Escorts', 'Models' and 'Masseurs', which, despite their innocent wording, offer sexual services to those who can break the simple code of the advertisers.

Preliminary work carried out at South Bank Polytechnic (subsequently funded by the AVERT (the AIDS Education and Research Trust) suggests that these types differ, both from each other and from the stereotypical street-walking prostitute in their modes of operation, their commitment to prostitution as a way of life and, most importantly from our current point of view, their potential role in the HIV epidemic. In what follows, we refer to information we have gathered from men currently or recently involved in prostitution and from their clients. We do not have direct information, and therefore do not comment on two other groups of prostitute, the model and the house boy.

The escort works for an agency, which takes a proportion of his earnings and offers a full range of sexual services in his own home or in that of the client. He tends to be better educated and more 'middle-class' than the street walker. The masseur, by contrast, is self-employed and while he too provides a full service in his own or the client's home, he is also required to practise the trade of his title. He too tends to be middle-class. Street walking, as the name suggests, is a more casual occupation in the sense that it does not require the paraphernalia of telephones, advertisements and premises before clients are contacted. The contract is made and may, sometimes, be fulfilled outdoors, in which case the range of sexual services provided is restricted to those that offer the opportunity of a quick getaway in the event of an intrusion. The street worker is more likely to be working-class, and it is in this scene that the teenage runaway is more likely to find himself. The generic term, 'rent-boys' sometimes refers to prostitutes as a class, but is also sometimes restricted in application to the last group, those who ply their trade on the streets.

Escorts

Escorts are distinguished from the other groups primarily by their employment by an agency. When an escort is recruited to the agency, the range of services that he is willing to provide is noted. Boys are often 'marketed' as particular types: the 'student' and the 'athlete' are common. He is expected to meet punters either in their own homes (or hotel rooms, etc.) or in his own.

The agency's role is that of intermediary between the client and the prostitute, matching the requirements of the punter to the availability of prostitutes. It relieves the escort of the need to contact his own punters and of most of the problems associated with hoax callers. The punter is offered a range of prostitutes and of services without the dangers of misalliance that a misleadingly worded advertisement might entail. For this service, the agency retains a third of the fee paid by the punter.

Escorts are expected to provide any and all of the 'big three': masturbation, fellatio and anal intercourse, all in either insertive or receptive mode. Although prostitutes claim rarely to fuck, punters claim regularly to do so with some prostitutes. It may be that a punter, in the bedroom, asks the escort for something 'out of the ordinary', that is, any of the more unusual or exotic sexual practices. This is seen as an opportunity by the boy to negotiate for extra cash, which, being free from the agency's subvention, is regarded as a double bonus.

Most of the clients are 'one-offs', making single or widely spaced visits to prostitutes, but our respondents reported that they had a few regular customers. These were regarded as useful in the winter: a time when casual punters are scarce. From the information that we have, it does seem that regular and casual clients differ in their sexual practices with the prostitutes.

Masseurs

Masseurs are freelance operators in the sense that they arrange their own publicity and manage their own administration. This frees them from the control of an agency and its *de facto* taxation at the expense of direct exposure to hoax calls and the problems of running what is, in effect, a small business. Apart from this, the service they provide is very similar to that provided by the escort. They too are expected to provide service either in their own homes or at the punter's preferred place and to provide a full range of sexual services.

Negotiation takes place directly between the prostitute and the punter, initially over the telephone. This means that negotiation over the type of service provided and its price has a flexibility that is absent in the case of the escort. The prostitute is free to negotiate higher and lower rates for particular practices, although these are set with at least an eye to the going escort rate. From the punter's point of view, this flexibility has to be weighed against the essential uncertainty involved in relying on the sexual compatibility of partners based on a description contained in a newspaper advertisement and the impression conveyed in a brief telephone conversation.

Moreover, whereas the escort is not frequently called upon to escort, the masseur is often expected to provide a massage, often to relax the customer prior to sex. Indeed, the gay press requires people advertising as masseurs to hold some qualification before accepting advertisements. It is said to be rare for clients to appear expecting only the massage. Some, however, do.

Street-Walkers (Dilly Boys)

What sets the dilly boy apart from the other groups is the public setting of his activities. This distinction, and the tendency for street-walkers to come from working- rather than middle-class backgrounds, creates a status ordering between private (escorting, masseuring) and public forms of prostitution (street-walking), a status ordering in which the dilly boy is deemed substantially inferior (See also Luckenbill, 1986). Working the streets almost inevitably exposes him to certain dangers — entrapment by the police, physical violence and contact with 'junkies' — which escorts/masseurs may more easily avoid.

Moreover, street prostitution is more accessible, demanding a minimum of capital outlay: the funds for accommodation and equipment which are essential to escorting/masseuring do not have to be met. It is this accessibility, as much as age, that makes the trade viable for the unemployed, the runaway and the low paid youngster, while access to the more prestigious forms of prostitution is restricted to the more affluent, better educated and, generally, older individuals.

Since the encounter between the street-walker and his client takes place in public, a whole set of covert manoeuvres and subterfuges has evolved (see Delph, 1978). The typical encounter can be regarded as taking place in three stages. First, the prostitute will position himself in a particular spot. He will then signal his availability and try to identify prospective clients. This is followed by a direct approach by one or the other player, which leads to a negotiation of the price, service and location. The sexual transaction, or the 'payoff', then takes place.

Some Caveats

Given the strictures we have addressed at those who have taken previous idiographic accounts of male homosexual prostitution to be representative of the whole universe under study, it is particularly important that we clarify the status of our description. We have tried to synthesize the accounts given to us by prostitutes and their clients. These accounts come from a small number of individuals who volunteered that information. Whether this description is an accurate reflection of the working practices of all or a majority of those working as prostitutes in London must remain unknown until further research is done.

Further research is also needed to clarify the relationship of this typology to others developed in the Netherlands (de Lagemaat, 1986) and in the United States (Marotta, Waldorf and Murphy, 1988). It may be that the differences reflect differences in social organization in the various centres, due to legal and other factors, or it may be that they are due to differences in approach by the researchers.

We have commented at some length on the moralistic and prurient squint of some writers on male homosexual prostitution that threatens to distort beyond recognition the experience of those involved in it. In our account, we have avoided talking about the prostitute as victim either of circumstances or of pathology. Prostitution is an economic choice made by individuals rationally and with dignity. It would be naive, however, to pretend that these choices are always made in circumstances of the prostitute's own choosing. We all have the choice of prostitution as a means of earning or supplementing our income: many of us count ourselves lucky not to have to consider that choice too seriously or too long. While there are some people (most frequently among the two 'professional' groups) who have chosen the profession from a position of economic security, for many, prostitution remains a choice made *in extremis*, the last means of paying the rent, the electricity bill or for food. For despite its manifold and oft-rehearsed disadvantages, it is possible for some, through prostitution, to make a relatively large amount of money in a relatively short time.

It would also be naive to imagine that the role of the escort agencies is always benign and altruistic. They are businesses, which exist to make money, but, despite the opprobrium often heaped upon them, it must be recognized that they provide an important service to the prostitute and the client, and we have heard of no brutal pimping such as seems to be more common with female prostitutes.

Prostitutes and HIV

What, then, is the role and the importance of the male homosexual prostitute in the HIV epidemic? It is important, first and clearly, to say that it is not, as is implicit in many discussions, even between *soi-disant* experts, as a 'pool of infection' or as a vector of disease. The view that infection by HIV, development of AIDS and death are not matters of concern when those involved are merely prostitutes and only become so when the lives, livelihoods or heterosexual pretensions of their clients are threatened is simply obscene. Such argument, whether made explicit or implicit, reinforces the tendency to equate HIV infection with blame, and is symptomatic of a naive individualism that ignores structural factors.

Second, it is important to clarify the role of identity and group affiliation in the transmission of HIV. Such factors are clearly and obviously irrelevant in the physical transmission of the virus: HIV does not distinguish between gay and straight. But identity may be crucial in the *prevention* of transmission. Someone who avows a gay identity or who regards himself as an injecting drug user will be more likely to take seriously and work through the issues involved in risk reduction than someone for whom homosexual sex or drug use (however frequent it may be) is dismissed as peripheral to their lives. Similarly, involvement in groups where that identity is shared and overt means that dissemination and discussion of risk reduction information and techniques is more likely than otherwise.

Let us, therefore, distinguish between the prostitute, a class of individual, and prostitution, a class of sexual acts. As Weeks has so clearly put it, ' . . . The crucial question then becomes: Would the transaction go on if goods and services were not exchanged? — a question involving self-concepts and identity as well as affection . . . ' (Weeks, 1980: 123).

Logically, therefore, there are two questions: what is the role of prostitutes in the transmission and the prevention of transmission of HIV; and what is the importance of prostitution? Taking these in reverse order, it is clear that the importance of prostitution, the exchange of money or favours for sex, is that it imports into the sexual negotiation an explicit inequality. As Richardson points out elsewhere in this volume (see Chapter 12), the assumption of much health education literature is that the negotiation of safer sex takes place between equals. This is rarely the case, but the negotiation between client and prostitute is one where that assumption is most sorely tried. This is not to say that the prostitute is always or necessarily powerless in the negotiation. The experienced prostitute can have a greater control over the sexual negotiation than his client, but the key is experience and the ultimate sanction of refusing to trade. When a prostitute is new to the job or desperate for money or a bed for the night, then the temptation to accede to demands for unsafe sex is greater. Nor is it the case that the punter will always try to have high risk sex. Many are aware of the need for safer sex and demand that from their prostitutes.

The role of prostitutes as a class in HIV infection is most nearly analogous to that of health workers, in that, for both, their work puts them at some risk of contracting the virus. The major difference is that, whereas the likelihood of, say, a nurse becoming infected in the normal course of duty is low, that of the prostitute is appreciably higher. The prostitute more often places himself (or herself) in situations where there is, at least potentially, a relatively high risk of transmission. For the health worker, accidental transfusion with HIV positive blood is the only real risk of contracting the virus. For the prostitute, many if not all transactions carry at least the possibility of semen to blood contact. If the role of health education with respect to HIV is to enable risk reduction, then it follows that the means whereby techniques of negotiation and sexual interaction can be learned have to be put in place.

It is only by retreating from the hegemonic images of homosexual male prostitutes which relegate them to the position of passive victim and instead recognizing this phenomenon in all its manifestations that health educators can find a way forward. For, in doing so, the actual or potential strengths which reside in the prostitutes' interactions — be it with friends, the gay scene, their agencies or their clients — can be seen as a conduit for empowerment. In this way, statutory and voluntary organizations can work with, for instance, the escort agencies, tapping their knowledge of and access to the prostitutes in order to enable collective decision-making and action. Thus, if prostitution is seen as the product not of psychic disorder but of rational choice, then the ultimate rational decision, to minimize activities likely to result in HIV infection, becomes a realistic goal.

References

BELL, A. P. and WEINBERG, M. S. (1978) *Homosexualities: A Study of Diversity in Men and Women.* London, Mitchell Beazley.

BENJAMIN, H. N. and MASTERS, R. E. L. (1964) *Prostitution and Morality.* London, Souvenir Press.

BOSWELL, J. (1980) *Christianity, Social Tolerance and Homosexuality.* Chicago, Ill., University of Chicago Press.

BRANDT, A. M. (1985) *No Magic Bullet: A Social History of Venereal Disease in the United States since 1880.* Oxford, Oxford University Press.

BRAY, A. (1982) *Homosexuality in Renaissance England.* London, Gay Men's Press.

BROWN, P. (1988) *The Body and Society: Men, Women and Sexual Renunciation in Early Christianity.* London, Faber.

BULLOUGH, V. and BULLOUGH, B. (1987) *Women and Prostitution: A Social History*. Buffalo, N.Y., Prometheus.

BUTTS, W. M. (1947) 'Boy Prostitutes of the Metropolis', *Journal of Clinical Psychopathology*, 8, pp. 673–81.

CORY, D. W. and LEROY, J. P. (1963) *The Homosexual and His Society: A View from Within*. New York, Citadel.

COXON, A. P. M. (1986) *Report of Pilot Study: Project on Sexual Lifestyles of Non-Heterosexual Males*. Cardiff, Social Research Unit Working Paper.

DE LAGEMAAT, G. (1986) 'The Making of the Modern Business Boy'. Unpublished paper, University of Utrecht.

DELPH, E. W. (1978) *The Silent Community: Public Homosexual Encounters*. Beverly Hills, Calif., Sage.

FOUCAULT, M. (1985) *The Use of Pleasure: Volume Two of the History of Sexuality*. Harmondsworth, Viking.

HARRIS, M. (1973) *The Dilly Boys: Male Prostitutes in Piccadilly*. London, Croom Helm.

HAUSER, R. (1962) *The Homosexual Society*. London, Bodley Head.

HOFFMAN, M. (1979) 'The Male Prostitute', in M. P. Levine (ed.), *Gay Men: The Sociology of Male Homosexuality*. New York, Harper and Row.

HOWARD LEAGUE (1985) *Unlawful Sex: Offences, Victims and Offenders in the Criminal Justice System of England and Wales*. London, Waterlow.

JACQUART, D. and THOMASSET, C. (1988) *Sexuality and Medicine in the Middle Ages*. Cambridge, Polity Press.

JAY, K. and YOUNG, A. (1977) *The Gay Report*. New York, Summit.

JERSILD, J. (1956) *Boy Prostitution*. Copenhagen, G. E. C. Gad.

KINSEY, A. C., POMEROY, W. B., and MARTIN, C. E. (1948) *Sexual Behaviour in the Human Male*. London, Saunders.

LEVINE, M. P. (ed.) (1977) *Gay Men: The Sociology of Male Homosexuality*. New York, Harper and Row.

LLOYD, R. (1979) *Playland: A Study of Human Exploitation*. London, Quartet Books.

LUCKENBILL, D. F. (1986) 'Deviant Career Mobility: The Case of Male Prostitutes', *Social Problems*, **33(4)**, pp. 283–296.

MAROTTA, T., WALDORF, D. and MURPHY, S. (1988) 'Males Doing Sex Work in the San Francisco Bay Area: A Typology and Description'. Unpublished paper, Institute for Scientific Analysis, San Francisco.

PITMAN, D. J. (1971) 'The Male House of Prostitution', *Transaction*, 8, pp. 21–7.

POMEROY, W. B. (1972) *Dr. Kinsey and the Institute for Sex Research*. London, Nelson.

REISS, A. J. (1961) 'The Social Integration of Queers and Peers', *Social Problems*, 9, pp. 102–19.

SEABROOK, J. (1976) *A Lasting Relationship: Homosexuals and Society*. London, Allen Lane.

VERSTRAETE, B. C. (1980) 'Slavery and the Social Dynamics of Homosexual Relations in Ancient Rome', *Journal of Homosexuality*, 5, pp. 227–36.

WEEKS, J. (1977) *Coming Out: Homosexual Politics in Britain from the Nineteenth Century to the Present Day*. London, Quartet Books.

WEEKS, J. (1980) 'Inverts, Perverts and Mary Annes: Male Prostitution and the Regulation of Homosexuality in England in the 19th and early 20th Centuries', *Journal of Homosexuality*, 5, pp. 113–134.

WEISBURG, K. D. (1984) *Children of the Night: A Study of Adolescent Prostitution*. New York, Lexington.

WEST, D. J. (1968) *Homosexuality*. London, Duckworth.

WEST, D. J. (1977) *Homosexuality Re-examined*. London, Duckworth.

Chapter 8

Variation in Sexual Behaviour in Gay Men

Ray Fitzpatrick, John McLean, Mary Boulton, Graham Hart and Jill Dawson

There is now substantial evidence that sexual behaviour among gay men has changed in response to AIDS. Rates of sexually transmitted diseases have declined in this group of men (Gellon and Ison, 1986). Rates of HIV infection in gay men attending genito-urinary medicine clinics have showed no indication of increasing in most recent years (Carne *et al.*, 1987; Evans *et al.*, 1989; Collaborative Study Group, 1989). Both clinic (Carne *et al.*, 1987; Evans *et al.*, 1989) and non-clinic (DHSS, 1987) surveys of gay men report important decreases in risky sexual behaviour. However, as substantial numbers of men still report high risk sex in all of these surveys, it remains an urgent task to understand variation in behaviour.

An early study of behavioural change in San Francisco found that gay men who know someone with AIDS were more likely to have made appropriate behavioural changes (McKusick, Horstman and Coats, 1985). A study of gay and bisexual men in Pittsburgh found that more regular condom use in high risk sex was associated with the view that condoms did not interfere with sexual pleasure (Valdiserri *et al.*, 1988). It has been argued that the Health Belief Model (Rosenstock, 1974) provides a useful theoretical framework for addressing questions of behavioural change in relation to HIV infection (Kotarba and Lang, 1986; Joseph *et al.*, 1987; Fitzpatrick, Boulton and Hart, 1989). The San Francisco and Pittsburgh studies illustrate two important components of the model. One central variable in the model is the individual's subjective appraisal of susceptibility or vulnerability to a health problem, which may facilitate taking appropriate health action. Knowing someone with AIDS may well have increased gay men's sense of vulnerability. On the other hand, the model argues that perceptions of the costs and benefits of taking appropriate health action will influence behaviour. Perceptions of the costs to sexual pleasure from the adoption of condom use may be just such a consideration.

One potential limitation of the Health Belief Model with regard to sexual behaviour change is that it focuses upon individuals' perceptions in isolation, whereas most sex is social action. Sex involves at least two individuals and some form of relationship. Research to date has given some small recognition to the different types of sexual relationship in which gay men may become involved. Most often this has involved describing gay men's sexual behaviour with 'casual' partners (Evans *et al.*, 1986, 1989). However, the importance that sexual relationships may have for an understanding of sexual behaviour has not been fully considered. This chapter considers some aspects of the Health Belief Model in relation to a study of sexual behaviour among men who describe themselves as gay, homosexual or bisexual in England.

The Study

The criterion for inclusion in this study was any man who has had sex with another man in the previous five years. The sample reported here comprises 356 men recruited from a diverse range of sources. One hundred and ninety-eight men (56 per cent) volunteered from gay pubs, clubs and gay organizations; eighty-two men (23 per cent) were recruited from genito-urinary medicine clinics; and seventy-six (21 per cent) were referrals from those already interviewed. Four main towns and cities were used to recruit the sample: London (52 per cent), Manchester (21 per cent), Oxford (13 per cent) and Northampton (5 per cent); a further 9 per cent were recruited from areas around these four centres.

Interviews focused upon sexual behaviour in the previous month and in the previous year. Information was gathered by means of a checklist of sexual behaviours, and respondents were asked, especially in relation to the last month, to describe their sexual behaviour with each of their partners in turn. Men were first asked about regular partners with whom they were currently in a relationship; they were then asked about other partners. Other sections of the interview examined attitudes, knowledge and beliefs in relation to HIV and AIDS, and social circumstances. The statistics used in this chapter are Student's test unless otherwise stated.

The mean age of the sample was 32.9 (sd 10.7), with a range from 16 to 67. The sample was predominantly middle-class, with 84 per cent of men in social class I, II, IIINM, according to the Registrar-General's classification of occupations. When asked how they preferred to describe their sexual orientation, 276 (78 per cent) chose gay, thirty-seven (11 per cent) chose homosexual, thirty-one (9 per cent) bisexual, and a further eight (2 per cent) preferred no designation. Men were asked to rate themselves on the Kinsey scale: 299 (84 per cent) described themselves as exclusively homosexual in terms of sexual activities, and 227 (64 per cent) as exclusively homosexual in terms of fantasies and attractions. The rest of the men described themselves in terms of varying degrees of both homosexual and heterosexual activity and feelings. Thirty-five men (10 per cent) were currently married, separated or divorced.

Sex in the Last Month

One hundred and fifteen men (32 per cent) had receptive anal sex in the month before interview; ninety-four (26 per cent) had receptive anal sex with a regular partner and thirty-three (9 per cent) with a non-regular partner; seventy-four (21 per cent) had receptive anal sex without a condom. Unprotected receptive anal sex much more commonly occurred with regular partners (fifty-nine men, 17 per cent) than with non-regular partners (eighteen men, 5 per cent).

A similar pattern is described by men with regard to insertive anal sex. One hundred and thirteen men (32 per cent) had insertive anal sex in the previous month; ninety-six (27 per cent) had insertive anal sex with a regular partner and thirty men (8 per cent) with a non-regular partner; sixty-three (18 per cent) had insertive anal sex without a condom. Unprotected insertive anal sex much more commonly happened with a regular partner (fifty-five men, 15 per cent) than with a non-regular partner (eleven men, 3 per cent).

Sex in the Last Year

Men were also asked about sex in the previous year. Two hundred and thirteen men (60 per cent) had receptive anal sex in the last year, more frequently occurring with regular partners (176 men, 49 per cent) than with non-regular partners (110 men, 31 per cent). Similarly, 224 men (63 per cent) reported insertive anal sex, more frequently occurring with regular partners (183 men, 51 per cent) than with non-regular partners (106 men, 30 per cent).

Men were also asked how regularly they used condoms in anal sex in the previous year. Men were equally likely to say they used condoms never, always or sometimes/often in sex with regular partners (Table 1). However, with non-regular partners, in both insertive and receptive anal sex, a majority always used a condom.

Relationships and High Risk Sex

From the interview data about sex in the last month, it was possible to distinguish five different groups in the sample. Ninety-one men (26 per cent) were currently involved in a regular exclusive relationship with one partner. A second group of forty-six men (13 per cent) was involved in a regular relationship which was not exclusive, as they

Ray Fitzpatrick et al.

Table 1. Use of Condoms in Last Year

	Always	Often	Sometimes	Never	Number of men having this kind of sex
				(percentages shown in brackets)	
Used in: Receptive anal sex — regular partners	76 (43)	18 (10)	28 (16)	54 (31)	176
Receptive anal sex — non-regular partners	63 (57)	6 (6)	23 (21)	18 (16)	110
Insertive anal sex — regular partners	77 (42)	10 (6)	33 (18)	63 (34)	183
Insertive anal sex — non-regular partners	68 (64)	1 (1)	20 (19)	17 (16)	106

had described themselves or their partner as having other regular relationships. Ninety-seven men (27 per cent) were involved in regular relationships but had also currently had sex with at least one non-regular partner. A fourth group of men (N = 67, 19 per cent) had only had sex in the last month with a partner who was not described as regular. Finally, fifty-five men (15 per cent) did not have any current sexual partners.

One important component of regular relationships compared with other current sexual partners may be that the former are more long standing. We asked individuals to date as accurately as possible how long ago they had first had sex with each partner they mentioned. The lengths of different kinds of relationship that emerged are shown in Table 2. There is some degree of overlap in the lengths of time for regular and non-regular partners. Some regular relationships had only been established shortly before the interview. Conversely, some men included in their non-regular relationships, partners with whom they had first had sex twelve years before the interview. On the other hand, there is a clear trend, shown by taking the median length of relationships, for regular relationships to last a great deal longer than those with other partners. Of the 319 current regular relationships described by men in the sample, 58 per cent had lasted for at least a year. By comparison, of the 377 current non-regular relationships described, 8 per cent lasted for at least a year. The median length of non-regular relationships was one month.

The highest rate of anal intercourse and of unprotected anal intercourse occurs in the group of men who reported being in exclusive regular relationships (Table 3). The lowest rates of these sexual activities are reported in the context of non-regular

Table 2. Median Length of Relationships for Different Kinds of Partner

Type of current partner	Regular	Non-regular
One regular exclusive partner	1 year 5 months (1 month–46 years)	—
Regular non-exclusive partners	2 years 1 month (1 month–28 years)	—
Regular and non-regular partners	1 year 3 months (1 month–22 years)	1 month (1 week–5 years)
Only non-regular partners		1 month (2 weeks–12 years)

partners. The ninety-seven men who had sex with both regular and non-regular partners in the month before the interview were twice as likely to report more risky forms of sexual activity with their regular partners. If men in exclusive regular relationships are compared with men having sex with only non-regular partners, the differences in sexual behaviour are very clear. Men in exclusive regular relationships were more likely to have receptive anal sex (Chi-square = 7.4, df = 1, p < 0.01), to have unprotected receptive anal sex (Chi-square = 11.3, df = 1, p < 0.001), to have insertive anal sex (Chi-square = 11.0, df = 1, p < 0.001) and to have unprotected insertive anal sex (Chi-square = 11.3, df = 1, p < 0.001).

Table 3. Types of Current Partner and Probability of High Risk Sex in Last Month

Sample grouped by type of current partner		Sexual activities (percentages shown in brackets)			
		Receptive anal sex	Receptive anal sex without condom	Insertive anal sex	Insertive anal sex without condom
One regular exclusive partner		39 (43)	30 (33)	42 (46)	28 (31)
Regular non-exclusive partners		20 (43)	12 (26)	17 (37)	10 (22)
Regular and non-regular partners	(R)*	35 (36)	17 (18)	37 (38)	17 (18)
	(NR)*	19 (20)	12 (12)	17 (18)	6 (6)
Only non-regular partners		14 (21)	6 (9)	13 (19)	5 (8)

Note: *Sexual activities with: (R) regular partners; (NR) non-regular partners.

We also asked interviewees to say how many male partners they had had sex with in the year before the interview. The median number of sexual partners for the sample as a whole was five, with a range from 0 to 248 partners. The five groups, distinguished in terms of their current sexual partners, reported significantly different mean numbers of male partners in the previous year (ANOVA F = 12.28, p < 0.001). Men currently in regular exclusive relationships and men with no current sexual partner reported the lowest numbers of male partners (5.0 and 5.5). On the other hand, men who currently had regular and non-regular sexual partners and men who had only non-regular partners reported much higher mean numbers of male sexual partners for the year (27.7 and 25.2).

The possibility was examined that men involved in different types of relationships might differ in whether or not they knew their HIV serostatus. Overall, 47 per cent of men had had at least one HIV test. There was no significant differences between men in the five subgroups in terms of whether they had had a test.

Age, Income and Sexual Behaviour

Men who reported receptive anal sex in the last month were younger than those who did not (p < 0.01). In addition, men who had receptive anal sex had lower incomes (p < 0.05). The relationships between age, income and risky sex were examined in the context of different kinds of partner men had reported in the previous month. Among men who had sex with a regular but not exclusive partner, those having receptive anal sex were of lower income (p < 0.05). Among men having sex with only non-regular partners, men having receptive anal sex were both younger and of lower income (p < 0.05). The relationships between age, income and receptive anal sex were examined by means of analysis of variance. For the sample as a whole, and for each subgroup by type of partner, the introduction of age as a covariate resulted in income differences no longer being significant. No significant differences for age or income were found in relation to insertive anal sex, either for the sample as a whole or for subgroups.

There were significant differences in age between the subgroups of men distinguished by the kinds of partner they described in the previous month. Men who had sex with regular but not exclusive partners and men who had no current sexual partner were older; men reporting both regular and non-regular relationships were younger (ANOVA, F = 2.67, p < 0.05). Analysis of variance revealed no significant differences of income between men reporting different types of current partner.

Perceptions of Risk

Men were asked to assess their personal risk in relation to HIV in a number of ways. In one question, they were asked to rate their personal position on a five-point scale in relation to the question, 'How risky do you think your current behaviour is in terms of the likelihood of being exposed to HIV — the AIDS virus?' The majority of men (71 per cent) regarded their behaviour as 'not very risky' or 'not at all risky'; 14 per cent of men were unsure how to judge their behaviour; only 15 per cent perceived their behaviour as either 'risky' or 'very risky'. A second question was put to the sample: 'How do you currently rate your chances of developing AIDS?' Again only 10 per cent rated their chances as 'highly likely' or 'likely'; the rest were either unsure (13 per cent) or thought their chances 'unlikely' or 'very unlikely' (77 per cent).

These ratings of risk were analyzed in relation to sexual activities in the previous month: 19 per cent of men who had unprotected anal sex and 22 per cent of men who had unprotected receptive anal sex with a non-regular partner rated their behaviour as risky. In other terms, 68 per cent of men having unprotected receptive anal sex and 78 per cent of men having unprotected receptive anal sex with a non-regular partner did not regard their behaviour as at all risky. A similar pattern of results was obtained in relation to the second question, so that, for example, only 11 per cent of men having unprotected receptive anal sex rated their chances of getting AIDS as at all likely. There was no evidence either that recent risky sexual behaviour led men to perceive their personal vulnerability to HIV infection as increased, or that raised levels of vulnerability were associated with reductions in risky behaviour. There were no age or income differences in these perceptions of vulnerability.

Views about Condoms

Men were asked a number of questions about their views on condoms. On all questions, a majority of men expressed positive attitudes and experiences (Table 4). Only 17 per cent did not regard condoms as acceptable in sex, and 11 per cent felt embarrassed using them. A larger minority (34 per cent) regarded them as messy and unpleasant to use in sex.

These attitudes appear to have some effects upon behaviour. Men were asked who normally suggested that a condom should be used in anal sex, when the respondent was both an insertive and a receptive partner. Many men saw this as something taken for granted between partners and not involving the need for anyone to have to make the suggestion. However, talking about anal sex in which the respondent was the insertive partner, 133 men described themselves and twenty-five men their partner as the person who normally took the initiative in suggesting a condom. Similarly, in talking about anal sex in which the respondent was the receptive partner, 102 men said

Table 4. Attitudes to the Use of Condoms

	Agree	Uncertain	Disagree
		(percentages shown in brackets)	
Condoms are now an acceptable part of sex for me	270 (75)	26 (7)	60 (17)
Personally I find using a condom embarassing	38 (11)	15 (4)	303 (86)
I find condoms messy and unpleasant to use	121 (34)	40 (11)	194 (54)
The interruption from putting on a condom puts me off sex	75 (21)	35 (10)	246 (69)

they took the initiative and twenty-eight that their partner took the initiative. The men whose partner normally had to suggest condoms in sex had consistently less favourable attitudes to condoms. Thus men whose partners took the initiative about condoms when the respondent was the receptive partner were less likely to regard condoms as an acceptable part of sex ($p < 0.005$), were more likely to find condoms embarrassing ($p < 0.05$), messy and unpleasant to use ($p < 0.05$) and to say that condoms put them off sex ($p < 0.05$). Similarly, men whose partners took the initiative over condoms when the respondent was the insertive partner had less favourable views about acceptability ($p < 0.001$) and were more likely to say condoms put them off sex ($p < 0.01$).

However, when the relationship between attitudes and *use* is examined, it appears that attitudes are less important. Among men reporting anal sex, insertive or receptive, in the last month or in the last year, attitudes to condoms were not significantly related to actual use.

Discussion

Evidence from a number of different sources indicates that sexual behaviour among gay men has changed since the earliest days of the AIDS epidemic. Our survey provides further encouraging results. The results can be compared with McManus and McEvoy's (1987) national survey of gay men by questionnaire via gay magazines, clubs and public houses carried out in 1984. In that survey, 8 per cent of gay men did not practise anal sex. In our results, 23 per cent of men did not have anal sex in the year before the interview. Similarly, although McManus and McEvoy's figures do not provide data on exact numbers of sexual partners, the median for their sample falls in the range of six to fifty partners in the last year, whereas the median for this survey is five partners.

The survey by McManus and McEvoy did not include questions about condom use. Carne *et al.* (1987) provide data on 100 gay and bisexual men attending a London STD clinic. In 1984 12 per cent of men always used a condom in receptive anal sex and 13 per cent in insertive anal sex. The investigators do not distinguish between types of partner, but, if their figures are compared with those reported by our sample for anal sex with regular partners (43 per cent and 42 per cent), then clearly a marked increase in use of condoms has occurred. It is quite possible that the 1984 clinic survey overestimated the amount of condom use among gay men at that time as their respondents were seen every three months in relation to a study of HIV infection and may have been particularly oriented to safer sex as a result.

On the other hand, other results in this survey may not provide such encouraging evidence. The DHSS survey of gay men (DHSS, 1987) found that in February 1987, 41 per cent of men reported having receptive anal sex in the previous year. In our survey, the equivalent figure is 60 per cent of men. Similarly, 55 per cent of men in the DHSS survey reported insertive anal sex compared with 63 per cent of men in this survey. In addition, the DHSS survey showed a small but steady decline in the proportion reporting receptive anal sex without a condom in the previous year in the successive waves of interviews, from 36 per cent in February 1986 to 29 per cent in February 1987. Our survey results for one year later indicate that 126 men (35 per cent) had receptive anal sex without a condom in the previous year. These figures might indicate that the rate of behavioural change may have slowed down most recently.

McManus and McEvoy (1987) observed that sexual practices changed with different partners in their 1984 survey, but provide no data in relation to their observation. Our results show quite clearly how large are the differences in sexual behaviour by men with regular and non-regular sexual partners. The most risky kind of sex — receptive anal sex — is reported to have happened in the course of the year by 49 per cent of the sample with a regular partner, and 30 per cent of the sample with a non-regular partner. The differences are greater if sexual behaviour in the last month is examined.

Levels of knowledge and awareness about HIV were as high in this sample as in other studies of gay men (Becker and Joseph, 1988): 98 per cent regarded it as unsafe to have unprotected receptive anal sex without a condom if one did not know the serostatus of one's partner. One major effect of these views is that unprotected receptive anal sex with a partner who is not well known appears to be regarded as risky and is less common as a result. On the other hand, in the context of a regular relationship, unprotected anal sex does not appear to be viewed by the majority of men in this way. Although it is possible that partners of the men in the sample were more likely to know their HIV serostatus, only 47 per cent of the sample had themselves had a test. Having a test was no more common among men in regular or exclusive relationships. Thus one must assume that confidence about risk from anal sex was often based on some other grounds than both partners having regularly and recently established by HIV test their serostatus.

Ray Fitzpatrick et al.

Views about condoms were generally favourable. Again, a major determinant of their use was having anal sex outside a regular relationship. In addition, favourable attitudes towards condoms were found to be related to taking the initiative in suggesting their use both in receptive and insertive anal sex. Of relevance to this finding is the evidence of Ross (1988a) that positive attitudes to condoms may be associated with personality traits of strong will and assertiveness among gay men. Such men, according to Ross, have the confidence to raise the issue of condoms without fear of rebuff.

However, attitudes did not influence use. This result quite strongly contrasts with the evidence of Valdiserri and colleagues' study (1988) of gay men in Pittsburgh and Ross's study (1988b) of gay men in Adelaide. Gay men in Pittsburgh who felt condoms spoilt sex were less likely to use them. In Adelaide, views about responsibility and comfort with condom use were associated with use. The difference between this study and the Pittsburgh and Adelaide studies may simply be the passage of time. Valdiserri *et al.*'s study was conducted in late 1986 and early 1987 and Ross's study in late 1986. Our interviews were conducted at least one year later than this. Attitudes may no longer be as strongly related to behavioural change in this group of men. Darrow (1974) notes that most complaints about condom use may be expressed by those who use them most. Above all, men with unfavourable attitudes to condoms will be having anal sex increasingly with men whose attitudes are favourable and who will take the initiative instead.

Younger men were more likely both to have non-regular partners and to have receptive anal sex with their non-regular partners. Within regular exclusive relationships, men having receptive anal sex were also younger. These results are consistent with the findings of McKusick and colleagues (1987) who found that younger men were more likely to have risky sexual behaviour in their San Francisco study of gay men. The current study, like most studies of gay men, has not interviewed many younger gay men and it is possible that the importance of this factor is underestimated in the current results.

Generally men in this study did not perceive themselves as particularly at risk of, or vulnerable to, HIV infection. This finding is consistent with other studies that have included this component of the Health Belief Model (Joseph *et al.*, 1987; Bauman and Siegel, 1987). Furthermore, the absence of any association between level of perceived risk and actual sexual behaviour is also consistent with other evidence (Joseph *et al.*, 1987; Siegel *et al.*, 1989). The tendency for men who are well aware of the general risks of particular sexual behaviours nevertheless to continue to have risky sex has been compared to the 'optimistic bias' found in other areas of health behaviour (Joseph *et al.*, 1987).

Above all, this study has indicated how important are the ways in which sexual behaviour appears to be contingent upon individuals' perceptions of their sexual partner. From an epidemiological point of view, the strategy of 'mutual monogamy', in which both partners are known to be absolutely concordant for HIV status, would represent a safer approach to the risks associated with particular forms of sex. However, many of the regular relationships in this study, in which risky sex was frequently reported, did not match such requirements. Because of enormous difficulties in tracking the underlying epidemiology of HIV, it is difficult to estimate how hazardous for individuals such sexual behaviour is. From a sociological point of view, the study reinforces further the need to question assumptions about the homogeneity of gay populations, which were so prevalent in the early American literature on AIDS. That much high risk sexual activity is clearly partner-specific is a finding which has implications for future health promotion, as are our findings in relation to age and income. Any future work in this area must recognize the significance of partner formation, and explore the social context in which expectations and attitudes arise, particularly in relationships which, it is anticipated, will endure.

References

BAUMAN, L. and SIEGEL, K. (1987) 'Misperceptions among Gay Men of the Risk of AIDS Associated with Their Sexual Behaviour', *Journal of Applied Social Psychology*, 17, pp. 328–49.

BECKER, M. and JOSEPH, J. (1988) 'AIDS and Behavioural Change to Reduce Risk: A Review', *American Journal of Public Health*, 78, pp. 394–410.

CARNE, C., WELLER, I., JOHNSON, A., et al. (1987) 'Prevalence of Antibodies to Human Immunodeficiency Virus, Gonorrhoea Rates, and Changed Sexual Behaviour in Homosexual Men in London', *Lancet*, 1, pp. 656–8.

COLLABORATIVE STUDY GROUP (1989) 'HIV Infection in Patients Attending Clinics for Sexually Transmitted Diseases in England and Wales', *British Medical Journal*, 298, pp. 415–18.

DARROW, W. (1974) 'Attitudes towards Condom Use and the Acceptance of Venereal Disease Prophylaxis', in M. RADFORD, G. DUNCAN and D. PRAGER (eds), *The Condom: Increasing Utilisation in the United States*. San Francisco, Calif., San Francisco Press.

DHSS (1987) *AIDS: Monitoring Response to the Public Education Campaign, February 1986–February 1987*. London, HMSO.

EVANS, B., DAWSON, S., MCLEAN, K. et al. (1986) 'Sexual Lifestyle and Clinical Findings Related to HTLVIII/LAV Status in Homosexual Men', *Genitourinary Medicine*, 62, pp. 384–9.

EVANS, B., DAWSON, S. MCLEAN, K., DAWSON, S., TEECE, S., BOND, R., MACRAE, K. and THORP, R. (1989) 'Trends in Sexual Behaviour and Risk Factors for HIV Infection among Homosexual Men, 1984-7', *British Medical Journal*, 298, pp. 215–18.

FITZPATRICK, R., BOULTON, M. and HART, G. (1989) 'Gay Men's Sexual Behaviour in Response to AIDS: Insights and Problems', in P. AGGLETON, G. HART and P. DAVIES (eds), *AIDS: Social Representations, Social Practices*. Lewes, Falmer Press.

GELLON, M. and ISON, C. (1986) 'Declining Incidence of Gonorrhoea in London: A Response to Fear of AIDS?' *Lancet*, 2, p. 920.

JOSEPH, J., MONTGOMERY, S., EMMONS, C., et al. (1987) 'Magnitude and Determinants of Behavioural Risk Reduction: Longitudinal Analysis of a Cohort at Risk for AIDS', *Psychology and Health*, 1, pp. 73–95.

KOTARBA, J. and LANG, N. (1986) 'Gay Lifestyle Change and AIDS: Preventive Health Care', in D. FELDMAN and T. JOHNSON (eds), *The Social Dimensions of AIDS: Method and Theory*. New York, Praeger.

McKusick, M., Horstman, W. and Coates, T. (1985) 'AIDS and Sexual Behaviour Reported by Gay Men in San Francisco', *American Journal of Public Health*, 75, pp. 493–6.

McKusick, M., Coates, T., Wiley, J. *et al.* (1987) 'Prevention of HIV Infection among Gay and Bisexual Men: Two Longitudinal Studies', in *Third International Conference on AIDS Abstracts Volume*. Washington, Conference Secretariat.

McManus, T. and McEvoy, M. (1987) 'Some Aspects of Male Homosexual Behaviour in the United Kingdom', *British Journal of Sexual Medicine*, April, pp. 110–20.

Rosenstock, K. (1974) 'The Health Belief Model and Preventive Health Behaviour', *Health Education Monograph*, 2, pp. 354–65.

Ross, M. (1988a) 'Personality Factors that Differentiate Homosexual Men with Positive and Negative Attitudes toward Condom Use', *New York State Journal of Medicine*, 88, pp. 626–8.

Ross, M. (1988b) 'Attitudes towards Condoms as AIDS Prophylaxis in Homosexual Men: Dimensions and Measurement', *Psychology and Health*, 2, pp. 291–9.

Siegel, K., Mesagno, F., Chen, J. and Christ, G. (1989) 'Factors Distinguishing Homosexual Males Practising Risky and Safer Sex', *Social Science and Medicine*, 28, pp. 561–70.

Valdiserri, R., Lyter, D., Leviton, L., *et al.* (1988). 'Variables Influencing Condom Use in a Cohort of Gay and Bisexual Men', *American Journal of Public Health*, 78, pp. 801–5.

Chapter 9

Needle Exchange in Historical Context: Responses to the 'Drugs Problem'[1]

Graham Hart

The history of the non-medical use of analgesic and psycho-active drugs is marked on the one hand by governmental, medical and judicial indifference — particularly in the nineteenth century — and on the other by frenetic activity in all these arenas. It is clear that at present we are, in historical terms, experiencing the second of these responses to drug use — near frenzied activity.

Until the mid-1980s, the 'threat' of the non-medical use of opiates, particularly heroin, lay in their potentially debilitating and dependency inducing effects on 'youth', particularly young working-class men and women on the country's council housing estates (Parker, Newcomer and Bakx, 1987). Whether smoking or injecting the drug, the individual physical deterioration and negative social consequences (crime, unemployability) associated with widespread heroin use were considered self-evidently dysfunctional and to be prevented, discouraged and, for those found transgressing, punished by heavy fines and custodial sentences. A series of health education campaigns targeting young people began in 1985; the 'Heroin Screws You Up' posters were one of the more public expressions of government concern in this area. In 1987 there were 221 deaths in England and Wales registered due to drug dependence or misuse. However, the decade has seen the appearance of a larger threat than drug use, and one which is associated with thousands rather than hundreds of deaths: AIDS.

In September 1988 the government announced that it was making £3 million available to health authorities in England purely for the purposes of preventing the further spread of HIV, the causative agent of AIDS, among injecting drug users. It would be naive to assume that these resources had been allocated only for the best interests of a highly stigmatized minority of people engaging in an illicit and health-threatening activity. Concern about the transmission of HIV from a predominantly heterosexual group of drug users to their non-injecting sexual partners, and subsequently into the heterosexual population as a whole (Moss, 1987) has been

133

sufficient to warrant what even the most critical observer would describe as a welcome addition to drug services.

This concern has had other outcomes. One of the most radical health interventions to occur in Britain in recent years in response to HIV infection among drug users has been the development of needle-exchange schemes. Sterile injecting equipment is dispensed free at the point of contact, as is advice on appropriate injecting sites, safer sex and condoms. How has a situation arisen such that, within a matter of years — some might say months — while the possession of street drugs remains illegal, the government has provided 'new' monies to ensure that the injection of these drugs is done with clean equipment? This chapter provides a short history of medical and government responses to drug use, from the nineteenth century to the present day, and then describes one needle-exchange and its clients. Finally, there is a discussion of the relationship between responses to drug use and HIV infection.

Responses To Drug Use: The Nineteenth Century

During the greater part of the nineteenth century the open sale of opiate-based products in pharmacies and even groceries indicates their general acceptability and use (Berridge and Edwards, 1987). Indeed, in the early years of the century opium poppies were cultivated for the express purpose of opiate production, with Mitcham in the 1830s proving to be a most congenial and successful farming area for the white poppy (*ibid*: 16). Most opium was imported, however, and traded in London in the same way as any other commodity.

Although 'infant doping' of working-class children — parents buying such products as Godfrey's Cordial and Dalby's Carminative — was a source of middle-class public health concern, the use of laudanum, an opium derivative, was prevalent throughout all social classes. In the fenlands of East Anglia, opium consumption was particularly high among working-class men and women, and variously used for self-medication and as an addition to beer purely for its narcotic qualities (*ibid*.: 38–40). Middle- and upper-class use was also widespread, with regular consumers including Elizabeth Barrett Browning, Gladstone's sister Helen and, undoubtedly for its medicinal qualities, Florence Nightingale (*ibid*.: 58–9). How, therefore, did opiate use become a social and medical problem?

Alongside the scientific development in bio-medicine which occurred at a rapid pace from the mid-nineteenth century onwards, the social role of medicine changed. Medical professionalization — a process of the definition of an area of expertise over which only one group could have control — occurred in tandem with and resulted in, changing notions of disease causation, its management and treatment. However, the 'clinical gaze', as described by Foucault, looked beyond what was pathological in individual cell cultures to what was perceived as socially pathological. Thus disease boundaries expanded to include behaviour that had previously been considered merely perverse, sinful or criminal (Rosenberg, 1986). 'Social problems' became equally amenable to the clinical gaze. Madness, sexual behaviour, alcohol and drug use all received their share of medical scrutiny and state control.

Throughout most of the nineteenth century opium was eaten or otherwise imbibed. However, from the 1860s onwards the hypodermic injection of morphine, an opium derivative, was popularized in the medical press as an optimal form of pain relief. From the 1870s however, iatrogenic addiction induced by doctors' liberal administration of morphia received widespread medical attention, with case histories appearing with increasing regularity. Who better to manage properly the care of the morphine addict than another member of the profession who had induced the state of dependency?

Middle-class concern regarding working-class sloth, lack of hygiene and inebriation found expression in a range of temperance organizations, in which medical men were active. Moral panics regarding 'infant doping', 'opium dens' and the 'discovery' of addiction as a disease amenable to treatment led to demands to regulate access to the drug and its derivatives, and by the end of the century, more as a result of pharmaceutical controls and a fall in popularity than due to government intervention, opium use declined.

Responses To Drug Use: The British System

Perceptions of opium use changed radically during the nineteenth century. During the first half of the century, as we have seen, it was both cultivated and used widely. As Berridge and Edwards (1987: 37) suggest, 'Opium itself was the "opiate of the people".' Towards the end of the century, however, the increase in subcutaneous and intravenous administration of morphine unwittingly produced so-called therapeutic addiction, with the majority of patients being middle-class. Overuse of the opiate derivative became the disease of addiction. From such a situation arose the so-called 'British system' of drug maintenance which developed during the twentieth century.

Stimson and Oppenheimer (1982: 205) have described the 'British system' as 'a loose collection of ideas, policies, institutions, and activities'. Its central tenet, since the deliberations of the Rolleston Committee on Drug Dependence in 1926 (HMSO, 1926), has been that addicts are patients suffering from a disease, not criminals. Arriving at this label was in no small part a consequence of the professional, indeed medical, status of many addicts; they were essentially respectable, if wayward, people (Ghodse, 1983). This labelling of addicts as patients was further reinforced by the first report of the Brain Committee on Drug Addiction in 1961 (HMSO, 1961) which affirmed that no special measures were required to treat addicts, although there had been a small increase in post-war years in non-therapeutic (i.e. non-iatrogenic) dependency.

From 1960 onwards the complacency of the British in relation to their 'system' was severely challenged by an increasing incidence of drug use, particularly amphetamines, barbiturates and heroin, among a wide range of young people. As with morphine in the late nineteenth century, injectable heroin was initially supplied by doctors. 'Patients' would visit private doctors, buy a prescription of heroin which far exceeded their immediate needs or for which they had no personal need at all, and sell on a black market the remainder of the drug. This generated further funds to visit once again their chosen practitioner to buy further prescriptions. This 'over prescribing by a few doctors' (Ghodse, 1983: 636) contributed to, but was not the single cause of, increased heroin availability and use in the 1960s.

The increase in heroin use and concern over its consequences led the government of the day to reconvene the Brain Committee. In its second report (HMSO, 1965), the committee radically changed its tune; it recommended, among other things: the compulsory notification of addicts by doctors to the Home Office; the restriction of the right to prescribe drugs such as heroin and cocaine to doctors licensed by the Home Office; and the setting up of clinics for the treatment of addicts.

The Dangerous Drugs Act of 1967, and later statutes, have ensured, in addition to these measures, heavy fines and prison sentences for the possession, production and trafficking of certain drugs; it is now also possible to have monies derived from the sale and distribution of controlled drugs seized by a court. As a result, the 'British system' now marries a medical model of addiction with a more obvious form of social control — the criminal justice system.

The 1970s saw the development of a limited number of Drug Dependency Units (DDUs) for drug addicts, with London attracting the largest number of resources. Dominated by psychiatrists in the early years of the decade, DDUs had what would now be described as liberal prescribing policies. Injectable heroin and Methadone, a manufactured opiate substitute (opioid), were prescribed, often on a maintenance basis which involved neither reducing or increasing dosage. Increased use of oral Methadone, however, and concerns about doctor-maintained addicts, resulted broadly in a change in prescribing policies. Reducing prescriptions had become the order of the day by the early 1980s, along with increased opportunities for psychotherapy, group work, access to social services and 'lifestyle modification'. Non-medical staff working in DDUs hoped this would end medical dominance and actively worked to de-medicalize the overall treatment and care of drug users.

'Heroin Screws You Up'

Drug Dependency Units have only ever seen a small fraction of drug users. Even if one restricts discussion to those who inject — rather than smoke, sniff or take drugs orally — and to those who primarily use heroin (rather than amphetamines or barbiturates), it is undoubtedly the case that the majority of drug users have no contact with treatment agencies (Hartnoll *et al.*, 1985; Power, Hartnoll and Daviaud, 1988).

The government's awareness of the existence of a mass of drug users not in contact with agencies, and the potential health threat posed by widespread use among young people, led them in 1985 to begin a campaign warning those who might be tempted to try heroin of the personal, health and social consequences of dependency. The first phase of the campaign had the theme 'Heroin Screws You Up'. This began in autumn 1985 and detailed the physical deterioration associated with addiction. The second phase, from summer 1986 to early 1987, encouraged young people to avoid peer group pressure to use heroin, and included television advertisements of a young girl being offered the drug at a party by her boyfriend and being ridiculed into accepting it ('Just say no'). The third phase, using billboards and the youth press, emphasized the immediate social consequences of frequent use. This included references to stealing from one's mother's purse, or taking her jewellery, and exchanging sex for money (see Power in MacGregor, 1989 for a discussion of these issues).

Unfortunately, it is said that these campaigns had negative as well as positive outcomes from a health education viewpoint. For example, the sallow youths appearing in the 'Heroin Screws You Up' posters were considered attractive enough to put on teenage bedroom walls alongside favoured pop stars. Much of the campaign was ignored by would-be users of amphetamines and barbiturates, and drugs with similar effects to heroin, such as pethidine and palfium. The campaign had been so firmly targeted to 'smack heads' (heroin users) that other drug use appeared relatively benign. However, events were overtaking such campaigns.

HIV Infection and AIDS

In 1981 the Acquired Immune Deficiency Syndrome was described and identified as a new medical condition. In 1984 the infectious casual agent of the disease was isolated, and it is now known as Human Immunodeficiency Virus. By the end of 1985 tests were available for the antibodies which develop as a result of infection.

Late in 1985 a general practitioner serving the Muirhouse Estate in Edinburgh — an area of substantial social deprivation and high prevalence of young injecting drug users — decided to use the HIV antibody test on blood samples he had collected and stored between 1983 and 1985 (Robertson *et al.*, 1986). The results indicated that there had been an epidemic of the infection among the practice's drug injectors, with 51 per cent of the sample showing HIV antibodies by 1985. A similar study reporting from Edinburgh early in 1986 gave a prevalence of 65 per cent (Brettle *et al.*, 1986). Both studies implicated the sharing of needles and syringes as the primary cause of infection, and pointed to an earlier epidemic of hepatitis B infection — also a blood borne viral infection — as further proof of the likely transmission function of the activity.

A coalition of Scottish medical and public health forces in 1986 put pressure on the Scottish Office to recognize the fact of an HIV epidemic. This resulted in a Scottish Home and Health Department Report, chaired by D. B. L. McClelland (SHHD, 1986). Apart from recommending easier access to prescribed substitutes to heroin, its most radical proposal was to make needles and syringes available to drug users on a one-for-one exchange basis. This was the first government commissioned report to acknowledge the potential value of needle exchange in preventing HIV infection.

Yet the government had not yet accepted the proposal unreservedly. Lord Glenarthur, Minister of State at the Scottish Office with responsibility for Health and Social Work, expressed the perceived contradiction which might result from increasing access to injecting equipment. In a press statement released with the report, he said: ' . . . Such a practice may have sound clinical advantages but it would have important implications for our policy on tackling another scourge of our times — drug misuse — to which we must also give high priority, at the same time as taking steps to prevent AIDS . . . ' (Press Release, SIO, 1986). Lord Glenarthur's dilemma, and that of many others, was how could central government suggest on the one hand that 'Heroin Screws You Up', and on the other provide the wherewithal to inject the substance free?

Needle Exchange

The introduction of needle exchanges occurred with remarkable rapidity. It is an example of government stomaching one 'evil' — distribution of needles and syringes to drug injectors — in order to obviate others. In this instance, these would be the heavy human and economic prices to pay for morbidity and mortality among drug users and possibly the heterosexual population as a whole from the further spread of HIV infection.

The change in policy which resulted in the setting up of needle exchange schemes is described fully by Stimson *et al.* (1989). Essentially, by 1987 fifteen pilot schemes had been incorporated into a national evaluation project directed by Gerry Stimson. Some schemes had started prior to receiving formal approval from government, notably those in Liverpool, Sheffield and at University College Hospital London, and evaluation of the latter had also begun. The national evaluation's findings have been reported (Stimson *et al.*, 1988a, 1988b) and so the remainder of this chapter examines the workings of one scheme alone — that which began at University College Hospital, London, subsequently transferred to the Middlesex Hospital, London and is known as The Exchange.

The Exchange is a shop-front street agency which is separate from the main Middlesex Hospital buildings. It is staffed by two drugs and health workers and several volunteers from local non-statutory drug agencies. The scheme's clients are predominantly white, men (the man-to-woman ratio is 4:1) and they are long-term drug users (see Hart *et al.*, 1989). Most began injecting at about 18, and their median age on entry is 32. Most inject heroin at least twice daily. The Exchange has proved popular with clients. From November 1987 to October 1988 the average number of clients attending per month was 257, and the numbers attending improved significantly over the course of the year (t-test, p = 0.0004). An average of 8,950 syringes were dispensed each month, and 6,918 were returned, an average return rate of 77 per cent. Returns improved significantly during the year; in November the return rate was 69 per cent but by October 1988 it was 78 per cent (Chi-squared trend test: p < 0.0001).

During interviews with a sample of clients one month and then again four months into the scheme, we found reductions in sharing needles and syringes (a) as compared to reported levels prior to entry to the scheme and (b) comparing first interview (< 1 month) to second interview (< 4 months). There was also a significant reduction in the frequency of injecting after four months (Wilcoxon signed rank test: p < .01).

We asked clients about their sexual behaviour in the last three months on first and second interview. The majority of the sample had had sex with another person during both periods (77 per cent, 74 per cent). There was an increase in the proportions having non-injecting sexual partners (45 per cent vs 56 per cent), a fall in the proportions with two or more partners (26 per cent vs 20 per cent) and reduced condom use (46 per cent vs 36 per cent). Seven of the seventy-nine men (9 per cent) who had been sexually active during the three months prior to the first interview had exchanged sex for money or drugs, compared to four of the twenty-three active women (17 per cent); all paying sexual partners were male. Those who had prostituted had a mean of thirty-eight sexual partners in the three months prior to interview (range 1–250); all but one used condoms during penetrative intercourse.

Overall, we consider the scheme to have been successful in a number of ways. Clients express satisfaction with a number of the scheme's features, and their health has benefitted from attendance. The proportion of clients experiencing recent abscesses — a frequent consequence of employing unsterile injecting equipment — fell during the period of the study. Although our data on clients' sexual behaviour are difficult to interpret, level of condom use is generally high compared to other predominantly or exclusively heterosexual populations (Sonnex *et al.*, 1989). However, this is just one scheme. As Stimson *et al.*, (1988b) have demonstrated, other schemes have not enjoyed such success. Punitive attitudes to clients, unduly strict attention to syringe return rates, inconvenient locations and opening hours have all contributed to the closure of schemes or dwindling support from the clients. The success of individual schemes can easily be contrasted with the relative failure of others.

Conclusions

For the greater part of the nineteenth century, opium was openly on sale in pharmacies, grocery stores and even public houses. For the greater part of this century, many of those dependent on opiates had either been introduced to drugs by doctors — therapeutic addicts — or were themselves medically qualified and had self-administered morphine. From the early 1960s, however, the number and social range of heroin users increased, and by the mid-1980s the British government was engaged in aggressive anti-heroin campaigns, backed by heavy legal sanctions. However, one life-threatening disease has changed the entire thrust of drugs-related health education and service provision.

With the appearance of HIV infection among the drug injecting population, a practice which occurred in a number of DDUs for a relatively short time in the 1970s began again. This was the provision of sterile injecting equipment. At that time, needles and syringes were either supplied directly or prescribed, along with heroin or ampoules of injectable Methadone (Physeptone), on the assumption that this would avoid the health problems — septicaemia, endocarditis as well as abscesses — associated with using other people's equipment. Indeed, such a practice also prevented infection with or the transmission of blood borne viral infections such as hepatitis B, which has similar transmission characteristics to HIV. However, with the movement away from an exclusively bio-medical model of addiction, and a de-medicalization of treatment and service provision which emphasized the social and psychological origins and consequences of dependency, drug maintenance regimens and the provision of injecting equipment declined. Drug workers and psychiatrists, along with Lord Glenarthur, did not wish to convey contradictory messages. A commitment to a treatment programme must mean a commitment to not using drugs, particularly by injection.

Such a view remains a tenet of much abstinence-oriented provision in the dependency services, statutory and non-statutory. Many people working in drug agencies are highly ambivalent about needle and syringe exchange, and psychiatrists in particular have yet to be convinced of the wisdom of increased availability (Ghodse *et al.*, 1987). As a result, few DDUs are involved directly in needle exchange; when they are so involved, it often takes place on premises separate from the dependency clinic or is undertaken on an outreach basis.

The policy impetus for needle exchange came from physicians, particularly those with an interest in communicable disease (SHHD, 1986). Often, however, non-medical drug workers have taken the lead or participated in setting up and later staffing needle exchanges. It is interesting to note that the de-medicalization of drug services, which began in the 1970s, may have come to a temporary halt. However interested in or concerned about the social and psychological aspects of dependency they may be, needle exchange workers are involved in a public health exercise which once again focuses attention on the physical realities of injecting drug use and indeed sexual behaviour. This can be interpreted either as medicalization with a return to a disease model of drug use — involving a virological rather than a psychiatric pathological agent on this occasion — or as a recognition that injecting drug users have pressing health needs in addition to, and as important *as*, their social and psychological requirements. It is too early as yet to determine the extent, costs or benefits of medicalization, the outcome being dependent in no small part on continued funding and support.

Finally, the present government, the most sympathetic observer of which might consider antipathetic to the best interests of drug injectors, has found itself in a remarkable situation. Allocations for the financial year 1989/90 for drug services are expected to be in the region of £17 million, doubling the amount provided in 1987/88 (Druglink, 1989). New initiatives in health outreach work are to be funded; there is political pressure for drug users in prisons to be offered treatment facilities; billboard posters entreat drug injectors not to share equipment; and needle exchanges hand out injecting equipment and condoms with alacrity. There appears to be an uneasy truce between government and drug users. The dilemma worrying Lord Glenarthur and others in government has been resolved, at least temporarily. Health education emphasizing primary prevention can continue to be directed to young people who may be *considering* hard drug use, whilst those who are presently involved in the activity receive a different message. Thus those who may be tempted by, but have not yet begun, recreational drug use are warned that 'Heroin Screws You Up', while those who, in the Department of Health's words, 'cannot or will not' end their drug misuse are discouraged from sharing equipment. AIDS has forced many to reconsider and reformulate attitudes and professional practice; it is to be hoped that the lessons learned in relation to drug use and HIV will not be forgotton in future policy and practice formation.

Note

1   An earlier version of this paper was presented at the Conference of the British Sociological Association, Plymouth, 20–23 March, 1989.

References

BERRIDGE, V. and EDWARDS, G. (1987) *Opium and the People: Opiate Use in 19th Century England.* London, Yale.
BRETTLE, R. P., DAVIDSON, J., DAVIDSON, S. J., *et al.* (1986) 'HTLV-III Antibodies in an Edinburgh Clinic'. *Lancet* 1, p. 1099.

DRUGLINK (1989) '£17m for Drug Services in 1989/90, *Druglink*, March/April'. London Institute for the Study of Drug Dependence.

GHODSE, A. H. (1983) 'Treatment of Drug Addiction in London'. *Lancet*, 1, pp. 636–639.

GHODSE, A. H., TREGENZA, G. and LI, M. (1987) 'Effects of AIDS Sharing of Injecting Equipment among Drug Abusers', *British Medical Journal*, 292, pp. 698–99.

HART, G. J., CARVELL, A. L. M., WOODWARD, N., JOHNSON, A. M. WILLIAMS, P. and PARRY, J. V. (1989) 'Evaluation of Needle Exchange in Central London: Behaviour Change and Anti-HIV Status Over One Year', *AIDS*, 3, pp. 261–65.

HARTNOLL, R., MITCHESON, M., LEWIS, R., and BRYER, S. (1985) 'Estimating the Prevalence of Opioid Dependence', *Lancet*, 1, pp. 203–5.

HIS MAJESTY'S STATIONERY OFFICE (HMSO) (1926) *Report of the Departmental Committee on Drug Dependence (Rolleston Committee)*. London, HMSO.

HER MAJESTY'S STATIONERY OFFICE (HMSO) (1961) *Interdepartmental Committee on Drug Addiction: Report*. London, HMSO.

HER MAJESTY'S STATIONERY OFFICE (HMSO) (1965) *Interdepartmental Committee on Drug Addiction: Second Report*. London, HMSO.

MACGREGOR, S. (ed.) (1989) *Drugs and Society*. London, Tavistock.

MOSS, A. R. (1987) 'AIDS and Intravenous Drug Use: The Real Heterosexual Epidemic'. *British Medical Journal.*, 294, pp. 389–90.

PARKER, H., NEWCOMBE, R. and BAKX, K. (1987) 'The New Heroin Users: Prevalence and Characteristics in Wirral, Merseyside'. *British Journal of Addiction.*, 81, pp. 147–57.

POWER, R., HARTNOLL, R. and DAVIAUD, E. (1988) 'Drug Injecting, AIDS and Risk Behaviour: Potential for Change and Intervention Strategies', *British Journal of Addiction,* 83, pp. 649–54.

ROBERTSON, J. R., BUCKNALL, A. B. V., WELSBY, P. D., et al. (1986). 'Epidemic of AIDS-Related Virus (HTLV-III/LAV) Infection among Intravenous Drug Abusers', *British Medical Journal*, 292, pp. 527–30.

ROSENBERG, C. E. (1986) 'Disease and Social Order in America: Perceptions and Expectations', *The Milbank Quarterly*, 64, pp. 34–55.

SCOTTISH HOME AND HEALTH DEPARTMENT (SHHD) (1986) *HIV in Scotland: Report of the Scottish Committee on HIV Infection and Intravenous Drug Misuse*. Edinburgh, SHHD.

SCOTTISH INFORMATION OFFICE (SIO) (1986) News Release, 24 September 1986: 'Publication of Scottish Committee Report on AIDS and Drug Misuse'.

SONNEX, C., HART, G. J., WILLIAMS, P. and ADLER, M. W. (1989) 'Condom Use by Heterosexuals Attending a Department of Genitourinary Medicine: Attitudes and Behaviour in the Light of HIV Infection', *Genitourinary Medicine*, **65**, pp. 248–251.

STIMSON, G. V., and OPPENHEIMER, E. (1982) *Heroin Addiction: Treatment and Control in Britain*. London, Tavistock.

STIMSON, G. V., ALLDRITT, L., DOLAN, K. and DONOGHOE, M. (1988a) 'Syringe Exchange Schemes for Drug Users in England and Scotland' *British Medical Journal*, 196, pp. 1717–19.

STIMSON, G. V., ALLDRITT, L., DOLAN, K., DONOGHOE, M. and LART, R. A. (1988b) *Injecting Equipment Exchange Schemes: Final Report*. London, Goldsmiths College.

STIMSON, G. V., ALLDRITT, L., DOLAN, K. and DONOGHOE, M. (1989) 'Syringe Exchange Schemes in England and Scotland: Evaluating a New Service for Drug Users', in P. AGGLETON, G. HART and P. DAVIES (eds), *AIDS: Social Representations, Social Practices*. Lewes, Falmer Press.

Chapter 10

Drug Injectors' Risks for HIV

Neil McKeganey and Marina Barnard

It is now widely recognized that the shared use of non-sterile injecting equipment by injecting drug users represents a major route of transmission for the spread of the Human Immunodeficiency Virus (HIV). As a result, a good deal of attention has recently focused upon encouraging injecting drug users to adopt strategies aimed at reducing their risks of becoming infected. While it is possible to provide drug injectors who are in contact with services of one kind or another with advice on the various ways in which they might reduce their risk, a major problem remains in providing similar advice to those drug injectors who are not in contact with services, and who undoubtedly comprise the majority of the drug injecting population. The importance for both practitioners and researchers of establishing contacts with a wide range of drug injectors has been further underlined by recent research which has identified higher levels of risk behaviour among those individuals who are not in contact with treatment agencies than among those who are (Coleman and Curtis, 1988; Power, Hartnoll and Daviaud, 1988; Stimson *et al.*, 1988).

This chapter presents data based on semi-structured interviews with 102 injecting drug users purchasing injecting equipment at a retail pharmacy in Glasgow, the majority of whom were not in contact with treatment agencies at the time of being interviewed. Our concerns centre on the age, sex, distribution and length of time injecting of individuals purchasing injecting equipment, the nature and extent of any equipment sharing between drug injectors and the extent of any sexual contact between drug injectors and others. Before looking at each of these areas, however, it is worth describing more fully the nature of our research and the methods of data collection employed.

Method

At present we are involved in a three-year Economic and Social Research Council funded ethnographic study looking in detail at drug injectors' lifestyles and risks for

HIV. The study is based in an area of Glasgow within which HIV has already been identified among the injecting drug using population and where injecting drug use itself is widespread. Our study area is characterized by high levels of unemployment and other classic indices of multiple inner-city social deprivation (McKeganey and Barnard, 1988).

Data are being collected through interviews at a number of key access points: drug rehabilitation units, needle exchange schemes, HIV clinics, counselling clinics and residential detoxification units. In addition, we are conducting observational work within those areas where drugs are bought and sold in order to collect first-hand data on topics such as the extent of needle and syringe sharing. As part of this study we have recently completed 102 interviews within the local retail pharmacy, well known in our area as a setting where sterile injecting equipment can be purchased at minimum cost. Some indication of the size of the local drug injecting population can be gauged from the fact that over the last year the pharmacy has been regularly selling between 3000 and 4000 sets of needles and syringes per month. The population within our study area at the 1981 census was estimated as 14,807. Although it is clear that not all of the injecting equipment was being sold to residents of our study area, nevertheless, our data would suggest that the majority of those individuals purchasing equipment were resident in the area surrounding the pharmacy.

The collection of data in a non-clinic-based setting inevitably imposes certain limits upon the kinds of data collected. Our main concern within the pharmacy was to minimize the potentially disruptive effect the research could have on the day-to-day running of the shop. From discussions with the pharmacist, it was decided that we should conduct short and seemingly informal 'chats' in a quiet corner of the shop with those drug injectors who agreed to participate in the study. Once the client had left the shop, the elicited information was then transferred onto a short standardized questionnaire.

Briefly, our questions covered the age, sex and length of time injecting of the respondents, their injecting practices and risks for HIV from shared use of unsterile injecting equipment, their cleaning of injecting equipment, the extent of their sexual contact with others, whether that involved other drug injectors or non-drug injectors, and whether condoms were used.

The brevity and informality of our interviews within the pharmacy were a tailored response to the exigencies of the research setting and the drug users themselves. The pharmacist, for example, has been careful to establish good relations with the injecting drug users such that they perceive the shop as 'a safe territory'. Transactions are quick, informal and made without judgment. Many of the drug injectors spoken to commented favourably on this aspect of the pharmacist's style of working. It seemed important in this study to avoid compromising the established good relations between the staff and the drug using clients in any way which might result in discouraging individuals from attending the shop. Further, it was noted that many of the individuals attending the pharmacy only purchased injecting equipment once they had already purchased drugs to be injected. It is known that the possession of drugs can itself precipitate withdrawal symptoms (Wikler, 1973) and, in the light of this, it seemed unlikely that very many individuals would agree to postpone their drug use to participate in a lengthy research interview.

In seeking to structure our data collection in this way, we have been limited in key respects. Because we have employed an informal, conversational format in our interviews, it has not always been possible to ask all of our questions of all of our sample. Where it was felt that to push for exhaustive coverage of each topic area would be to compromise the goodwill of the interviewee, the former was sacrificed in favour of the latter. It would, therefore, seem more appropriate to describe the data presented here as comprising a quantitative analysis of qualitatively elicited material rather than as a statistical analysis of a standardized data set.

Age and Sex

The average age and sex of men and women injecting drugs in our sample were calculated separately. For women, the average was 22.9 years; for men, it was 24.6 years (see Table 1). Although Table 1 shows a total of thirty-two drug injectors falling within the 16–20 age range, the majority of these were clustered at the upper end of the scale. Most respondents reported having started injecting drug use when they were 16 or 17 years of age. When one considers Table 2, which shows the length of time injecting reported by individuals, it is clear that there is an underrepresentation of younger drug users with a short history of injecting.

Table 1. Age and Sex of Sample

	16–20	21–25	Age 26–30	31–35	35 +	Total
Men	24	23	20	8	3	78
Women	8	11	3	2	–	24

Average age of women = 22.9 years
Average age of men = 24.6 years
Male-to-female ratio = 3.25:1

Table 2. Length of Time Injecting

	<2 years	2–4 years	Time 4–6 years	6–8 years	8 + years	Total
Men	10	19	15	8	19	72
Women	8	8	2	3	–	21

Average length of time injecting for men = 6.19 years
Average length of time injecting for women = 3.24 years

The reasons for this underrepresentation of younger and more recently initiated drug users are likely to be complex. One possible explanation might be that younger drug injectors are reluctant to signal their drug use by purchasing equipment. In addition, it is known that individuals tend to be initiated into drug injecting and drug use generally in social situations within which drugs are offered by family members or close friends (Pearson, 1987). Within such circumstances, it is likely that the social nature of initiation will extend also to the sharing of injecting equipment. Indeed, it seems very probable that it will be only after a period of use, of uncertain duration, that an individual will make the shift from using other people's injecting equipment to purchasing their own equipment, thereby revealing the importance of drug injecting in their own eyes and in the eyes of others. It seems highly likely that younger, more recently initiated drug injectors may be at increased risk of using injecting equipment that has previously been used by others and thus at increased risk of HIV infection.

The male-to-female ratio of drug injectors in our sample is 3.25:1. However, in addition to our interviews we asked the staff of the chemist to record the age and sex of all people purchasing injecting equipment over an eighteen consecutive day period. Analysis of these records shows that here the sex ratio was 2.2:1. This indicates that our interview sample is somewhat weighted in favour of men. Two main factors may account for this: first, there is some evidence that more men than women were asked if they would be interviewed; and, second, more women than men declined to be interviewed.

The fact that men outweigh women in both our interviewed sample and in the record of all purchases is likely to have a number of causes. It may, for example, indicate that there are more men than women injecting drugs, and certainly a sex ratio of 2:1 is not unusual in relation to other studies. However, this sex ratio may also indicate a division of labour within heterosexual drug injecting couples such that the purchasing of injecting equipment is regarded as the man's rather than the woman's responsibility. From interviews conducted elsewhere in our research, there appears to be some evidence of such division of labour occurring:

> ...I share all the time with my girlfriend, but I don't share with anyone else and she doesn't share with anyone else. See, I have to hit for her — aye, I buy them, she won't even go into the chemist. See, she doesn't even think she's a junkie, she is though.... (21-year-old male drug injector interiewed in Needle Exchange, 3 February 1989)

We have also identified a reluctance among some women to be seen purchasing equipment:

> ...It's funny you should ask that [about purchasing injecting equipment]. Up until eight months ago I used to stand by the railings, you know, near the chemist and wait until someone I knew came down...street. Sometimes I'd be standing there half an hour or so but I wouldn't go in

there . . . then finally one day I came out of the Post Office and I just flew across the road. I don't know, I must have been strung out but I went in. I had a bright red face the first time but I just said 'A set of blue and orange 2 ml syringes'. It was alright after that . . . . Even now, I'd never go in there when it was full, no way, the only way I'd go in is when it's empty . . . . (24-year-old female drug injector interviewed in Residential Drug Detoxification Unit, 10 December 1988)

The obvious sense of embarrassment which this drug injector experienced on purchasing injecting equipment seemed to be felt even more poignantly by young women with children, for whom the purchasing of equipment could be read both by themselves and by others as tantamount to their failure not only as a woman but also as a parent.

Rosenbaum (1981) has sensitively analyzed the particular disapprobation society reserves for women with children who inject, and it seems highly likely that this will have an impact upon individuals' preparedness to purchase sterile injecting equipment. The practical result of such negative social imagery may be a greater propensity to share other people's injecting equipment on the part of some women, placing them at particular risk of HIV.

The Shared Use of Injecting Equipment

There is some evidence that the sharing of unsterile injecting equipment carries a greater risk of HIV transmission among injecting drug users than does sexual contact (Des Jarlais *et al.*, 1987). Reported findings from different populations of injecting drug users suggest a strong correlation between the frequency of shared use of injecting equipment and HIV infection (Des Jarlais *et al.*, 1987). In Edinburgh, for example, it is reported by Robertson and his colleagues that gatherings of between ten and twenty injecting drug users were not uncommon during 1983. This may partially explain the high incidence of the HIV infection among Edinburgh drug users at this time (Robertson *et al.*, 1986). However, there is some difficulty in assessing the relative risks of transmission through shared use of equipment as against the risks of sexual transmission, not least because some of the people injecting drugs are also in sexual contact with each other. The available data suggest that heterosexual transmission, although an additional risk factor for injecting drug users, is not so significant for transmission of the virus as the sharing of non-sterile injecting equipment. Recent reports by Cowan and colleagues estimate that, in Scotland at least, heterosexual transmissions may be three to five times less likely than from shared use of unsterile needles and syringes. However, as they note, this figure is by no means negligible (Cowan, Flegg and Brettle, 1989).

There has been a good deal of discussion on the role of sharing of injecting equipment in the spread of HIV infection. However, the term 'sharing' collapses two activities, lending and borrowing, which differ markedly in terms of the level of personal risk and in their risk of further transmission of HIV (McKeganey, Bloor and Watson, 1988; McKeganey, Barnard and Watson, forthcoming). Lending occurs when an individual is asked to make available his or her injecting equipment to another person. As such, it is a practice which carries with it little or no personal risk to the lender so long as he or she sterilizes it prior to re-use or refuses to accept its return. Many of the individuals interviewed in our study reported that they would not accept the return of equipment which had been lent to another individual. Lending is a practice which carries with it little or no risk to the lender, but is of high risk to others if the lender is HIV seropositive; this behaviour could spread infection to all those to whom equipment is lent. 'Borrowing', by contrast, is an activity which involves high personal risk for the individual concerned but is of relatively low risk epidemiologically as it is only the borrower who becomes infected. We have examined the differential practices of lending and borrowing in Table 3. The data here show an ongoing preparedness to lend injecting equipment when requested to do so. From these data, it is clear that such requests are not infrequent.

Table 3. Lending and Borrowing Behaviour

	Men N = 74	Women N = 23	Total N = 97
	(Percentages shown in brackets)		
Report being asked to lend needles and syringes	43 (58.0)	15 (65.0)	58 (59.0)
Report having recently borrowed or being prepared to borrow others' used injecting equipment	20 (27.0)	4 (17.3)	24 (24.7)
Report having recently lent or being prepared to lend injecting equipment	40 (54.0)	15 (65.2)	55 (56.7)
Report not being prepared to borrow or lend	23 (31.0)	5 (21.7)	28 (28.8)

Among this sample of injecting drug users we noted a marked discrepancy between an individual's willingness to lend injecting equipment on the one hand and preparedness to borrow on the other. Less than a third stated that they would borrow another's injecting equipment, but over half said they would lend needles and syringes if so requested. Only a minority reported an unwillingness to lend or borrow injecting equipment. Nevertheless, quite a few individuals drew a distinction between regular and emergency sharing, commenting that if they had drugs to inject but no needle and syringe of their own, they would make use of others' equipment. This is illustrated by the comments of a 34-year-old male drug injector: ' . . . when you're choking for a hit and you've not got any works, you'll use anyone's . . . . If there's a nail with a hole in it you'll use it . . . . Everyone shares then, even though they say they don't . . . .'

There appears to be a multiplicity of reasons why needle sharing continues, despite an awareness of the risks involved and a high level of provision of sterile injecting equipment. These reported reasons have been detailed elsewhere by McKeganey (1989), but it seems worthwhile to outline them briefly here. First, it may take place in situations where there is a general lack of availability of clean equipment, for instance late in the evening or on a Sunday when the pharmacy is closed. Second, it may occur in situations of specific unavailability, where clean injecting equipment is not available in the immediate situation in which drugs are being used. Third, sharing may take place in situations where an individual may be anxious or embarrassed at being seen acquiring sterile injecting equipment. Fourth, it may occur in situations where the sharing of injecting equipment signals friendship or family ties. Fifth, it can be found in situations where individuals are unconcerned as to the risks they are taking by sharing needles and syringes. Sixth, it may occur in situations where a drug injector may feel an obligation to another drug injector who requests the use of her/his equipment. Finally, it may take place in situations where the drug injector is already HIV antibody positive and sees no further risk accruing to her or himself from using non-sterile equipment.

There can be little question that the provision of clean injecting equipment is an essential component of any risk reduction strategy enabling drug injectors to make the behaviour change required to avoid HIV infection. It seems unlikely, however, that provision of sterile injecting equipment will, in itself, be sufficient for drug injectors to minimize their risks of HIV infection arising from the shared use of injecting equipment. What seems necessary is a cultural and behavioural change within drug using subcultures, whereby it becomes socially unacceptable for individuals to request the use of each other's injecting equipment. This point has been made by Des Jarlais and colleagues (1986) in the context of the New York drug using subculture, and also by Stimson and colleagues in their evaluation report on the risk behaviours of clients attending needle exchanges in Britain (Stimson *et al.*, 1988).

Sexual Transmission

Among a wide variety of policy-makers, practitioners and researchers, there is a growing concern that the main transmission route for HIV infection to pass into the heterosexually active, non-drug using population may be as a result of sexual contact with drug injectors (Des Jarlais *et al.*, 1987; Chaisson *et al.*, 1987). Moss has described the spread of HIV infection among drug users as constituting 'the real heterosexual epidemic' (Moss, 1987). In New York City, it would seem that injecting drug users are the transmission source for the majority of cases in which heterosexual activity is the apparent mode of transmission and also in the majority of cases of maternally transmitted infection (Des Jarlais and Friedman, 1987).

Recent reports on the situation among injecting drug users in Edinburgh support the view that it is the sexual partners of current or former drug users infected with HIV who are most at risk of contracting the virus (Robertson and Skidmore, 1989). Even in areas of a low prevalence of HIV, as is the case in Glasgow, there is a good deal of concern as to the potential for future epidemic sexual transmission where sexually active adults are in contact with individuals who are, knowingly or unknowingly, seropositive for antibodies to HIV. Data on risk factors for male to female transmission of HIV indicate that a seropositive person may be differentially infectious during the natural course of the illness, and that it is the 'clinical state of the carrier' which is the prime risk factor rather than the longevity of the relationship and the frequency of sexual contacts (European Study Group, 1989).

In the light of such concern, there appears a clear case for investigating the extent of drug injectors' sexual activity and for identifying the degree to which this activity involves other drug injecting or non-drug injecting individuals (see also the chapter by Hilary Klee elsewhere in this volume, Chapter 11).

The data collected on sexual behaviour of drug injectors presented in Table 4 relate to only a proportion of our sample. However, the table is revealing since it shows that many of our drug injectors were in ongoing active sexual relationships with non-drug using partners. Indeed, many of the men interviewed firmly stated a disinclination to become involved with women who inject drugs. This was sometimes explained in terms of an economic rationale, it being more difficult to cater for two drug habits than for one. It was more often accounted for in terms of a moral

Table 4. Sexual Transmission

	Men	Women	Total
		(percentages shown in brackets)	
Partner drug injector	5 (11)	3 (50)	8 (16)
			(N = 51)
Partner non-injector	40 (89)	3 (50)	43 (84)
			(N = 89)
Having sex: Yes	63 (87.5)	10 (59)	73 (82)
No	9 (12.5)	7 (41)	16 (18)
			(N = 85)
Condoms used	10 (14)	8 (50)	18 (21)
Not using condoms /not prepared to use condoms	59 (86)	8 (50)	67 (79)

disapproval of female drug use: ' . . . I don't know why but I don't like to see a girl using, you know, putting a needle in her arm. I don't think a girl should do that. I suppose a man shouldn't either but somehow it's worse in a girl . . . ' (20-year-old male at Needle Exchange).

The potential for spread of the virus into the non-drug using population would, therefore, seem to be considerable, particularly when one also considers that the majority of drug injectors in this sample were unaware of their actual HIV status and were not using any form of barrier contraception.

The majority of drug injectors we interviewed were aware of the risks of HIV associated with the use of unsterile injecting equipment. Their understanding of the dynamics of sexual transmission seemed, however, to be much less clear. In responding to the questions regarding sexual transmission, many of the drug injectors stated that they were not concerned as to this possibility, and explained this lack of concern in terms of the fact that their partner 'does 'nae sleep around'. It would seem, therefore, that many of our interviewed sample interpreted the questions relating to sexual transmission as having to do with their risk of *contracting* the virus from their partner rather than the risk that they might themselves be the agents for *transmitting* the virus to their partner. It was also clear that the majority of drug injectors in our sample interpreted sexual risk as having to do with the issue of frequent partner change.

There has been a good deal of promotion for condom use as a means of preventing HIV infection. However, for some individuals in our sample, the introduction of condom use into long-term, often marital relationships was interpersonally problematic for them. Greater success in promoting the widespread use of condoms might be possible if they were more clearly dissociated from 'promiscuity'. However, prior to any wider promotion of condom use, an awareness of the risks of sexual transmission needs to be developed. It is this, in particular, which appears to be lacking at present.

Policy Implications

In view of the research findings presented here, it seems appropriate to end this chapter by considering some of the policy implications of our work. From our interviews, it is clear that despite the proximate availability of sterile injecting equipment and evidence of concern regarding risks for HIV, the sharing of previously used needles and syringes continues to occur. We have identified younger, more recently initiated drug users and also women as being those least likely to make use of the facilities offered by the pharmacy. The reasons for continued sharing appear to be as much social in character as pragmatic. Thus, although one approach might be to provide a twenty-four-hour supply of needles and syringes, it seems likely that some sharing will inevitably continue, particularly while it remains socially acceptable to do so.

The provision of sterile injecting equipment is an important part of any strategy which aims to reduce the risk of HIV transmission among injecting drug users. Of equal importance, however, is encouraging the kind of cultural change among drug injectors which would render it unacceptable either to lend or to borrow another's injecting equipment. It is worth noting that some of the drug injectors participating in this study were already beginning to devise ad hoc interactional strategies for coping with requests to make their injecting equipment available to others. Some individuals, for example, regularly carried a spare needle and syringe which they would not use themselves but which they would provide to others on request. Other individuals stated that they responded to such requests by concealing the fact that they might have a needle and syringe on their person. Although not all such strategies may be equally successful at reducing transmission of HIV, nevertheless they indicate an attempt on some drug injectors' part to reduce their personal risk within a particular social milieu. There may be some value in drug injectors receiving social skills training aimed at developing such strategies further and enabling them to decline requests to make injecting equipment available to others without at the same time compromising their standing in the eyes of other drug injectors.

Any such changes in the drug using subculture are unlikely to take place overnight. It would, therefore, seem prudent to place equal emphasis on the sterilization of injecting equipment in situations where it is to be re-used by others. This measure has been implemented with some success in many American cities where the sale of needles and syringes is prohibited by law (Watters, 1987).

Many of the drug users spoken to had little sense of their risks of HIV transmission through sexual activity. This signals a need to promote much greater awareness of the risks of sexual transmission rather than just through shared use of injecting equipment. There is also a need in any future health education and media campaigns to focus attention upon the sexual partners of injecting drug users and to encourage an awareness of the risks of HIV, as well as the various ways in which these may be reduced (Bradbeer, 1989). The evidence from Edinburgh suggests that unprotected heterosexual sex as a risk factor is now more common than exposure to needle sharing (Robertson and Skidmore, 1989). Thus it is important to encourage a sense of responsibility among drug injectors not only as far as their own health is concerned but also for that of their sexual partners.

References

BRADBEER, C. (1989) 'Women and HIV', *British Medical Journal*, 298, p. 342.
CHAISSON, R. E., MOSS, A. R., ONISHI, R. OSMOND, D., *et al.*, (1987) 'Human Immunodeficiency Virus Infection in Heterosexual Intravenous Drug Users in San Francisco', *American Journal of Public Health*, 77, 2, pp. 169–72.
COLEMAN, R. M. and CURTIS, D. (1988) 'Distribution of Risk Behaviour for HIV Infection amongst Intravenous Drug Users', *British Journal of Addiction*, 83, pp. 1331–4.

COWAN, F. M., FLEGG, P. J. and BRETTLE, R. P. (1989) 'Heterosexually Acquired HIV Infection', *British Medical Journal*, 298, p. 891.

DES JARLAIS, D. C. and FRIEDMAN, S. R. (1987) 'HIV Infection among Intravenous Drug Users: Epidemiology and Risk Reduction', *AIDS*, 1, pp. 67–76.

DES JARLAIS, D. C., FRIEDMAN, S. R. and STRUG, D. (1986) 'AIDS and Needle Sharing within the IV Drug Use Subculture', in D. A. FELDMAN and T. M. JOHNSON (eds), *Social Dimensions of AIDS: Method and Theory*, New York, Praeger.

DES JARLAIS, D. C. WISH, E., FRIEDMAN, S. R. STONEBURNER, R., *et al.* (1987) 'Intravenous Drug Use and the Heterosexual Transmission of the Human Immunodeficiency Virus: Current Trends in New York City', *New York State Journal of Medicine*, May, pp. 283–6.

EUROPEAN STUDY GROUP (1989) 'Risk Factors for Male to Female Transmission of HIV', *British Medical Journal*, 298, pp. 411–14.

MCKEGANEY, N. P. (1989) 'Drug Abuse in the Community: Needle Sharing and the Risks of HIV Infection', in S. CUNNINGHAM-BURLEY and N. P. MCKEGANEY (eds), *Readings in Medical Sociology*, London, Routledge.

MCKEGANEY, N. P. and BARNARD, M. A. (1988) 'A Statistical Comparison of the Study Area and Other Neighbouring Areas', *Glasgow, Social Paediatric and Obstetric Research Unit Report*, Glasgow.

MCKEGANEY, N. P., BARNARD, M. A. and WATSON, H. (forthcoming) 'HIV Related Risk Behaviour among a Non-Clinic Sample of Injecting Drug Users', *British Journal of Addiction*.

MCKEGANEY, N. P., BLOOR, M. J. and WATSON, H. (1988) 'Risks of Sharing Injecting Equipment', *British Medical Journal*, 297, p. 1472.

MOSS, A. R. (1987) 'AIDS and Intravenous Drug Use: The Real Heterosexual Epidemic', *British Medical Journal*, 294, pp. 389–90.

PEARSON, G. (1987) *The New Heroin Users*. London, Basil Blackwell.

POWER, R., HARTNOLL, R. and DAVIAUD, E. (1988) 'Drug Injecting, AIDS and Risk Behaviour: Potential for Change and Intervention Strategies', *British Journal of Addiction*, 83, pp. 649–54.

ROBERTSON, J. R. and SKIDMORE, C. (1989) 'Heterosexually Acquired HIV Infection', *British Medical Journal*, 298, p. 891.

ROBERTSON, J. R., BUCKNALL, A. B. V., WELSBY, P. D., ROBERTS, J. J. K., *et al.* (1986) 'Epidemic of AIDS Related Virus (HTLV-III/LAV) Infection Among Intravenous Drug Abusers', *British Medical Journal*, 292, pp. 527–9.

ROSENBAUM, M. (1981) *Women on Heroin*. New Brunswick, N.J., Rutgers University Press.

STIMSON, G., ALLDRITT, L. J., DOLAN, K. A., DONOGHOE, M. C., and LART, R. A. (1988) *Injecting Equipment Exchange Schemes, Final Report*. London, University of London, Goldsmiths College.

WATTERS, J. K. (1987) 'A Street Based Outreach Model of AIDS Prevention for Intravenous Drug Users: Preliminary Evaluation', *Contemporary Drug Problems*, Fall, pp. 411–42.

WIKLER, A. (1973) 'Dynamics of Drug Dependence: Implications of a Conditioning Theory for Research and Treatment', *Archives of General Psychiatry*, 28, pp. 611–16.

Chapter 11

Some Observations on the Sexual Behaviour of Injecting Drug Users: Implications for the Spread of HIV Infection

Hilary Klee

The sharing of contaminated injecting equipment by some injecting drug users has led to a marked increased in reported HIV seroconversions in Europe and the United States. The high prevalence of HIV infection among injecting drug users has implications for the welfare of a much wider population, and the potential risk to the non-drug using heterosexual population of further transmission through unprotected sexual activity has caused considerable disquiet. To what extent is such concern justified?

Very little is known about the sexual behaviours of drug users and the extent of their contact with non-drug users. The high level of concern shown by governments and health authorities is understandable; drug misuse is a problem that is escalating in many developed nations, and injecting as a method of administering drugs is increasingly employed. Those who inject do not always use sterile equipment. The repeated use of injecting equipment by different people without sterilization is a highly effective way of passing on any blood borne infection, and is a serious risk to health.

There are other reasons for concern. In the absence of new needles and syringes, equipment that has been used is not always adequately cleansed. Appropriate hygienic measures may be abandoned under certain conditions, for example, when in the throes of withdrawal. The temptation to accept others' equipment will be strong when a user is in possession of drugs but not of the means to inject. Some users will not carry needles and syringes with them when out buying their supplies (scoring) for fear of interception by the police. They may be 'caught short' if some delays have occurred. Others may find themselves in a social context that exerts pressure to share with others in the interests of solidarity. Passing on used equipment may be seen as a favour to others in need and regarded as involving no risk at all if the giver is seen as 'clean'. A common view among injecting drug users is that the recipient has to take responsibility for his or her own actions. On the other hand, refusing used equipment may be construed as an indication of mistrust. There is, in any case, a fatalistic attitude common among long-term users that risk-taking is part of the lifestyle. Furthermore, along with tobacco smokers and those persisting with high levels of alcohol use, many drug users tend to ignore exhortations to change their lives for the sake of their health. Is it to be expected that health education messages concerning AIDS will suddenly take effect? There may be more factors to add to the list that would contribute to the level of risk activity among drug users (Power, 1989). The concern of governments and health professionals seems well justified the needs to be met by appropriate research that establishes the nature and extent of current risk activity and the reasons for it.

The research described here attempts to answer some of these questions. It is incomplete, however, and the results available at this stage have been generated by preliminary interrogation of the data. Though more subtle influences that affect risk behaviour will undoubtedly emerge as a result of analyses of data at the end of the project, these data may be useful indicators of general patterns.

Location

The project is located in the north-west of England, an area with a particularly acute drug problem (Home Office Statistical Bulletin, 1989), and an area where the growing demand for drugs is apparently easily met by drug suppliers. The study covers the inner-city areas of Manchester and Liverpool, their suburbs, coastal towns on the western seaboard and inland towns such as Chester, Bolton, Preston and Bury. The region thus provides considerable heterogeneity in culture and wealth. It is an area well served in terms of statutory and non-statutory treatment agencies, many of them forward-looking and employing vigorous harm minimization strategies.

Aims

The overall aim of the study is to investigate those activities that may lead to the contracting and transmission of HIV infection among injecting drug users and their contacts. The variables operationalized in the first phase interview schedule have included not only details of current sexual and drug-related behaviour, but also any potential factors that may bear upon risk activity. They are inter alia: drug history and current drug use; funding of drug use and illegal activity; sexual, peer and family relationships; attitudes and behaviours associated with health and hygiene; personality characteristics connected to control and self-image; perceptions of personal vulnerability to AIDS infection; and AIDS beliefs and knowledge. The focus of this chapter is on the sexual activity of injecting drug users and their relationships with non-drug users.

Methods

The investigation is in two phases. The first phase is now complete and the data presented here have been selected from it. Just over 300 injecting drug users were interviewed between April and December 1988 by trained interviewers. The interviews were semi-structured in nature and lasted on average an hour and a quarter. They were all recorded on tape with the respondents' permission. The second phase involves the completion of a questionnaire, administered by research assistants, between six and nine months after the first contact, and focuses on key issues such as changes in drug use, sharing and sexual contacts.

Our 303 respondents were recruited in a variety of ways. These included out-patient treatment facilities (37 per cent), outreach activity in which 'snowballing' techniques were used to reach users not in contact with agencies (32 per cent), in-patient treatment facilities (20 per cent), the probation service (6 per cent) and, finally, a small number through non-statutory agencies (5 per cent). Approximately half are under 25 years of age, and seventy-eight of the 303 (26 per cent) respondents are women. The main drug of preference is heroin (75 per cent), with 13 per cent injecting amphetamine sulphate, 9 per cent Methadone and 3 per cent crushing and injecting prescribed drugs or injecting a variety of different drugs.

The Effects of Drug Use on Sexual Activity

Respondents were asked about the effects of their drug use on their sexual activity. Regular administration of heroin is reputed to have a deleterious effect (Mirin *et al.*, 1980), whereas amphetamine sulphate has the reputation as an enhancer of both social and sexual interactions (Holbrook, 1983). The consequence most frequently mentioned by heroin users was of decreased interest (62 per cent). In contrast, this was reported by only 15 per cent of amphetamine users, who tended to report either no effects (33 per cent) or greater interest (31 per cent). Better performance was claimed by 9 per cent of heroin users, and this matched the numbers reporting worse performance. This paradox is explained by different interpretations of what is 'better' in performance terms. Delays in ejaculation are seen by some as a positive benefit, by others as extremely tiresome. Of some interest are the comments from users being maintained regularly on Methadone, a heroin substitute prescribed in many treatment agencies. Of this group, 48 per cent reported less interest, 15 per cent reported better performance and 13 per cent no effects. The differences between Methadone and heroin are well described by one male user (age 23): 'If I'm on heroin, it kills all my senses. On Methadone, if I can keep it fairly lowish, I've got most of my senses . . . maybe I've not got so much sex drive as if I wasn't using any at all though.' Dosage-related impairment of sexual function by Methadone has already been noted in the literature (e.g. Crowley and Simpson, 1978). Whether these differences are due to pharmacological effects, to relatively restricted dosages of Methadone or the more settled lifestyle of maintained users is uncertain at this stage, but they have implications for the levels of sexual activity to be predicted in different groups of drug users.

Given that the majority of our sample professed less interest in sex, a question that naturally follows is whether this is borne out in behavioural terms. Within the week prior to the interview, 31 per cent had engaged in sexual intercourse. Extended to the month before interview, this rises to 54 per cent, to six months before interview to 81 per cent and to a year before interview to 88 per cent. These levels are similar to those found by the Monitoring Research Group in their national survey of injecting equipment exchange schemes (Stimson, 1988). The numbers of different sexual partners reported by our respondents for the six-month period prior to interview were also comparable to the national study: 18 per cent reported no contacts, 50 per cent one contact and 32 per cent two or more contacts.

Sexual Interactions with Regular Partners

About half of the respondents (51 per cent) have regular sexual partners, and, of these, 56 per cent are themselves drug users; the majority (71 per cent) also inject their drugs. Thus 23 per cent of the whole sample have an ongoing sexual relationship with non-drug users. We have anecdotal evidence from the first phase interviews that many male drug users prefer non-drug using partners. This is being followed up more specifically in the second phase and will be reported at a later stage.

An analysis of the level of sexual activity of opiate users (heroin/Methadone) with regular partners was performed. Too few amphetamine users had regular partners to permit a meaningful analysis of this group. Tables 1 and 2 identify significant differences in sexual activity according to the drug status of the partner. Those

Table 1. The Frequency of Sexual Intercourse in Opiate Users with Regular Drug Using or Non-Drug Using Sexual Partners

	Once per week or more	Once per month	Less than once per month	Total
Drug user	32	24	19	75
Non-drug user	38	10	11	59
Total	70	34	30	134

Chi-square = 6.60, df = 2, p < .05

respondents with non-drug using partners report more recent and more frequent sexual activity. These data have considerable implications for the potential spread of infection into the non-drug using population. Presumably decreased interest in one partner because of opiate consumption is an effect ameliorated by the expectations and needs of the other partner.

Table 2. The Recency of Sexual Intercourse in Opiate Users with Regular Drug Using or Non-Drug Using Sexual Partners

	Less than one week	Two to four weeks	More than one month	Total
Drug user	30	24	18	72
Non-drug user	31	7	12	50
Total	61	31	30	122

Chi-square = 6.80, df = 2, p < .05
(N.B. The disparity between Tables 1 and 2 in overall totals is due to missed data on the recency of sexual intercourse).

Casual Sexual Encounters

Pilot work established a definition of casual sex acceptable to respondents as transitory sexual interactions with little emotional involvement. A different pattern was discernible between opiate and stimulant users (see Table 3). Proportionately more opiate users than amphetamine users report having no casual sex in the six months prior to interview. Differences in the effects of drugs on sexual arousal may not be the only factor here. We have found critical differences in social relationships between the two groups in terms of their relative sociability. Amphetamines are a potent central nervous system (CNS) stimulant capable of decreasing fatigue and producing behavioural arousal. Mood is elevated, a feeling that contrasts sharply with the drifting feeling induced by opiates which 'increases emotional distance from external stimuli and internal responses' (Zinberg, Harding and Apsler, 1978). The more isolating effects of heroin, therefore, may inhibit social interactions that are the context for

Table 3. Opiate and Stimulant Drug Users' Reports of the Incidence of Casual Sexual Encounters in the Six Months Prior to Interview

	Casual sex		Total
	Yes	No	
Opiate users	98	158	256
Stimulant users	23	17	40
Total	121	175	296

Chi-square = 5.29, df = 1, p < .05

many potentially sexual contacts. An alternative hypothesis would be that the preference for opiates indicates a need to detach oneself from the world, so an inherent disposition to withdraw from society is enhanced by the use of the drug.

Predictably, more respondents with regular partners (39 per cent) reported never having casual sex than respondents without partners (20 per cent), though 5 per cent of the former also reported sexual relationships elsewhere.

It seems that despite reporting a decreased interest in sex, most of the sample are engaged in sexual activity, with either a regular partner or a casual contact. To allow further investigations, respondents reporting less interest in sex were extracted from the sample. Of these, 63 per cent reported never having casual sex, but 10 per cent reported having such contacts frequently and 27 per cent periodically. In terms of the frequency and regularity of sexual intercourse, 52 per cent had sex within the last month and 45 per cent were having sex once a fortnight or more frequently. There are undoubtedly many factors that contribute to a particular level of sexual activity and only one will be arousal potential. For example, in our sample, many males with regular partners who complained of the effects of their drug use upon their sex lives felt the need to 'make an effort' for the sake of their partners.

The Use of Condoms

The incidence of sexual activity between injecting drug users and their partners is of minor concern if safer sex practices are observed. An index of safer sex that is most easily monitored is the use of condoms. The AIDS epidemic has radically altered public attitudes to open discussion of previously taboo topics connected with sex. Widespread use of the contraceptive pill relegated barrier contraceptives to the stone age of sexual enlightenment. They are now back on the public agenda not as contraceptives but as prophylactics against a variety of sexually transmitted infections, of which HIV is seen as the most serious. As yet no major effort to promote their use has been mounted. They are discussed openly, however, are easily available and inexpensive. They are free to users of drug clinics.

A range of questions concerning the use of condoms was included in the first phase of the project. Most respondents (70 per cent) had tried them at some time in the past, and most (78 per cent) felt they were easy to obtain. Current use, however, was low and seems unlikely to rise. Of those whom we know were sexually active within the last year before interview (88 per cent), 75 per cent never used them currently, 13 per cent used them occasionally and 12 per cent used them every time. The majority of regular users were prostitutes. The reasons for such avoidance were revealed by questions about their acceptability. This differed for men and women (see Table 4). Men, in particular, were not well disposed towards them; 62.5 per cent of male respondents disliked them or disliked them intensely. Neutral attitudes were held by

37 per cent, and one man liked them. Of the eight women who also liked them, seven are prostitutes.

Table 4. *Positive-Negative Affective Responses to Condoms by Male and Female Respondents*

	Extreme dislike	Dislike	Neutral	Like
		(percentages shown in brackets)		
Males	31 (14)	108 (48.5)	82 (37)	1 (0.5)
Females	3 (4)	23 (31)	40 (54)	8 (11)
Total	34	131	122	9

More critical, perhaps, are responses from those respondents without regular partners who report having casual sexual contacts. This would be the group most likely to carry condoms if they knew and were concerned about the sexual transmission of infections. Seventy-two per cent of this group do not carry condoms. This is not because they do not feel at risk of HIV infection through unprotected sex. The majority (83 per cent) of them report that they feel at risk. However, there is a significant relationship between the perception of risk and carrying condoms; those who feel at high risk do tend to carry them.

The picture is not much brighter with respect to the prospective use of condoms. Respondents were asked whether they thought they would use them with a new partner in the future. Thirty-seven per cent said they would. However, when related to whether they carried them currently, it seems that some would be unprepared. The majority of men (61 per cent) do not carry them and would not use them, 27 per cent do not carry them but say they would use them, 11 per cent carry them and would use them and a mystifying 2 per cent apparently carry them but say they are not sure they will use them.

The unpopularity of condoms, despite the perception of risk and the perceived seriousness of the disease professed by almost all of our respondents, raises questions about the likelihood of a change in attitude. We have data that suggest there is some reduction in the incidence of needle and syringe sharing. Awareness of the risks associated with sharing seems to have behavioural outcomes. However, the risks associated with sexual transmission of the virus are, in contrast, barely considered. This is a feature of the thinking not only of drug users themselves, but also of those who are concerned for them. The present construction of harm minimization by many drug agencies understandably focuses upon the major risk and leaves condoms to collect dust on the shelves. Given the extent of interaction betwen injecting drug users and non-drug users, perhaps an equally vigorous approach to safer sex would be advisable.

The alternatives to the use of condoms in order of effective prevention of HIV infection are: celibacy; non-penetrative sex; delay of some months before sexual intercourse but after an antibody test; serious checking up on the prospective partner's history; and less detailed evaluations based on reputation.

We asked respondents how they would approach a prospective sexual contact now that AIDS is around. As with several other areas of questioning in the interviews, the topic was likely to elicit socially desirable rather than frank responses unless handled with care. A way that seemed to work with our sample was to set up scenarios in which doing the 'wrong' thing would be understandable. In this case, the desirability and willingness of the prospective partner were mentioned and an amenable environment that was conducive to sex. Ten per cent refused to make any kind of prediction on the grounds that their relationships with their long-term partners ensured they would not find themselves in a position; 11 per cent said they would be unconcerned, since the risk was minimal anyway; 21 per cent were not concerned because they used condoms; 18 per cent said they would be concerned, but would not feel able to handle any checking up; 16 per cent would attempt some check on past history; 10 per cent would defer penetrative sex until a deeper relationship was established; 6 per cent would be influenced by the person's reputation; and 4 per cent would be influenced by the person's appearance. The residue of respondents referred to a mixture of checking, reputation and appearance. Thus about a third would be seriously at risk with new contacts. Judgments about partners that are based on strategies of a fairly superficial nature are of dubious value but would be used by another quarter of the respondents.

Prostitutes

A small number of our respondents (nineteen) fund their drug use through prostitution. Seventeen are women and two are men. The drug of choice for all the women and one of the men is heroin, the other using amphetamine sulphate. All but one carry condoms regularly, the exception being a woman who reports that she is attempting to come off drugs and is no longer working the streets. Predictably, this group has attitudes towards condoms that are rather different from those of our other respondents. Both men and seven of the women feel quite neutral about them, three women dislike using them and seven like using them.

Ten women have regular partners and they distinguish between the use of condoms with clients and their use with partners. The majority only use them with clients. It was apparent from several interviews that condoms are as much was psychological barrier as a physical one, reducing contact and effectively distancing clients from the emotional mainstream of the women's lives. All of them are well aware of the risk of disease. As one woman put it, 'No, I like to use them . . . I don't like having something inside me that I don't know where it's been.'

Offers of additional money to have sex without condoms were common, though few said they accepted them. However, there may have been underreporting here despite our efforts to reduce the social unacceptability of an affirmative response. A more detailed study of drug using prostitutes could reveal more fully the circumstances under, and extent to which, they are persuaded to accept unprotected sex. The need to obtain money to buy drugs can reach desperate levels, and those who reported accepting offers said they did so in a state of withdrawal. More money means less delay before acquiring sufficient funds to stop work and buy drugs. Thirteen of the women said that they had worked the streets when withdrawing. Normally, however, they all worked when under the influence of a recent 'fix', either soon after administration and therefore 'high', or having achieved a stable state and therefore 'straight'.

The financial rewards were often considerable, as they would need to be with a daily habit of heroin use. Eleven of the women spent many hundreds of pounds a week on their supply of heroin. This is typical of the whole sample of heroin users. The male prostitutes needed less money. They are weekly users and therefore buy less, and an amphetamine user benefits because the drug is cheap. Six of the sample estimated that they had money to spare from their activities that more than covered their purchase of drugs; the rest said they made enough. If caught by the police, they were unlikely to receive a prison sentence, unlike other more prevalent ways of funding a drug habit such as shoplifting. Thus, despite the very real dangers from attack, there are sufficient advantages to prostitution that will ensure that some drug users will be willing to take it up.

The sexual behaviour of prostitutes in the context of the AIDS epidemic is likely to be informed by their knowledge and concern about the disease. A high proportion of this group was deemed to have an excellent level of knowledge concerning transmission of the virus, a level higher than the total sample. Thirteen were rated excellent, six were rated good. Most thought that AIDS was a more serious threat than other health problems. Their concern was shown by the high number who had been tested for the virus. Both men and fourteen women had been tested; one person had been found to be antibody-positive. A further three women were considering having the test. The reasons for deciding to be tested were divided equally between past sharing activities and past sexual interactions. In comparison, 50 per cent of the total sample had been tested, the majority because of sharing. Perhaps because they felt they had been cleared by the test, nine prostitutes felt they posed no risk at all to others, three felt they might and five were not sure.

Theoretical Considerations

Serious consideration of implications for theory will not be attempted before the completion of the project. However, some aspects of the data can be placed fairly easily into the framework of certain theories that are applied to health issues and may point up some areas worthy of further exploration. One potentially useful approach is that of Rogers (1975, 1983). In his Protection Motivation Theory of fear appeals and attitude change, health messages give rise to certain types of cognitive responses in the audience. In determining the level of motivation associated with self-protective behaviour, three are critical: an appraisal of the severity of the disease in question; the expectancy of exposure to it; and a belief in the efficacy of the recommended coping responses. These are similar to key concepts in the Health Belief Model (Becker, 1974), for example, the perceived susceptibility to the disease and its seriousness, and the benefits of preventive action. In Rogers' theory, the recommended behaviour will not occur if values on any of the three variables are zero. In one test of the model, Rogers and Mewborn (1976) found that the efficacy of the coping response was more critical in determining behaviour than other components.

With reference to the data presented here, it seems that the expectancy of exposure may be a variable that is more important than response efficacy. When asked about the costs associated with the use of condoms, only eight of our 303 respondents doubted their reliability, and when asked about their benefits, over three-quarters named the prevention of infection as their prime benefit. The product of a cognitive evaluation was a belief in the effectiveness of condoms. The emotional response to them is less positive. This lack of correspondence is important. The affective and cognitive components of attitudes should be distinguished, according to Ajzen and Timko (1986). In their study of students' attitudes to health, they found that health behaviour was predicted more accurately from affective rather than from cognitive measures of attitudes.

The data here point to expectancy of exposure as a prime determiner of behaviour. Messages conveyed by the media and other sources of health education focus upon the sharing of injecting equipment, emphasizing this as the major way for drug users to contract the virus. Sexual contact is not often mentioned in communications directed at drug users. Thus, while expectancy of exposure is felt to be high by some injecting drug users, the source of that exposure is not sexual interaction. It might be predicted that any protective action that occurs will relate to sharing and not to safer sex.

In addition to response efficacy in dealing with the threat of the disease, Beck and Lund (1981) and Rogers (1983) suggest that personal efficacy should be taken into account. This is the expectation of being able to perform the recommended action. The value of personal efficacy as a predictor of behaviour was supported by Ajzen and Timko (1986) who found that perceived control over health-related actions was strongly associated with self-reports of those actions. There are correspondences again here with the Health Belief Model, and the concept can be translated in the model to one of the perceived barriers to action. However it is named, it may well assume some importance in determining condom use. It is far from certain that many young people feel able to deal with the introduction of condoms into their sex lives. The common term 'passion killers' conceals real fears, made explicit by some of our male respondents, that they will cause detumescence at a critical moment. In terms of a Health Belief Model analysis, the costs of using condoms are perceived to outweigh the benefits and thus decrease the probability of such behaviour.

In the Theory of Reasoned Action (Fishbein and Ajzen, 1975), the influence of significant others (the subjective norm) is balanced against beliefs about the outcome of issue-relevant behaviour. Either may be weighted to form an attitude that underpins any overt intention. For many young people, the peer group is of considerable importance and can exert much influence. Whether this is so for longer-term drug users is uncertain. They tend to report losing their friends as their drug careers progress, although other drug users may constitute a new peer group. The ease with which most of our respondents talked about condoms, and their negative feelings towards them, suggest that such views are prevalent in their reference groups. The subjective norm will support the continuation of antipathy towards condoms, and where peer influence is strong and combined with beliefs about negative outcomes associated with their use, the intention is unlikely to be to use them. It seems that only among prostitutes is there evidence of real concern about risks associated with sex and a consequent acceptance of condoms; the norm is to use them and prostitutes are skilled at using them. They are more aware of the dangers of sexually transmitted diseases, particularly since such infections could prevent them from working. They do feel at risk and thus are likely to take preventive action. From the perspective of the Theory of Reasoned Action, the strong belief in infection as an outcome of unprotected sex and the group's acceptance of condoms will combine and lead to the intention to use them. From a Health Belief Model perspective, the real question in relation to drug using prostitutes is whether the benefits of using a condom will always outweigh the costs.

The tendency to comply with advice on health will be strongest among those who believe themselves to be greatly at risk, who believe in the seriousness of the disease, who believe in the effectiveness of the recommended protective action and who feel capable of performing it. When asked about the degree to which they felt personally at risk of HIV infection through unprotected sex, our respondents in the main reported that they felt at some risk. A small proportion felt at high risk and it was they who tended to carry condoms. Thus, in general, perceived susceptibility to the disease through sexual behaviour was low, perceived seriousness was high, perceived efficacy of condoms was high and personal efficacy low.

Given the problems associated with the use of condoms in the minds of most of our respondents, the more likely immediate outcome of an increase in perceived threat of the virus through sex is a reduction in casual sex and more careful selection of partners. This poses less of a threat of losing face, embarrassment and loss of self-esteem than inept handling of condoms.

Hilary Klee

Conclusions

It is clear from these data that, despite the negative effects upon interest in sex that are claimed for opiates, there is nevertheless a considerable amount of sexual activity among their users. Levels of sexual activity in users with regular partners are affected by the drug status of the partner, non-drug using partners being associated with a higher frequency of sexual intercourse. Since approximately a quarter of the respondents are in steady relationships with non-drug users and many also report that they try to avoid drug users for casual sex, the degree of sexual activity with non-drug users is high. As the prevalence of seropositivity increases among drug users, the incidence of HIV through sexual transmission to non-drug users will also increase, unless protective measures are employed. While our respondents are aware of the risks of unprotected sex, most do not see the use of condoms as providing an answer.

The activities of amphetamine users may prove to be of major concern, since they appear to differ markedly in their social and sexual behaviour from opiate users. At this stage of the analysis, it is uncertain whether their higher level of casual sex is associated with other forms of risk behaviour such as sharing equipment or unprotected sex.

Prostitutes indicate their concern at the risk of infection by regularly using condoms, but the application of this self-imposed rule is not without rather dangerous exceptions. They may be particularly vulnerable to offers of money for sex without condoms because of their need for drugs.

The prediction of health-related behaviours is notoriously difficult and it may be that currently competing models will need some modification before predictions specifically related to certain types of risk behaviour in drug users can be made. There are variables that are generally regarded to be of importance to protective behaviour, notably the perceived seriousness of the disease, perceived vulnerability to it, the effectiveness of the recommended action and the personal capacity to perform it. Such variables, and any others that assume importance in the context of AIDS-related risk activity, need to be combined in a way that will yield a predictive measure.

The data emerging from this investigation are unlikely to alleviate concern as they suggest an alarmingly low uptake of advice about safer sex. Emphasis upon the risks involved in sharing has diminished the perceived importance of sexual transmission of HIV infection among drug users; this needs to be addressed by government and health professionals when planning harm reduction strategies.

Acknowledgments

The project is funded by the Economic and Social Research Council. The senior investigators are the author and Jean Faugier, and the research assistants are Cath Hayes and Tom Boulton.

References

AJZEN, I. and TIMKO, C. (1986) 'Correspondence between Health Attitudes and Behavior', *Basic and Applied Social Psychology*, 7, 4, pp. 259–76.

BECK, K. H. and LUND, A. K. (1981) 'The Effects of Health Threat Seriousness and Personal Efficacy upon Intentions and Behavior', *Journal of Applied Social Psychology*, 11, pp. 401–15.

BECKER, M. H. (ed.) (1974) *The Health Belief Model and Personal Health Behavior*, Thorofare, N.J., C. B. Slack.

CROWLEY, T. J. and SIMPSON, R. (1978) 'Methadone Dose and Human Sexual Behavior', *The International Journal of the Addictions*, 13, 2, pp. 285–95.

FISHBEIN, I. and AJZEN, I. (1975) *Belief, Attitude, Intention and Behavior: An Introduction to Theory and Research*, Reading, Mass., Addison-Wesley.

HOLBROOK, J. M. (1983) 'CNS Stimulants', in G. BENNET, C. VOURAKIS and D. S. WOOLF (eds), *Substance Abuse: Pharmacological, Developmental, and Clinical Perspectives*. New York, John Wiley.

HOME OFFICE STATISTICAL BULLETIN (1989) Area Tables.

MIRIN, S. M., MEYER, R. E., MENDELSON, J. M. and ELLINGBOE, J. (1980) 'Opiate Use and Sexual Function', *American Journal of Psychiatry*, 137, 8, pp. 909–15.

POWER, R. (1989) 'Methods of Drug Use: Injecting and Sharing', in P. AGGLETON, G. HART and P. DAVIES (eds), *AIDS: Social Representations, Social Practices*. Lewes, Falmer Press.

ROGERS, R. W. (1975) 'A Protection Motivation Theory of Fear Appeals and Attitude Change', *Journal of Psychology*, 91, pp. 93–114.

ROGERS, R. W. (1983) 'Cognitive and Psychological Processes in Fear Appeals and Attitude Change: A Revised Theory of Protection Motivation', in J. CACIOPPO and D. R. PETTY (eds), *Social Psychophysiology*, New York, Guildford Press.

ROGERS, R. W. and MEWBORN, C. R. (1976) 'Fear Appeals and Attitude Change: Effects of a Threat's Noxiousness, Probability of Occurrence, and the Efficacy of Coping Responses', *Journal of Personality and Social Psychology*, 34, pp. 54–61.

STIMSON, G. V. (1988) *Injecting Equipment Exchange Schemes: Final Report*. London, University of London, Goldsmiths College.

ZINBERG, N. E., HARDING, W. M. and APSLER, R. (1978) 'What Is Drug Abuse?' *Journal of Drug Issues*, 8, pp. 9–35.

Chapter 12

AIDS Education and Women: Sexual and Reproductive Issues

Diane Richardson

The majority of public education campaigns about AIDS and HIV have so far tended to assume that people are capable of making personal choices about safer sex and drug use (Vass, 1987). This reflects the dominant ideology underlying health education practice in general, where health is normally regarded as something over which the individual has personal control (Naidoo, 1986). Within this framework, the goals of health education are, first, to ensure that people have access to information concerning their health, and, second, to encourage them, on the basis of this information, to make healthy choices. Ultimately, however, responsibility for good health lies with the individual, insofar as it is their decision as to how they choose to live their lives. This individualistic approach to health education has characterized the British government's response to AIDS which began in earnest towards the end of 1986. One of the early campaigns, entitled 'AIDS: Don't Die of Ignorance', included advertisements on billboards, television and radio, as well as in newspapers and magazines. While this welcome initiative demonstrated that the government had at long last accepted some responsibility for AIDS education, the campaign's central message was that AIDS is preventable through the individual's choosing to act responsibly on the basis of the information they had been given. A free government leaflet advising people how to avoid infection with HIV was distributed to 23 million homes in January 1987. It concluded that: 'Ultimately defence against AIDS depends on all of us taking responsibility for our own actions' (DHSS, 1987). Similar messages can be found in more recent advertising campaigns. For example, one advertisement produced in 1988 has a picture of a condom with the words, 'Life insurance for 15p'. The slogan underneath reads: 'You Know the Facts, the Decision is Yours.'

A major criticism of this kind of approach to AIDS prevention is that it presents advice about risk reduction in a social vacuum. It fails to acknowledge that 'choices' and 'decisions' concerning safer sex, and safer drug use, will be shaped not only by what we know but also by our fears and prejudices about AIDS, as well as by the limitations on our means to act on the advice we are given. This is particularly important when we are considering AIDS education programmes aimed at women. For instance, articles and pamphlets advise on the importance of safer sex and the use of condoms, but hardly ever do they address the difficulties women may encounter in trying to get their male partners to use condoms and to have safer sex. Nor do they usually analyze why such difficulties occur and how women might respond in such situations. To do this, it is necessary first to set sexuality in a socal context and ascertain what certain sexual acts mean to those engaged in them. AIDS education has, for the main part, failed to do this.

Safer Sex: Rights

In our society, it is impossible to talk about sex without also talking about power. As part of their socialization, boys learn that sexual activity, but more especially heterosexual intercourse, is an important means of proving their masculinity, with all the privileges, status and rewards that implies. To become a 'real man', they must strive for a form of sexuality 'where they are always the active partners in sexual encounters. It is they who have to take the initiative, make things happen, and control the event' (Jackson, 1982). Just as boys learn that sex is something they are expected to do to girls, girls learn that sex is something that is supposed to happen to them. The view of women as sexually passive is a common theme in representations of women. It is also present in many of the laws relating to sexual activity.

While acknowledging that not all women and men accept prevalent notions about female and male sexuality, for others, such beliefs are highly important in shaping their responses to safer sex advice. For instance, a girl who is 'prepared' for sex by carrying condoms may be perceived as 'easy', and on the lookout for sex. We do not call boys names if they 'sleep around', but if a girl does this, she risks her reputation. Similarly, a girl who suggests using a condom or mutual masturbation, or other forms of non-penetrative sex, may also risk her reputation, as well as possibly losing her boyfriend. She may, for instance, be blamed for making him feel sexually inadequate because she has gone beyond her expected role by taking the sexual initiative (Pollack, 1985).

In addition to beliefs about how women and men are expected to behave sexually, there may be economic or cultural reasons why a woman may feel unable to negotiate safer sex with a male partner. Within some marriages, for example, sex may almost be a bargain, part of what a husband expects of a wife in return for supporting her and any children they might have. The perception of sex as a man's right and a woman's duty within marriage is sanctioned in various ways, most notably in current rape law which allows that it is legal for a man to rape his wife. Fear of how their male partner may react is clearly an issue for some women, who may be at risk of being beaten up or raped if they were to insist on safer sex practices.

Most advice about safer sex, in assuming individual choice and personal responsibility, has ignored those situations where sex is not an experience between 'consenting partners'. Most obviously, this includes women who are raped and sexually abused. But it also includes women who are under all sorts of subtle, and in some cases not so subtle, pressures to have sexual intercourse as a result of their social and economic dependence on men (Richardson, 1989).

In future it is important that AIDS prevention efforts acknowledge that, in many cases, women do not have the power to act on the knowledge they have; they are constrained — albeit to varying extents according to their class position, age, sexual orientation, and racial and cultural background — by the degree of control they have within heterosexual relationships. It is not just ignorance which could put their lives at risk, but lack of power and sexual equality. Having said that, it is, of course, important for women to have access to information about AIDS. However, if they are to be effective, AIDS health promotion programmes will need to address both women's specific educational needs and their relative powerlessness.

At one level, what is needed are ways to help women feel more assertive and say what they expect and need from sex. However, the danger in regarding this as the 'solution' is that once again the focus is on individual behaviour change. No amount of groupwork, assertiveness training or self-empowerment exercises will be enough. AIDS education programmes can only assist women in exploring what they want from sex and relationships, as well as attempting to make them feel more confident about asserting their needs within the limitations of their social and economic situation. Many women at risk of HIV infection lack the economic and social power to protect themselves from infection. Consequently, it will be necessary to develop resources and to introduce new social policies so that individual behaviour change can be sustained. As Shaw (1988) comments: 'New economic resources, housing, drug treatment centres, battered women's shelters, accessible health services and childcare, as well as legal resources, are probably necessary for women in specific communities to stay off IV drugs and be safe in their sexual relationships.'

Equally, one could argue that if men adopted a different attitude to sex, women would not be in the position of having to assume responsibility for safer sex. What is also required, therefore, are measures which will encourage men to consider risk and not leave the responsibility for safety of sex to women. Paradoxically, it would appear that attempts at preventing the spread of HIV infection by the government, media and medical profession have so far done just the opposite.

Safer Sex: Responsibility

The government's AIDS campaign, as indicated above, has called on individuals to act responsibly on the basis of advice given about safer sex and condom use. Yet despite exhortations to 'take responsibility for our own actions' underlying most preventional efforts, there appears to be a tacit acceptance of the assumption that men are 'naturally' less able to exercise self-control when it comes to sex than are women. One consequence of this is that women are, once again, expected to shoulder the responsibility for making sex free from risk. For example, during 'AIDS WEEK' in February 1987, all four television channels broadcast a series of programmes on AIDS. Time and time again girls were asked if they would carry condoms, whereas boys were asked if they would agree to use them. More recently, in March 1989 the Health Education Authority launched their first advertising campaign targeted at women, with the aim of encouraging women to ask their male partners to use condoms. While the campaign drew attention, long overdue, to AIDS as an issue for women, in the absence of a similar campaign directed at heterosexual men, it served to reinforce the belief that women are responsible for safer sex. Similarly, a popular educational film for teenagers, 'Sex, Drugs and AIDS', offers another example of how current campaigns often place the burden of responsibility for risk reduction on women. The film shows a group of girls discussing how they approach getting their boyfriends to wear condoms. What the film does not show is a similar scene of boys discussing why they will use condoms (Wofsy, 1987).

The recent development of a 'female condom', which is inserted into the vagina and fits over a woman's external genitalia, also raises questions about responsibility. On the one hand, one could see this as giving women greater control. Instead of having to ask a male partner to agree to use a condom, a woman could decide for herself to use a condom if she had vaginal intercourse. Equally, one could ask who has this new condom been developed for, and why only now? Is it so that men can have intercourse without having to wear a condom themselves and can continue to leave responsibility for safer sex to women?

As Coward (1987) comments, there are some cruel ironies in this, not least in the fact that, as suggested above, women are frequently prevented from practising safer sex, however motivated *they* are, by their relative powerlessness when confronted with male sexual demands. There is also a contradiction in expecting women and girls to carry condoms and encourage their use when traditionally it is men who are supposed to initiate, seek out and be prepared for sex. As Scott (1987) observes, 'public permission for women to carry condoms urges us to declare an interest in and a preparedness for heterosexual penetrative sex, which women have always been supposed to deny.' Women who carry condoms, insofar as they challenge such beliefs, may risk being labelled an 'easy lay', another reason why women may find it difficult to insist that their male partner wears a condom if they have intercourse.

The assumption that women are more responsible than men has important implications for notions of blame. It would seem, Alexander (1988) suggests, that 'when women or gay/bisexual men get AIDS it is their fault, but if heterosexual men come down with the disease, it is the fault of the women and gay/bisexual men.' As the expected gatekeepers of male sexuality, it is primarily women who are deemed responsible for preventing heterosexual transmission of HIV. For instance, in a report entitled 'Many Single Women Forego Condoms in *Defiance* of AIDS' (emphasis added), we are told that:

> Many single women having sex with a new man are still not insisting they use condoms, despite the publicity campaigns to prevent the spread of AIDS.... Fifty-seven per cent of the 21,000 women who answered a questionnaire in Cosmopolitan magazine said that they had not made their new man use a condom. (*Guardian*, 1988: 7).

What is lacking in the report is any discussion of the reasons why women might not feel able to insist on condoms and, also, why they should have to. Men and their responsibility for the safety of sex are conspicuously absent.

In much the same way, it is prostitutes and not their male clients who are being scapegoated for the spread of AIDS, despite the fact that studies show that in the West, unless they share equipment to inject drugs, women who work as prostitutes are unlikely to be HIV positive.

AIDS prevention campaigns, such as the promotion of condom use, must not be targeted on women alone. Men must also be strongly encouraged to take responsibility for protection against HIV infection, as well as contraception, in heterosexual relationships. Undoubtedly, this will not be easy. During this century, the majority of men have not had to think about sex as a possible danger to themselves in any serious way, while women have always had to be in fear of unwanted pregnancy, of rape, of health risks associated with contraceptive use or of loss of reputation.

The reasons for this are complex and relate to the meanings associated with sex in our culture. As part of the social construction of male sexuality, many men come to believe that sex is both more important and more uncontrollable for them than it is for women, that men and not women should take the sexual initiative, and that what counts as sex is penetration of the vagina by the penis. One reason men may be unwilling to alter their sexual behaviour in the light of AIDS is that they do not regard safer sex as sex, and assume they will not enjoy it. While some men may be willing to agree that satisfying sex need not imply intercourse, others will not. For them, safer sex may seem dull or uninteresting sex, a poor substitute for the 'real thing', which would impose too many restrictions on their sexual pleasure. Another possible reason is that such changes would represent a threat to male identity and self-esteem. In our society, having sex, but more especially having unprotected vaginal intercourse, is a central aspect of the social construction of being masculine: a 'real man'. It is a way, for men, of achieving status and also power over others.

Although many men may be resistant to changing their sexual habits, it is possible. Studies indicate that over the last few years many gay men have changed their sexual practices in line with risk reduction guidelines (see Fitzpatrick *et al.* elsewhere in this volume, Chapter 8). If gay men can change, so too can heterosexual men. Unlike gay men, however, many heterosexual men appear to lack the motivation to change. They either do not see AIDS as affecting them, or, if they do, deny it because they are afraid that by acknowledging their concerns they might be thought of as gay or bisexual. Men who refuse to practise safer sex for such reasons may be putting both women and themselves at risk. How can they be encouraged to act responsibly?

Workshops on eroticizing safer sex and the production of safer sex pornography are examples of attempts within the gay community to change sexual attitudes and behaviour (although, from a feminist perspective, the use of pornography to promote changes in male sexual practices is problematic). Apart from selling the idea to men that safer sex can be fun, exciting and satisfying, condom use will also have to be sold to men through public advertisements on TV and radio, in the cinema, and in newspapers and magazines. The way some manufacturers have approached this is to associate wearing a condom with being masculine. For example, the advertising slogan of a brand of condoms called Jiffi was 'Real men come in a Jiffi'. In the United States, slogans such as 'Are you man enough for safer sex?' represent a similar attempt to appeal to a desire among men to prove themselves to be masculine.

This approach to encouraging men to take responsibility for sexual pleasure free from risk may persuade some men to use condoms. What it will not do, however, is challenge the fundamental association between masculinity and sexual performance which so often creates problems for women in heterosexual relationships and, as already suggested, can make it difficult for them to negotiate sex on their terms. Nor will it go any way towards challenging the homophobia which allows many heterosexual men to deny their own risk of HIV infection.

Another contradiction in AIDS prevention efforts is the emphasis on the correct use of condoms as the best way of preventing AIDS. Just as the 'naturalness' of men's resistance to self-control is assumed, so is the necessity of heterosexual intercourse (Scott, 1987). You are most at risk of contracting HIV through sex if you engage in anal or vaginal penetration. Despite this, AIDS education campaigns have, by and large, uncritically accepted a view of sex as intercourse. Safer sex advice is centred on recommending fewer sexual partners and being told, 'Always use a condom.' There is very little discussion of non-penetrative sex, and what there is, is very often apologetic. 'Obviously the more people you sleep with the more likely you are to become infected. But the answer doesn't just mean fewer sexual partners. It also means using a condom, or *even* having sex that avoids penetration' (Health Education Authority advertisement, December 1988; emphasis added).

Why is this? As indicated above, the dominant definitions of sex associate 'normal' or 'natural' as well as satisfying sex with vaginal intercourse. To advocate non-penetrative sex as a less risky and potentially very enjoyable way of making love poses an important challenge to this view of sexuality, a view which is enshrined in the law and in religious teachings and informs many people's ideas about sex. Not only might it encourage a shift in the meaning of sex, especially in relation to women, from sexual reproduction to sexual pleasure, but it would also legitimate the experience of many women who prefer non-penetrative sex to intercourse. It would underline the fact that this is neither 'abnormal' nor a problem, but a valid form of sexual expression and pleasure for both women and men.

These are not new issues. Feminists, both earlier this century and more recently, have been concerned with the issue of sexual responsibility and safer sex (in particular, the prevention of unwanted pregnancy, health risks associated with contraceptive use and sexual abuse). There is consequently a certain irony and not a little anger involved in observing the way in which the government, media and the medical profession have responded to the 'AIDS crisis'. It seems as if only now, when men's health is at stake, do we need to consider sexual risks and responsibilities. Why was there no campaign for safer sex ten or fifteen years ago? The answer that AIDS is a life-threatening condition is not a sufficient explanation. Safer sex has a major role to play in the prevention of deaths from cervical cancer. Similarly, taking birth control pills and other forms of contraceptives can be associated with serious side effects, which in some cases can be fatal. None of these is associated with condom use or non-penetrative sex (Richardson, 1989).

Pregnancy and AIDS

Another area in which AIDS particularly affects women is in relation to reproduction. Women infected with HIV can pass on the virus to the foetus during pregnancy, via the placenta, or possibly during birth. How likely this is, is not yet clear. Preliminary reports from various studies suggest that the risk of an infected mother giving birth to an infected child may be between 20 and 35 per cent (Mok *et al.*, 1987). The probability of transmission may be related to the length of time a woman has been infected or whether she has developed HIV-related illness. Some researchers have also suggested that pregnancy might escalate progression of HIV-related illness in women who are infected, but more research is needed to ascertain whether this is the case and, if so, why.

Because of the possible risk of transmission during pregnancy, medical advice in the United States and most European countries is that women who think they may have been infected should be tested and, if positive, delay having children until more is known about perinatal transmission and the effects of HIV on pregnancy. Those who are already pregnant should consider having an abortion.

Such advice is unrealistic for many women. It is a popular misconception that because modern methods of birth control are highly reliable, women nowadays are relatively free to choose whether or not to have a child. This is both oversimplified and, very often, inaccurate. Pregnancy is not necessarily a choice over which women have control. Apart from the enormous social pressures, especially on married women, to bear children, women's ability to postpone motherhood will also depend on how able they are to prevent, or terminate, an unwanted pregnancy, that is, on their access to contraception and abortion. But, as Roberts (1981) points out, it is the medical profession which to a large extent controls women's reproductive choices in this respect. The pervasiveness of male control of women's fertility is also exemplified, as stated earlier, by the structure of heterosexual relationships and differing rights and responsibilities for women and men. In other words, reproductive freedom also depends on being able to say no to men who would ask and, in some cases, force a woman to have unprotected intercourse.

The relationship between pregnancy and AIDS could help to bring about improvements in services for women, such as better contraceptive advice and access to information about abortion, which are old demands and not specific to AIDS. But it could also lead to further restrictions in women's reproductive rights. If we take the term 'reproductive rights' to mean the right to decide when and if to have children, and the right to health services to back up our decisions, the question is, how are these affected by AIDS?

In some cases, it means discussing the right to have an abortion and the right to effective and safe contraception to prevent an unwanted pregnancy. This particularly applies to HIV antibody positive women living in countries such as Ireland, where abortion is illegal, and where access to information on how to obtain and use contraceptives — or on how to obtain an abortion elsewhere — is restricted. In countries where abortion is legal, AIDS-related discrimination may also restrict women's access to abortion. There are reports, for instance, of some London clinics refusing to carry out abortions for women deemed to be 'at risk', or who are known to be infected (O'Neill, 1987).

In other contexts, the debate about reproductive rights and AIDS is about the right to have children. Does a woman who is HIV antibody positive have the right to begin or maintain a pregnancy? According to some, all women who test HIV antibody positive should be sterilized or, if they are already pregnant, be made to have an abortion. Sterilization is one 'solution' to those opposed to abortion. This is in spite of the fact that not all babies born to HIV antibody positive women are infected, and that, in other circumstances where the foetus is 'at risk', parents are counselled in order that they may decide whether or not to continue with the pregnancy.

Concern has already been expressed that in some hospitals doctors are doing 'directed counselling', in which HIV antibody positive women are being told that they *should* have an abortion or sterilization. In August 1988 it was reported that in Scotland, which has the largest number of HIV positive women in Britain, at least six had been forced to have abortions (*Guardian*, 17 August 1988). This has led, in some cases, to these women waiting until very late in the pregnancy before going to see a doctor, for fear of being told that their pregnancy would have to be terminated.

Some pregnant women who test positive do decide to have an abortion, others continue with the pregnancy. For some women, deciding not to have a child, whether this involves having an abortion or not, will be difficult. For many women, becoming a mother is an important aspect of how she sees herself and her future, a view which society strongly encourages in the importance it places on women wanting and being able to have children, especially if they are married. For women who inject, pregnancy may be one of the few times they feel good about themselves and have an incentive to change their drug-taking behaviour.

There are also issues of race and ethnicity to consider. It is one thing for a doctor to advise a white woman who is HIV antibody positive not to have children, it is another to say this to a black woman. Historically, black women have been subjected to forced sterilization and coerced family planning decisions.

The routine screening of pregnant women for HIV antibodies also raises questions about women's reproductive rights. In some countries, Norway and Sweden for example, the HIV antibody test is already given routinely to all women who are pregnant. In Norway, it is also given routinely to all women seeking an abortion. By August 1987, in Norway, 71,583 pregnant women had been tested, of whom seven were found to be HIV antibody positive. Four of these were known about already.

Mandatory testing means you have to take the test. Routine testing means that you are given the test after you have been told that testing will be done. Theoretically you have the right to refuse, but the onus is on you to say if you do not want the test. Voluntary testing is where you decide you want to take the test. Although taking the test may be 'voluntary', it is not always with informed consent. Women are often tested without being given any counselling. In one clinic in Norway, the only information was a card on the wall announcing that the HIV antibody test was one of the tests that would be given routinely. What if you cannot read, do not see the card, or do not speak the language in which it is written?

Even if a woman is told that the HIV antibody test is one of the tests she will be given, and this is explained to her, she may find it hard to say no. Some women may be afraid that if they refuse to take the test they will not get the treatment they need. For instance, how many women seeking an abortion are going to feel that their reproductive 'choices' may be affected if they said no to the test? Also, in Norway, if you say no to the test you are treated as if you are positive, with all the negative implications this can have. For example, it may mean being put into an isolation ward for the birth and having one's baby treated as HIV antibody positive. The question then is, how far is it consent if a woman says yes to taking the test? Many women will feel obliged or may simply not be aware they are being given the test, or what the test results mean.

There is not *national* programme in Britain, as yet, to test routinely pregnant women for HIV antibodies. However, some local authorities have approved routine testing, and the British Medical Association acknowledges that elsewhere, in some hospitals, pregnant women are being positively encouraged to take the test. There have also been reports of pregnant drug users being tested without their knowledge, consent or adequate counselling (O'Neill, 1987).

The British government intends to test 20,000–30,000 pregnant women in 1989, in three different areas of the country, in order, it claims, to monitor the prevalence of HIV infection in the UK. The General Medical Council and the British Medical Association are both opposed to the singling out of pregnant women for testing primarily because they are available. They are also concerned that women should have the right to say no and receive proper counselling about the test and the significance of a positive result *before* being given a test. Given the numbers, it is a legitimate concern to ask how many of these 60,000–90,000 women will receive adequate counselling in already busy ante-natal clinics? Even if they do, will they feel they have a right to say no to the test without being penalized? These are important questions, but we must also remember that even with adequate counselling and the right to say no, testing is not necessarily going to prevent perinatal transmission of HIV. A woman who tests negative early in the pregnancy may become positive at a later stage, or may not yet have developed antibodies to the virus. Related to this, it is interesting that no one has suggested testing men who want to become fathers.

While it is important for women to have access to safe, low or no cost abortion, and to accurate information and adequate counselling about the meaning and consequences of taking the HIV antibody test, this must be offered on a voluntary and not a routine basis. Women need to be fully informed of the facts about pregnancy and AIDS and supported in the decisions *they* make about whether to take the antibody test or, if they are pregnant, whether to have an abortion. This needs to be provided in a manner that is appropriate to a woman's age and educational level, and with sensitivity to her ethnic and cultural background. It is also important to try to provide women with this information *before* they become pregnant, and well-woman and family planning clinics obviously have an important role to play in this respect. Finally, those women who decide to continue with the pregnancy, or who have no choice, should be counselled to plan for the care of a potentially infected child, as well as dealing with the emotional aspects of possibly giving birth to an HIV antibody positive baby (Hauer and Dattel, 1988).

References

ALEXANDER, P. (1988) 'Prostitutes Are Being Scapegoated for Heterosexual AIDS', in F. DELACOSTE and P. ALEXANDER (eds), *Sex Work*, London, Virago Press.

COWARD, R. (1987) 'Sex after AIDS', *New Internationalist*, March, pp. 20–21.

DHSS (1987) *AIDS: Don't Die of Ignorance*. London, DHSS.

Guardian (1988) 'Many Single Women Forego Condoms in Defiance of AIDS', 26 September, p. 7.

HAUER, L. B. and DATTEL, B. J. (1988) 'Management of the Pregnant Women Infected with the Human Immunodeficiency Virus', *Journal of Perinatology*, 8, 3, pp. 258–62.

JACKSON, S. (1982) *Childhood and Sexuality*. Oxford, Basil Blackwell.

MOK, J., *et al.* (1987) 'Infants Born to Mothers Seropositive for Human Immunodeficiency Virus', *Lancet*, 1, pp. 1164–8.

NAIDOO, J. (1986) 'Limits to Individualism', in S. RODMELL and A. WATT, *The Politics of Health Education*. London, Routledge and Kegan Paul.

O'NEILL, S. (1987) 'Women in the AIDS Trap', *New Society*, 22 May, p. 5.

POLLACK, S. (1985) 'Sex and the Contraceptive Act', in H. HOMANS (ed.), *The Sexual Politics of Reproduction*. London, Gower.

RICHARDSON, D. (1989) *Women and the AIDS Crisis*, 2nd ed., London, Pandora Press.

ROBERTS, H. (1981) 'Male Hegemony in Family Planning', in H. ROBERTS (ed.), *Women, Health and Reproduction*. London, Routledge and Kegan Paul.

SCOTT, S. (1987) 'Sex and Danger: Feminism and AIDS', *Trouble and Strife*, 11, pp. 13–18.

SHAW, S. N. (1988) 'Preventing AIDS among Women: The Role of Community Organizing', *Socialist Review*, 100, pp. 76–92.

VASS, A. (1987) 'The Growing Threat from AIDS to Victims of Rape and Sexual Abuse', *Social Work Today*, 4 May, pp. 8–9.

WOFSY, C. (1987) 'Human Immunodeficiency Virus Infection in Women', *Journal of the American Medical Association*, 257, 15, pp. 2074–6.

Chapter 13

AIDS Prevention Strategies in Europe: A Comparison and Critical Analysis[1]

Hans Moerkerk with Peter Aggleton

While opinions differ on many of the scientific, medical and social issues associated with HIV infection and AIDS, on one thing experts and politicians seems to agree: prevention was, is, and for the next few years will be, the most important means by which we can respond to the challenge of a viral infection with often devasting consequences. In this chapter, we will review some of the different approaches to AIDS prevention that have been employed throughout Europe, and the efforts of various international organizations to support them. Of necessity, the account will be oversimplified and incomplete. Nevertheless, we hope to identify a typology of responses which may provide the foundations for more detailed future comparative analysis. We will begin by describing key features in the epidemiology of HIV infection and AIDS across Europe.

When we speak of Europe, we should not have in mind a single united continent, since within it there are considerable differences in political structure, cultural background and social development. In some countries, such as the Republic of Ireland, sex between men is still illegal, while in others, such as the Netherlands, the advent of AIDS has in some respects provided further impetus for gay emancipation. Differences between countries such as Greece, Albania and Iceland are considerable. It is, therefore, crucial not to view Europe as a single entity but as the sum of many different cultures and political structures which have responded inconsistently and unevenly to the advent of HIV infection and AIDS. All this needs to be borne in mind when considering the ways in which different countries have responded.

Western and northern European countries are characterized by the fact that the majority of reported cases of HIV infection and AIDS consist of men who have sex with men. On average, this comprises about 70 per cent of reported cases in this part of Europe, although this proportion is decreasing with the growth of infection among injecting drug users. Heterosexually acquired infections that are not linked to injecting drug use are still relatively rare in these parts of Europe.

In southern Europe, on the other hand, there are higher proportions of injecting drug users among people with HIV infection and AIDS. This is particularly the case in Italy and Spain. However, it is important to recognize that less efficient reporting in southern European countries may mean that the numbers of gay and bisexual men who are affected are underreported at present. In southern European countries there has also been a more rapid increase in reported cases of HIV infection among children and among heterosexuals.

In eastern Europe, HIV and AIDS have only recently been identified as potential problems, and governments are now beginning to move beyond an initial response which suggested that AIDS was a sickness confined to African students or gay capitalists. Nevertheless, the impression continues to be given that HIV is a virus which can, and should be, stopped at the border.

Given the cultural, social and political diversity of Europe, it is little wonder that there has been a variety of preventive responses. While individual nations may be aware of the need for international or supranational cooperation, present arrangements within Europe mean that a consistent response is difficult to achieve. For example, a number of European countries are united in international associations within which the political and administrative competences are increasingly being transferred to supranational authorities, such as the European Community. Others participate only in economic alliances, such as COMECON or the EFTA. Most northern, western and southern European countries work together on a social or cultural level in the Council of Europe, and the European region of the World Health Organization unites them all, but its power to implement a general policy on AIDS prevention, and its opportunities to do so, are severely limited.

Varieties of Response

We will now examine the ways in which different European countries have tried to organize their AIDS prevention activities. While recognizing that in many countries non-governmental organizations (NGOs) and AIDS Service Organizations (ASOs) are very active, and have sometimes been the initiators of activities on a national scale, we will begin by looking at 'official' policy developed by government bodies charged with AIDS control. It is possible to identify four types of countries in relation to the ways in which primary prevention activities have so far been organized and coordinated, although, as we will see later, the picture is complicated by the fact that the citizens of some countries may have access to more than one set of prevention initiatives (Figure 1).

Type 1:	Pragmatic responses
Type 2:	'Political' responses
Type 3:	Bio-medical responses
Type 4:	Emergent responses

Figure 1. Varieties of Official Response to HIV Infection and AIDS

First, there are those that have adopted a largely pragmatic approach. Examples of such countries include Norway, Denmark, the Netherlands and Switzerland. Most of these involved themselves in AIDS control fairly early in the epidemic, usually as far back as 1983–84, and developed strategies in which the emphasis is on information and education to bring about a favourable response from particular groups or the population in general. Mid-term and long-term strategies have been developed in which the emphasis has been as much on preventing hostility against, and discrimination towards, affected groups as it has been on providing people with the facts about transmission and risk reduction. The emphasis in these countries has not been on prohibition or on other coercive forms of control, but on planning, evaluation, pragmatism and consensus. In situations where this kind of approach has been adopted, NGOs and ASOs have often been afforded considerable room for manoeuvre, and the actions they have taken have, on the whole, had little consequence for the grants they have continued to receive.

Second, there are countries in which AIDS policy has been developed in accordance with what is politically possible or politically desirable. Examples here include Britain and the Federal Republic of Germany, although policies and interventions in Austria, Ireland, Finland, Iceland and Sweden have to some extent been influenced by such concerns. In these countries, governments have usually dictated the strategies to be adopted; frequently, pragmatism and anti-discrimination have been eschewed in favour of approaches in line with the political stance of the government of the day. Thus, in Britain, AIDS prevention activities have been complicated by the passing into law of Section 28 of the 1988 Local Government Act which prohibits local authorities from promoting homosexuality. While activities which are concerned with 'treating or preventing the spread of disease' are specifically excluded by the legislation, the climate of anxiety and fear created by this law has done much to hamper the development of effective AIDS prevention strategies for men who have sex with men.

In countries which fall into this second category, the law is often seen as an instrument by which human behaviour can be regulated and the epidemic controlled. This creates severe problems for prevention programmes since it means that the state is likely to interpret AIDS prevention narrowly in terms of the behaviours it considers desirable. Strategies such as these are unlikely to prove effective, as unsuccessful efforts to regulate prostitution by similar means clearly demonstrate.

A third group of countries are those in which AIDS is regarded primarily as a problem which is amenable to bio-medical solutions. In these countries, which include Belgium, France, Spain, Italy and Greece, governments have displayed only short-term interest in the issues. Instead, established medical institutions have been charged with determining official policies and interventions. NGOs and ASOs generally have a marginal role to play in these contexts, and there has been little participation by community groups in the planning and implementation of AIDS prevention activities. Given the lack of strategic planning that is evident in these countries, one might be forgiven for supposing that government involvement is largely cosmetic, being concerned more with impression management than with dealing with the problems.

Finally, there are those countries in which HIV disease has only recently been identified as a serious concern. Most eastern European states fall within this category. The majority of these countries have as yet to formulate an adequate basis for medium- and long-term planning, and many have in the interim resorted to the use of existing legislation as a means of AIDS control. The position is complicated by the fact that many of these countries are undergoing a degree of political liberalization. This may afford NGOs a more important role in determining future policy and practice. Developments of this kind are particularly evident in Hungary, the German Democratic Republic, Czechoslovakia and Yugoslavia. Only Albania adheres rigidly to the view that right thinking socialists do not give in to the 'sins of the flesh', and therefore are unlikely to acquire HIV infection.

This typology is over simplified and schematic, and within any one country, there will be a variety of responses, some in line with 'official' policy, others at odds with it. Nevertheless, identifiable differences do exist, raising important questions for those who would seek unproblematically to develop a coherent European response to HIV infection and AIDS. It is also important to recognize that differences between countries exist in respect of the health education messages promoted through the media. This can be particularly confusing for those living in countries such as the Netherlands where there may be access to television from countries such as Britain, Belgium, France and the Federal Republic of Germany, as well as the Netherlands itself. This kind of situation also creates problems for refugees, migrant workers and tourists who may be given different advice depending on the country they are in. Towards the end of this chapter we will examine some of the ways in which these challenges can be taken up, but before that we will look at some specific responses.

A Pragmatic Response

One of the best illustrations of a largely pragmatic response to HIV infection and

AIDS can be seen in the Netherlands. Here, since 1983 there has been a policy of AIDS control which is largely uncontentious in its twofold concern to stop further infection and to prevent unnecessary anxiety and social disturbance. While in recent months there has been some growing distance between the medical profession and others concerned with legal and ethical questions over the issue of anonymous seroprevalence studies, the relationship between central government and NGOs has been largely supportive and facilitative.

Prevention activities began in 1983 and were initially directed towards those at greatest risk of HIV infection. These included men who have sex with men and injecting drug users. Subsequently, other groups have been included, such as prostitutes and their clients, young people at school, migrants and refugees, tourists visiting Holland and professional workers who may be able to make information about HIV infection and AIDS more widely available through their work. Following a large national campaign in 1987, more focused activities were developed in 1988 on topics such as AIDS and work, AIDS and young people and so on. Every year the Dutch STD Foundation has been involved with prevention activities during holiday periods.

Distinctions have always been made in this work between health information and health education. While the facts may lay the foundations for behaviour change, additional focused interventions are needed to support people in the changes they and their partners may need to make. AIDS prevention activities in the Netherlands are coordinated by the National Commission on AIDS Control, an independent organization with its own executive. The National Commission on AIDS Control also has a key role to play in advising the government and, in particular, the Secretary of State for Health.

Attention is currently being given to an evaluation of the health education programmes that have so far taken place. This will involve social researchers in a wide range of projects, including those that will examine knowledge levels and patterns of behaviour. Efforts will also be made to identify problems that have arisen over the past few years and ways of dealing with them.

A 'Political' Response

Sweden fits well within the category of countries making a political response. The government has developed a comprehensive and committed AIDS policy as part of a pre-existing system of social and public health. For many years, and in accordance with reformist and neo-pluralist principles, efforts have been made socially to engineer 'desirable' solutions to a wide range of health problems. As a consequence, substantial resources have been made available for public education and health care. Such state involvement in health issues generally has had important consequences for AIDS prevention activities.

Overall, Swedish policy is informed by the view that the state should regulate and set clear boundaries on human behaviour, and legislation is seen as an important instrument in the attainment of this politically formulated objective. It is not surprising, therefore, that HIV antibody testing has become one of the most important components of prevention programmes, with current legislation requiring anyone suspecting that they might have been infected by HIV to undergo examination by a doctor. The so-called 'treating doctor' has the responsibility of prescribing how the patient should behave. Together with a well developed system of contact tracing, these measures constitute an important part of Swedish AIDS prevention policy.

Within Sweden, there have also been efforts to de-homosexualize the issue of AIDS. The majority of public information campaigns have emphasized that AIDS is everyone's problem, and gay men have hardly been mentioned at all, except in posters of a young man who, we are to presume, is HIV antibody positive, which carry the caption, 'He visited a Copenhagen gay club a few months ago' — a message which hardly proved popular with the Danish government!

One of the most important questions to be asked about this particular approach is the extent to which it is compatible with the minimization of social disturbance. In particular, it will be important to enquire into the extent to which anti-gay sentiment is enhanced by an approach which seeks to use punitive measures to control sexual expression and behaviour. It should, of course, be recognized that other strategies have been adopted by statutory and grass-roots agencies in Sweden. Some of these have been more focused in their interventions, and some have taken more seriously equal opportunities and social emancipation concerns.

A Bio-medical Response

An illustration of a bio-medical approach is offered by official responses to AIDS in Belgium. Belgium has a complicated political structure and is divided by ideologies which impede a common effort in the struggle against AIDS. Financial support for preventive action, and especially the encouragement of NGOs and ASOs, has been quite inadequate. The emphasis instead has been on medical institutions and a 'curative' approach.

In December 1986 a National AIDS Committee was established, composed only of doctors responsible mainly for testing and research. Only later was a High Council to Fight AIDS created, which included lawyers and specialists in ethics. Until February 1987 the advertising of condoms was banned, and it was not until that year that every household received information about HIV and AIDS via a leaflet and television publicity. The unevenness of official responses is demonstrated by the fact that later in 1987 over 5000 condoms promoted for use in anal sex were confiscated by the state.

In the Flemish-speaking part of Belgium, the bulk of the AIDS work has so far been carried out by NCOs supported by a few medical institutions which are aware that AIDS prevention needs careful organization and planning. The regional government and the medical establishment as a whole have not supported these activities, so that initiatives such as the 'AIDS bus', the 'Gay Service Project' and the 'Hot Rubber Project' have had to be cancelled. In despair, some Flemish organizations have applied for subsidies from their northern neighbours. This is not to deny the important work that has been done by several NGOs such as the AIDS Telephone, the Centres for Family Planning and Sexual Education and the Red Cross.

In many respects Belgium is a typical example of a country with a relatively high level of political apathy and only a short-lived interest in AIDS prevention on the part of the authorities. Focused mainly on traditional medical aspects, few preventive actions have so far been systematically planned or evaluated.

An Emergent Response

Prevention strategies in Hungary provide an example of an emergent response. In Hungary there has been little by way of a sustained programme of public information other than a leaflet drop to households in 1987. Specific groups such as gay men, prisoners and students from outside Hungary have been addressed via the medical authorities, and HIV antibody testing has been widely promoted as an effective approach to prevention. So far, health education strategies have been relatively simplistic, with an emphasis on leaflets and posters. These have tended to use 'fear' as a prevention strategy, and have operated from the premises that legislation can control the epidemic and that the 'authorities' are best placed to take charge.

The relationship between NGOs and the state remains underdeveloped in Hungary, although there is now an active gay group concerned with AIDS and STD prevention in Budapest. At the end of 1987 the Hungarian AIDS Foundation was created and is now very active, making contact with prostitutes and injecting drug users. It also runs a telephone information line. The National AIDS Committee, which is government controlled, has as yet no coherent planning model, nor have there been sustained attempts to evaluate AIDS prevention activities, other than in epidemiological terms.

It remains to be seen whether the Hungarian government will make efforts to involve NGOs more fully in the development of medium- and long-term strategies. It remains also to be seen whether efforts will be made to move beyond a narrowly medical and legislative response, to embrace issues of prejudice and social inequality. In many ways, Hungary provides an illustration of a country which has recently identified the full nature of the problem and which is attempting to find its own way.

International Organizations and European AIDS Prevention Strategies

We will conclude by reflecting on the role of international organizations in European AIDS prevention. The important question here is the extent to which international or supranational cooperation can enhance the activities currently underway in individual countries. That such a goal is desirable seems beyond question when conflicting information is available in different countries. For example, on the issue of safer sex, the Dutch currently advise, 'when you have been monogamous with one partner for five years, your sex is always safe', the British, 'it is safest to stick to one partner', and the Belgians, 'it is safest to select one loyal partner.' Only the Norwegians and the Danes have a positive approach, with the advice that 'when you have changing sexual contacts, always protect yourself and your partner by using a condom.' Similarly, only the Netherlands and Switzerland classify oro-genital contacts as relatively safe, but even here the advice given is different. Thus, you are advised not to 'get semen in your mouth' in Holland, but to 'be careful that semen does not enter your throat' in Switzerland.

It should be clear from what has been said so far that AIDS prevention strategies vary considerably among countries. This raises important questions about the extent to which a common approach is possible, or even desirable. Indeed, it may be better to aim for what can be described as condition-creating activities concerned with AIDS prevention rather than to seek to develop uniform (and possibly monolithic) prevention programmes. These might include the setting up of information services that cross national boundaries, as well as the establishment of a common set of ethical and legal principles relating to the rights of people with HIV infection and AIDS. It would also seem important that international cooperation should be facilitative rather than restrictive in its effects. This is made all the more complicated by the diversity of organizations that already exist. The European Community, the Council of Europe and the European region of the World Health Organization all have their own aims and objectives. Efforts will need to be made to clarify the roles and responsibilities of each of these bodies if a clear and unambiguous set of priorities is to be established.

The European Community

The European Community occupies an important position when it comes to decision-making in respect of political and social issues. This is true insofar as non-member countries are concerned too, in that the actions of the European Community are central in climate-building throughout the continent. Already declarations about HIV/AIDS have been made by European government leaders (1987) and the Council of Ministers of Health (1987, 1988). It is important now to turn these statements of principle into deeds. This is where problems are likely to arise, particularly in a body in which the main lines of policy are largely shaped by political considerations. This is certainly true of public health, which is not mentioned explicitly in the Treaty of Rome, and in which strong nationally oriented traditions exist. On the other hand, there have been sustained efforts to develop a European Community stance on health protection and environmental issues. The major question now is: in what respect and to what extent is AIDS prevention policy a matter that falls within the competence of the European Commission?

The Council of Europe

Twenty-three northern, western and southern European countries are currently active in the Council of Europe, particularly in respect of cultural, educational and ethical matters. In 1986 this organization designated AIDS as one of the areas in which it would become active, and in November 1987 detailed plans for prevention programmes were announced, along with a series of statements concerning the legal position of people with HIV infection and AIDS. In 1988 further recommendations were made concerning AIDS and prisoners and AIDS and work, and in the summer of 1989 statements on the social and ethical implications were published. The emphasis so far has been on declarations and statements of principle. It remains to be seen whether these will be followed by legislation requiring the development of consistent approaches.

The World Health Organization

The World Health Organization's role in the development of AIDS prevention activities across Europe has so far been relatively low key, being confined to the facilitation of expert meetings and consultations, and the support of limited programmes of research and development. In many ways it would seem quite inappropriate for a European equivalent of WHO's Global Programme on AIDS to be developed, since this would run the risk of duplicating existing patterns of provision. Nevertheless, there is important work to be done in facilitating better communication between eastern and western European countries, and European nations themselves have an obligation to continue to support WHO activities to do with AIDS prevention in the third world.

Conclusion

In the months and years ahead, a more consistent and coordinated approach to AIDS prevention in Europe will need to be developed, recognizing that different groups may have different needs. If prevention activities are to have long-term success, they will need to offer people positive and acceptable options. Desirable changes in behaviour cannot be brought about by coercive and legalistic interventions; rather, they must be taught, encouraged and supported. This will require a sophisticated package of prevention measures informed by insights from a wide range of social research into sexual motivations and behaviours. Only by doing this will it be possible to deal effectively with the complex bio-medical and social challenges that HIV and AIDS present.

Note

1   This is an edited version of a paper given at the International Workshop on the Prevention of Sexual Transmission of AIDS and Other STDs, sponsored by the Dutch STD Foundation and the World Health Organization and held in Noordwijkerhout in May 1989. The proceedings of this conference are to be published by Swets and Zeitlinger B. V., Amsterdam.

Chapter 14

The Social Organization of HIV Counselling

David Silverman

> In many ways AIDS is like many other illnesses which devastate individual
> lives. What is remarkable about AIDS, however, is not simply its virulence,
> but the weight of symbolic meaning that it carries. (Weeks, 1989: 18)

The rapid growth in numbers of people with HIV infection and with AIDS (PWAs)
has been perceived as generating a 'crisis' in health care systems. Contemporary crises
occupy a number of familiar sites, including the economic, the administrative and the
scientific. In the case of AIDS, the perceived 'crisis' has produced questions for each of
these sites: how to meet the cost of hospital care, how to reorganize welfare and
medical services, and how to find a vaccine or a cure.

As Weeks points out, however, what is remarkable about the AIDS 'crisis' is the
symbolic meaning that saturates it. The marginality of many people with AIDS (gay
men, injecting drug users, Haitians and Puerto Ricans) has allowed them to become
the target of a 'moral panic' associated with perceived threats to symbolic boundaries.
Here were 'foreign bodies' invading the sacred temple of 'the family' with its 'pure'
and 'clean' moral order. This demanded what Weeks (1989: 5) calls 'rituals of
decontamination': cleaning a swimming pool after one HIV seropositive man swam in
it, and burying the dead in specially built 'secure' coffins.

While the public responses to AIDS occupy familiar economic, administrative
and scientific sites, we must contextualize the response within each site, and the overall
conception of an 'AIDS crisis', against an understanding of the symbolic order which
was perceived to be put at risk. For instance, the current preoccupation with the threat
to 'the general population' constituted by injecting drug users and bisexual men
intermingles the objective danger of cross-infection with a shock at breached symbolic
boundaries.

What, then, do we know of the current epidemiology and its likely future
course? At present, Britain and Sweden are towards the lower end of western
European incidence, below France and considerably below the United States.

However, such figures tell us nothing about the pool of HIV infection in each country and so the likely future course of the epidemic. Unfortunately, in predicting the future there are many imponderables.

The economic burden of the epidemic looks likely to be severe. In Sweden, one estimate predicts an increase in costs from 350 million SEK in 1987 to 700 million SEK by 1990 (Herlitz and Brorsson, 1988). One London hospital is currently spending over 5 per cent of its budget on HIV disease including AIDS, and it is estimated that the lifetime medical costs of one person with AIDS currently exceed £20,000 (Green, 1988). In both Britain and Sweden, even a 'low' estimate suggests that the number of beds required for AIDS patients will increase three- or four fold between 1987 and 1991 (Green 1988).

However, once we try to predict the longer-term future, we are on dangerous ground. Take the case of the so-called 'explosion' of HIV infection into heterosexuals who do not inject drugs. According to a recent newspaper report, the normally sober actuarial profession estimates that AIDS cases among heterosexuals could exceed those among homosexuals by the year 2005 (*Independent*, March 1989). On this prediction, it is claimed that compulsory testing among single people may 'become commonplace'. Understandably, the protectors of the assets of pension funds and insurance companies may want to take a 'worst case' view. Fortunately, current evidence of the spread of the epidemic among heterosexuals who do not inject is less worrying (see Table 1).

Table 1. Overall Percentage of Positive HIV Tests in STD Clinics, 1986/87

Country	Positive HIV Tests
Sweden	0.4[1]
United Kingdom	0.25[2]–1[3]
United States	0.7[4]–3.8[5]

Sources: 1 Lidman *et al.*, 1988.
2 PHLS, 1989.
3 Loveday *et al.*, 1989.
4 Hull *et al.*, 1988 — voluntary testing only.
5 *ibid.* — anonymous testing.

If we assume that people attending clinics for the treatment of sexually transmitted diseases (STDs) may be at a relatively high risk, these figures give room for hope, if not complacency. The apparently low prevalence of HIV infection is underlined by the British Public Health Laboratory Service which only discovered thirty-six positive heterosexuals from a sample of 14,000. All but one of these were associated with injecting drug use or contact with a country where heterosexual transmission is common.

Further evidence of the spread of the epidemic in Europe is found in the limited transmission of the virus to female partners of HIV seropositive males. A recent study found that three risk factors were crucial in transmission: the presence of STDs in the women, anal sex and the index case having full-blown AIDS. Where none of these factors was present, only 7 per cent of partners seroconverted, and only where two or more factors were found did a majority become HIV positive (European Study Group, 1989).

These recent figures underline Padian's (1987) contention that the extensive heterosexual spread of the virus in the African continent may be due to local circumstances. Given this and the continuing decline in rates of seroconversion among gay men (see Miller, 1987; Winkelstein *et al.*, 1987), we can at least say that some predictions of the future course of the epidemic have been exaggerated. However, a grave problem remains in needle sharing among injecting drug users, particularly in certain regions (see Stimson *et al.*, 1989; Mulleady *et al.*, 1989), while the lay beliefs of many young people (Warwick *et al.*, 1988) and the knowledge and behaviour of some poorly educated people (US National Center for Health Statistics, 1989) may be a continued source of concern.

Varieties of Response

Given this mixed evidence, we can look briefly at how governments have responded. In Britain and Sweden, health education campaigns have been developed which have been far less reticent about discussing sexual practices and condoms than in similar interventions within the United States. In both countries, the confidentiality of HIV test results has been stressed — although the Swedish practice is far from libertarian, as we shall shortly note. The needle exchange scheme for injecting drug users is an important initiative by the British government, although it has yet to convince some drug workers that a 'least risk' policy is acceptable (Stimson *et al.*, 1989). Blind spots remain over the spread of HIV infection in prisons, while stumbling efforts are being made to develop health education strategies to address the needs of particular audiences. The Swedish response is unique in that:

> Each doctor caring for an HIV positive patient is required to give legally binding instructions to the patient to prevent the further spread of the infection. With the co-operation of the patient, the doctor must also perform contact-tracing. If the doctor finds that the patient does not follow the instructions, or if contacts refuse to appear for testing, these persons are reported to the responsible Medical Officer of Health with full identity. (de Ron *et al.*, 1988).

These authors argue that this response will contain the epidemic; Henriksson (1988), in contrast, is less optimistic and argues that interventions such as these should be seen as evidence of Sweden's 'strong' if misguided belief in the efficacy of formal methods of social control.

From a different national culture, the appeal to policing and to compulsory isolation of recalcitrants looks authoritarian. Moreover, it appears to contravene the Council of Europe Foreign Ministers' Recommendation on this issue which clearly rejects 'compulsory screening of either the general population or of particular population groups' (Massarelli, 1988). It is also possible that such a policy may stop people seeking HIV antibody tests and may drive index cases and their contacts underground. Both courses of action are unlikely to encourage the practice of safer sex. Furthermore, they shift the focus away from the 'general population' (who, if they are sensible, will take precautions with new partners) to a supposedly 'deviant' already infected group invested with the sole responsibility for preventing further infection. This seems a heavy price to pay for a system which so far has only managed to trace five people previously unknown to be HIV positive (Lidman et al., 1988). State policing of health issues such as that in Sweden is unknown in most of Western Europe and the USA, although South Carolina has attempted mandatory reporting of the names and addresses of HIV seropostive persons, a move which has driven people away from clinics (Johnson, 1988).

Increasingly, however, 'safer sex' is being defined in both western Europe and the USA in the context of what we may call 'partner policing' (see Biggar et al., 1988; Hearst and Hulley, 1988). This strategy is based on the idea that each person should take responsibility for the risks they encounter in their sexual relationships with others. Unfortunately, by stressing the interrogation of one's prospective sexual partners and by implying that legal action may be taken if 'lies are told, it introduces a legalistic/contract version of human relationships which many find distasteful' (Watney, 1989). The alternative is to avoid needless enquiries into sexual history and to act as if a new partner is HIV seropositive.

These are some of the ideological assumptions made in current debates about the nature of health education about HIV and AIDS. However, even if we know what to say to people, how should its delivery be evaluated? Aggleton (1989) has recently pointed to the understandable resistance of some health educators to spend time evaluating their HIV/AIDS education. To them, evaluation may represent prevarication in a situation where they are *in situ* having to cope right now. Some health educators may also feel that evaluation is overtheorized, whereas they are the practitioners whose practical expertise should be respected. Where evaluation does take place, much emphasis tends to be laid on health education as information-giving. An assessment of effectiveness is usually made by survey research focusing on outcomes. However, simply having more information about a health issue does not necessarily lead to behavioural change. Moreover, even where intervention is successful if we focus on outcomes alone, we do not know how or why such interventions work.

Consequently, Aggleton calls for *process evaluation* focusing on social organization. This will mean a concern with the learning processes that people go through, the competing interests around health education and the unintended consequences of educational interventions. Therefore, in future work we need to pay more attention to relating health education to a broader cultural, social and, perhaps, political context. We might also consider studies of risk modification in other areas. A great danger in this field is to assume that in HIV/AIDs education we are dealing with entirely different phenomena, thus forgetting things that have been learned in other health initiatives. In particular, we might learn from a ten-year research project in Finland concerned with reducing risk for coronary heart disease reported recently by Nelkin (1987). The Finnish study, and other similar investigations, reveal that people can be induced to change their behaviour providing that five key conditions are met. First, they need to get their information from credible sources, in particular from groups with whom they identify and whom they trust. Second, this information should not be based on moral arguments. Third, the new information should correspond to that already received. Fourth, it needs to be reinforced by people's social situation and their reference groups. Finally, Nelkin argues, behaviour change is most likely when health education interventions are supported by adequate community and counselling services.

Nelkin goes on to call for two types of study. The first of these are studies of the risk perceptions of different groups. Survey research tends to suggest that people underestimate familiar risk and overestimate risks that are unfamiliar, involuntary, invisible and catastrophic. Second, we need to map the confused multiplicity of national and local agencies now involved in health and social policies relating to AIDS. In doing this, we need to examine interprofessional relations and situations where institutional fragmentation is counter-productive. It is within this context that the study of HIV counselling provision reported in this chapter was carried out.

The 'Safer Sex Study'

The 'safer sex study', funded by the English Health Education Authority is assessing counselling especially about safer sex. Two interrelated areas are focused on. The first is the social organization of institutions (particular STD clinics). Of interest here is who is doing the counselling and what relations do they have with other people both within their own institution and outside? The second related area of interest is the process of counselling itself. This is being examined via audio recordings of actual counselling sessions, supplemented by video recordings of work at the Royal Free Hospital, London (Haemophilia Centre and District AIDS Unit).

It appears that at present about 30 per cent of HIV antibody tests done in Britain are requested by general practitioners (GPs). Yet studies indicate that GPs are far from experienced in talking about sexual behaviour. There is also a problem of confidentiality here because, if someone visits a GP for an HIV antibody test, the consultation is likely to appear in their notes, and if an insurance company subsequently consults the GP, the doctor will have to give whatever information is available, providing the patient has signed the release. Moreover, it has been suggested that because GPs probably only get one true positive out of 50,000 tests, they are likely to steer clear of the whole area and hence of safe sex advice.

Conversely, STD clinics are a significant site for identifying people who are HIV antibody positive, staff have the experience of talking about sex and are used to issues of confidentiality. But STD clinics are often understaffed and overstretched, particularly when it comes to giving health advice, and the services they provide vary widely. Moreover, particularly during government sponsored information campaigns, clinics are saturated with patients. This generates a cyclical pattern of patient load which makes forward planning difficult.[1]

A recent report by the British Department of Health on 'Advice, Support and Counselling for the HIV positive' (Chester, 1987) notes the *ad hoc* arrangement of services and suggests that, as a solution, certain staff only should be involved in HIV antibody test counselling. However, although this may maximize staff resources, lack of continuity of support and care may be a problem. The report also suggests that support for people with HIV infection and/or AIDS should make more use of the skills of social workers. However, it must be remembered that British social workers usually work in the local authority sector, while those who work in STD clinics, including health advisers, are health service employees. This can be a recipe for suspicion, lack of coordination and possibly conflict.

It has been estimated that there are about 400 health advisors in STD clinics, with widely different salaries and training (Sadler, 1988). Some are nurses, some (especially in the north of England) are health visitors, some are ex-contact tracers.[2] Some have had no more than a one-week course at one of the three National AIDS Counselling Training Centres. Some have the sole contact with the patient from the pre-test stage to breaking the news of the test result. Some only see patients assigned to them by doctors who themselves do pre-test counselling and give the results.

The safer sex study aims to put this confusing picture into an institutional context and to relate that context to an analysis of actual episodes of counselling. So the aim, as it were, is to look 'up' to the institutional structures in which people do counselling or receive it, and to look 'down' in fine detail at the unfolding of individual counselling sessions. This chapter reports on preliminary findings from the study as a whole.

The Institutional Context

HIV infection is the site for a complex sets of relations (economic, political and cultural) between the state, the professions and the potential recipients of care. Since the issue of the state is dealt with effectively elsewhere (Watney, 1987, 1988, 1989), this chapter focuses on the relations within and between professions and their patients or clients. Four areas will be sketched: the competition for resources; client-professional relations; interprofessional conflicts; and intraprofessional differences over theories of care.

Competition for Resources

As I have commented elsewhere, genito-urinary medicine and allied medical practices have moved, almost overnight, from being 'Cinderella' specialisms to well funded, high status work (Silverman, 1989). Before the 1980s, STD work was poorly resourced and had little political impact. Doctors could expect to produce simple cures with antibiotics and were rewarded with dingy 'special clinics', often secluded from the rest of the hospital. Frequently, they had no status enhancing beds for in-patient care. Counselling and social work back-up were unknown or very limited and routine 'contact-tracing' was one of the few points of entry into the outside world. Today doctors working in this field find themselves in an unexpected spotlight, sought by the media, in control of considerable resources and in the midst of prestigious drug trials. Their role has become as much political as clinical: fighting to get anti-viral drugs from their health authority, sitting on government bodies and acting as gatekeepers for medical and social scientific research.

Counselling for HIV infection and AIDS in British hospitals thus takes place in a political context where the increase in resources has generated a continuing struggle over resource allocation. For instance, it is important for professionals working in genito-urinary departments to maintain their central role in dealing with the crisis. So doctors stress the need to locate HIV 'within the spectrum of other STDs',[3] while Health Advisers underline the importance of their ethics of confidentiality and their experience with contact-tracing. Different battles may be fought over the care of in-patients. Just as genito-urinary medicine may sometimes fight with virology for out-patients, so it can struggle for beds for AIDS patients with, say, chest physicians. As one London doctor put it, 'Whose virus is it?'

Client-Professional Relations

In Britain, these relations have been shaped by the sequence of the impact of HIV infection on different groups. Early in the course of the epidemic, the gay community mobilized its own organization to respond to AIDS through health education campaigns, through establishing 'buddy' systems of support for people with AIDS, and through fighting for welfare and housing benefits. In London, and to some extent in other major cities, the word speedily got about that certain hospitals were the place to be tested (once the availability of treament made it worthwhile to know one's HIV serostatus). Usually in London — which itself helped to preserve anonymity, unlike 'local' hospitals — these clinics were valued because the staff were widely perceived as 'non-judgmental', with a good deal of experience with HIV. Even though relations are good between several of these hospitals and organizations like the Terrence Higgins Trust, both sides recognize the political tensions involved. Community activists still complain, for instance, of hospitals 'dumping people with AIDS on them for crisis support.'[4]

Conversely, in the regional hospitals, client-professional relations appear to be relatively de-politicized. Workers here seem much less worried about the implications of giving researchers access to clients, and clients themselves more readily assent to participate in research. As one health professional said in such a centre: 'We don't get the militant element here'.[5] Nevertheless, some centres seem to have incipient conflict. For instance, a doctor's claim that his STD clinic had good relations with the local gay community was contested by a local community worker who argued that this relationship was limited to one or two middle-class gay men. He suggested that he knew many young, gay men who felt punished or judged at this clinic — which he also described as 'test-happy'.[6]

The relations between injecting drug users and health workers in the context of HIV have been discussed at length elsewhere (see Stimson *et al.*, 1989); here two comments are pertinent. First, injecting drug users largely lack the community organizations available to lesbians and gay men. Second, there is evidence that many existing forms of health provision will be unacceptable to them. For instance, it was suggested by a community worker that one provincial hospital was largely out of touch with the needs of injecting drug users, lacking experience because in the past the latter had not come into much contact with STD clinics. Hence the main conduit for testing in the area seemed to be an infectious diseases clinic.[7]

Outside the gay community and injecting drug users, we are largely faced with unorganized, frightened and apolitical individuals who expect help from hospital services but who are often intimated by the aura of an STD clinic. Two issues currently concern health workers here: coping with a flood of 'worried well' who may demand a series of HIV antibody tests and deny the validity of negative results, and, conversely, negotiating with STD patients about an HIV test for the current Public Health Laboratory Service (PHLS) study of the incidence of HIV infection. An illustration of the de-politicized atmosphere in clinics outside London was provided by the fact that, on one two-day visits to one such clinic, no patient declined to enrol in the PHLS study.

Interprofessional Conflict

A common complaint among patients, community groups and health professionals themselves is that in HIV antibody test counselling staff only want to 'talk' to clients, nobody wants to engage in the battles to obtain welfare and housing benefits. These complaints can be seen most clearly in the overt and covert conflict between health advisors and social workers. These tensions are best illustrated via two ideal type composite accounts generated following interviews with a number of health advisors in sexually transmitted diseases and a number of social workers.

According to many health advisors interviewed, what social workers should do is 'social work'. This means sorting out practical problems, such as benefits and housing. Instead, all they want to do is to talk to patients. They think they know all about counselling but they lack the clinical background and so give the wrong advice. Moreover, they do not pay sufficient attention to confidentiality — the very ethos of STD clinics. They are cut off from clinics and reveal too much at their case conferences. They may even inform the police when they think a crime has been committed. According to this perspective, social workers should let health advisors do the counselling and stick to routine welfare issues.

Social workers on the other hand perceive themselves as able to offer clients long-term care by the same person often in their own home. By aiming to develop a special relationship with their clients based on their past training and experience, they feel able to deal more adequately with emotions and fears. In their view, it is these emotions that are central to professional-client relations in the field of HIV. Consequently, unlike other professionals, who may be satisfied with brief advice-based interviews, 'information-giving' defines the social worker role in far too perfunctory a way. Professionally qualified in counselling, social workers perceive themselves as the proper people to help clients cope with HIV and AIDS. Indeed, their very distance from doctors gives them a more independent perspective.

It is important to stress that we are dealing here with 'ideal types' — these accounts would not necessarily be told in the same way by all such workers. Here, each side stresses its strong points: clinical experience and respect for confidentiality in the case of the health advisors; experience of relevant casework and psychological training in the case of social workers. What is perceived as a strength by one profession, working within a clinical environment in the case of health advisors, is perceived as a deficit by the other, with social workers stessing the independent hierarchy of authority to which they are responsible. Moreover, each invokes its own magic formula: health advisors stress that their patients' anonymity is uniquely protected by an 'Act of Parliament'; social workers emphasize that they too are governed by 'statutory requirements'. Like the battle for the possession of the virus by medical specialities, indeed like sociology's on-and-off struggles with psychology and social policy, we are confronted with the politics of territory.

David Silverman

Intraprofessional Differences

It would be wrong to assume that professions are monolithic groups. For instance, as we shall shortly see, a health advisor may adhere to a mode of counselling remarkably close to that advocated by many social workers. Others, faced with a heavy patient load for pre-test counselling, may concentrate on conveying accurate information in order to obtain informed consent. Still others, with lower patient loads, may manage pre-test counselling sessions of up to forty-five minutes, based on theoretical models that may be fundamentally at variance with individualized, psycho-pathological theories (see, for example, Miller and Bor, 1988). From the preliminary fieldwork I have carried out, there is material which gives us a glimpse of how such theories work out in practice.

Counselling in Practice

This section focuses on five instances of pre-test counselling. All except one of the extracts chosen focus on the issue of 'safer sex'. It should be stressed that at this early stage of the research, no claim is being made about the representativeness of these extracts, either in relation to the usual work of the individuals concerned or to that of their institutions. The aim is simply to identify and illustrate the existence of certain styles of pre-test counselling.

The Information-Giving Model

In this example, the Counsellor (C) is a health advisor in an STD clinic. The Patient (P) is a heterosexual man in his 20s. Before the extract begins, C has explained what the HIV antibody test means. This has focused on what antibodies are and how long they take to develop. The rest of their conversation is concerned with the giving of information.

> C: When someone is told that they're HIV positive there are various things that are really common sense if you think about it that they need to do/
> P: /yeah
> C: If someone is injecting drugs then we preferably try and get them to stop injecting or if not make sure that they've got sterile equipment at least but the most important thing is that they then (0.5) adopt safer sexual practices. Do you know what we mean by safer sex?
> P: Yeah, you mean a condom
> C: Right what else

P: Er not going well not having more than one sexual partner.

C: /yeah

P: And the rest of the — I mean I've had all the ( )

C: /right, um, obviously.

P: /coughs/

C: /you know, full sex isn't everything although obviously over the last few years this is what has come to be accepted. We also ask people to consider doing things like that — massage, mutual masturbation, that kind of thing, um, without necessarily going the whole hog and having penetrative sex (1.0) as I said earlier, people who've got a negative test you know if they've got to repeat it later on or even if they're not it's an idea from that point, you know, to look after themselves (0.5)/

Before this extract began, the counsellor stayed within the information-giving mode (offering a mini-biology lesson on antibodies). She maintains the same approach when telling the patient what an 'HIV positive' person 'needs to do'. However, via two questions, she tries to enter into the patient's sense of the phenomenon at hand ('safer sex'). Yet the patient's answers are not explored, and the counsellor then launches into an advice-format once more, based on what 'we'd advise'.

For the purposes of this chapter, this brief extract serves as an example of a paramedical method used in STD clinics. The stress throughout is upon getting informed consent to the HIV antibody test. Much emphasis is, therefore, placed on understanding body functioning and on civil rights issues such as confidentiality and insurance. The danger with this approach is that the standardized agenda may result in an information overload for the patient. The transitions from information-giving to questioning about the patient's understandings and back again are abrupt, and it is doubtful whether the information given engages with the patient's own understandings and practices. It may also be the case that, no doubt unintentionally, the patient is getting the confusing and politically dangerous message that 'safer sex' is something for people who are HIV antibody positive, whereas a negative test result means that you simply need to 'look after' yourself.

The Medical Model

In many centres, especially in London, pre-test counselling is done by doctors and only those patients perceived to be at high risk of a positive test result are referred to health advisors. The standard format in thse situations often involves a history-taking sequence followed by a physical examination. Both of the following extracts re-enact the medical model found in many other consultations.

C: Um and we'll see you next week with the results of those and with your blood test result (0.5) now then if I can just say in general terms, there's a little bit more advice. Obviously you *had* a casual episode of intercourse and it's worried you enough to come along . . . .

P: Mmhmm/

C: /and have the test taken, umm, and what we are really trying to advise all people to do not talking just specifically to you but in general, that really do do have to advise people to be very careful about any sort of casual intercourse.

P: Mmhmm

C: The sensible rule is *no risk sex*. No risk sex means having *no penetrative* intercourse with anybody about whom you don't know enough

P: Mmhmm

C: To be certain that they aren't going to pass on some infection and I'm not just talking about HIV infection, although that is of course a cause for a lot of concern. We're actually seeing a lot of other sexually transmitted infections a lot of *warts* and things like that again are trans . . . you know are transferred, umm, sexually. Now if you're going to have intercouse with people about whom you really don't know about, then it *is* important that you use a sheath. But a sheath *isn't a foolproof method* of avoiding an infection *so* don't be conned into thinking that if you use a sheath you are all right, you're not at risk. You are still at risk of certain infections. The *basic* rule is to *try* to stay as much as you can within *one permanent* faithful *relationship* and if you're not in that sort of relationship and you're having relationships all over, then *avoid* penetrative intercourse.

Here, unlike in the previous example, no attempt is made to ground the advice (given here to a single woman in her 20s) in the patient's own understandings. Later a question time may be granted, but, as one might expect, the patient only asks for more details of attending for the test result. It is dangerous to assume that doctors *cannot* for some reason, perhaps because of their training or perceived interests, talk in any other way to patients. The following extract shows an alternative approach used by a doctor with a gay man in his 30s:

C: You've come along for HIV testing have you?

P; Yes.

C: Oh right (0.5) what's prompted . . . ?

P: Umm, I just feel that I've got . . . I've just got to the stage where I feel I'd like to know either way

C: Right have you been getting *problems* at all?

P: No.

C: /shuffling papers (0.5) Right, and have you had contacts in the past that have been *risky*?

P: Ahh, no.

C: You're a gay man.

P: Yeah.

C: Do you have a regular partner?

P: No.

C: (long pause) And you practice safe sex normally?

P: *Yes*

C: What does safe sex mean to you?

P: (0.5) Umm (2.0) no fucking.

C: Right, non penetrative.

P: Yes.

C: Do you still have oral sex?

P: Yes.

C: /(1.0) *and* do your partners ejaculate into your mouth when/they

P: /no.

C: Right (0.5) so it sounds like you practice safe sex (17 seconds) Right and how's your health been?

P: It's fine, fine.

Taken from the start of the consultation, this extract shows how the doctor begins by giving the patient the opportunity to state what his understandings are. Unlike the exhortations to the doctor's notion of safer sex in the previous extract, we find here approval being given to the patient's own account of these practices.

The Systems Model

The patient-tailored information given by the doctor in the following extract best illustrates the kind of counselling which Miller and Bor (1988) describe as systems-counselling. Based on family therapy, it seeks to identify patients' understandings and practices in the context of their support systems within the community. In the following extract, a clinical psychologist is using this method with a heterosexual man in his 30s.

C: You've not had HIV testing before

P: No (6.0)

C: Have you ever received blood at all?

P: No.

C: And have you ever given blood?

P: No.

C: No. Do you know why I asked those questions?

P: For in relation to HIV?

C: Mm

P: Mm

C: (?) what is it or (?) tell me/

P: /it's one of the ways it can be transferred, so certainly if I received blood I could receive HIV infected (0.5) blood.

C: Right and that's why I was asking about sexual partners as well.

P: Mm

C: Because it can have transferred um during sexual intercourse — anal or vaginal/intercourse

P: /mm . . .

C: What do you understand about your own (0.5) risk for HIV?

P: Well, hhh, I suppose I'm in one of the high risk categories because I've had a lot of partners (0.5) I don't know what to call a lot certainly over a hundred.

Notice here the three opportunities that the patient is given to offer his own version of the risks of HIV infection. Later on, the counsellor will elicit the patient's network of family and friends and, using material from his previous answers, will generate his sense of how significant others would respond to this present situation and possible diagnoses. In this counselling framework, this leads to a discussion of 'dreaded issues' which aims to clarify for the patient his support network and makes it unlikely that he will become overdependent on clinic-based support.

The systems model seems to offer a well thought out, easily learned analytic basis to counselling which avoids paternalistic advice-giving and patient overdependence. It also generates a method whereby patients can ask questions about themselves, with possible unintended consequences, however, that will be considered later.

The Psycho-Pathological Model

'Questions concerning the client's sexuality may raise profound feelings of anger as well as relief . . . . Anger may also reflect transference issues stemming from the client's perception of the question as a negative parental injunction' (Shernoff, 1988). Many social workers define HIV/AIDS counselling in terms of emotions and fears (see above). Occasionally, as in the comment above, social work practice is located within an explicit neo-Freudian model. However, we are not dealing here with discrete theories 'owned' by particular professions. This psycho-pathological vocabulary, coupled with the contemporary themes of 'empowerment' and building up 'self-esteem', is popular among community groups who offer counselling. Moreover, as the following extract shows, some health advisors want to enter into an exploration of emotions and fears. This is more likely to happen where counsellors are freed from routine pre-test counselling and have the time to pursue these issues if they choose. The following conversation is thirty minutes into the consultation. The patient is a heterosexual man in his 20s who has just been referred by a doctor because he is perceived to be 'at risk':

> C: Umm you've been through the support bit and the confidentiality bit right. umm.
> P: Umm.
> C: Right yes, umm, I think there's one thing that we may not have looked at in great detail is some of the fear that may be around, umm, it's fine to sort of say that well yes I was at risk for this area and this this this and this and actually what's happened to all the feelings inside you. Have you had times when you've panicked about it?
> P: (?) how I feel about it (1.0) well umm let's think/footsteps sound/I do have fear
> C: Right
> P: Umm (4 seconds) because I I umm being an ex-statistician .
> C: heh heh
> P: And study statistics I do understand the the odds and I. (0.5) so I know it it's fairly unlikely at least I think it's probably very unlikely that I've got it.
> C: Humm
> P: But I do have fear umm because I don't particularly like I've thought I'm a bit of a hypochondriac
> C: Umm
> P: I don't particularly like the idea knowing really how all of this is coming on
> C: Uhuu
> P: I don't think anyone does
> C: Uhh

This sequence is set up by the counsellor's questions about 'fear', 'feelings' and 'panic'. Unlike the 'information-giving model', this approach is compatible with eliciting patients' own versions of their experience and practices, and provides patient-tailored information. However, in comparison with the 'systems model', two tensions arise. First, it may individualize patients by looking at them in terms of a pathological model unlocated in a social context. Second, if used 'successfully', it may offer more than it can give, by encouraging overdependence. Depending on which way you look at it, it may be an advantage or a disadvantage that the patient in the above extract asks if he can come back soon to talk again.

Policy Implications

As a researcher in this field, I have been impressed by the commitment and enthusiasm of the counsellors I have observed, many of whom work within severe time constraints. There is no absence of goodwill on the part of staff, nor is there any evidence that there is any one *wrong* professional background for counselling. Nevertheless, certain directions for policy are beginning to emerge from the study, sometimes supported by other research.

First, in the clinics I visited most pre-test counselling is now sought by heterosexuals. This follows the American pattern, both in New York (Grabau and Morse, 1988) and in San Francisco (Evans *et al.*, 1988). Although the vast majority of test results are negative, most of those seeking the test have engaged in risky behaviours in a wide range of social contexts. This underlines the need to emphasize risk reduction behaviour, regardless of HIV antibody test results (Kageles *et al.*, 1988). Safer sex can be discussed in an individualized way which diversifies the options available to patients (Sankary, 1988), while clarifying the specific nature of the problems that a particular patient is facing (Bor and Miller, 1988a).

Second, the professional field in which counsellors have been trained is not significant in terms of the quality of their work (Pacharzina *et al.*, 1988). We saw in connection with the medical model how two doctors used different methods to discuss risk reduction. Again, as in the context of the psycho-pathological model, there are sometimes similarities between the theories used by different professions.

Third, one of the major problems of pre-test counselling is the danger of information overload. The need to obtain informed consent often leads to extended 'lectures' on biology and confidentiality. Two possible solutions suggest themselves. First, by encouraging patients to display their knowledge and fears, staff can shorten their turns at talk and tailor information to the client. Second, the amount of information that still has to be absorbed, together with the strain of presenting oneself for an HIV antibody test, may mean that pre-test counselling is not a very efficient site for exploring risk reduction. Post-test counselling, providing the result is negative, may be a far more effective time to discuss safer sex.

Fourth, many of the counselling sessions I have observed face problems of integrating service provision with counselling. As noted earlier, few workers relish attending to such nitty-gritty issues as welfare benefits and housing. One tempting solution is to allocate counselling around the HIV antibody test to health advisors and to allocate social workers only to those who are HIV antibody positive or who have AIDS. After all, they are the ones who will need such services (Chester, 1987). However, as Chester himself recognizes, provisions like this run the risk of sacrificing continuity of care, implying that relationships have to be re-created afresh at each transition point in the trajectory of care. Given this, it may be preferable to see organizational structures created where there is not such a rigid separation as at present between counselling and service provision.

Fifth, as Freudenberg *et al.* (1988) argue, 'institutional factors such as time availability, patient flow and management's perceived commitment to AIDS prevention strongly influence how effectively AIDS counsellors use newly acquired skills.' In a British context, one might add that an additional institutional problem is the present lack of a clear career structure for health advisors. Apart from the institutional solutions that are required here, one remedy might lie in methods of counselling which reduce patient dependency on the counsellor, while offering a way of establishing the patient's major concerns (see Bor and Miller, 1988a; Miller and Bor, 1988).

Sixth, there is a danger of assuming that risk reduction can be raised as a topic only through mass media campaigns or through counselling, usually at STD clinics. Gay men have shown the important role of locally generated dicussion, particularly in the context of videos which eroticize safer sex (D'Eramo *et al.*, 1988). Street work with prostitutes in Plymouth (Roberts, 1989) and interventions in 'pick-up' bars in San Francisco (Stall and McKusick, 1988) suggest the value of non-hospital-based work. Family planning clinics may also offer an underutilized site for risk reduction counselling (Bowen *et al.*, 1988).

A Counselled Society?

'[In the counselling exchange] we learn what we are like, what our experience is, how things are with us' (Taylor, 1986: 78). This chapter concludes with an aside which readers are invited to read or ignore as it pleases them. It is based not on an evaluation of styles of counselling but upon a reflection of the cultural significance of its increasing use for all kinds of personal problems.

I begin by returning to the extract cited in connection with the psycho-pathological model and noting the facility with which the patient is able to formulate his fears and feelings. It is tempting to discount this, given that he is middle-class and admits to being 'a bit of a hypochondriac'. But here is another more forceful example.

C: Right we've got about half an hour together so how best do you want to use this time

P: Well I'd forgotten why I was coming because of what's happened since

C: Mm

P: Umm, hhh, no, originally I wanted to come and see you because I thought (?) I was at the stage I could sensibly start thinking about (0.5) AIDS

C: Mm

> *P*: Rather than um depression.
>
> *C*: Mm
>
> *P*: I thought I'd got through that and was strong enough to think about it and talk about it and in my diary and this is without a word out of (?) I've written in today's entry/for my appointment.
>
> *C*: /mm
>
> *P*: (name of counsellor excised) where do we go
>
> *C*: Mm, do you still feel strong enough today to talk about AIDS/sensibly
>
> *P*: /yeah/the question's still there
>
> *C*: Mm what would you consider sensibly?
>
> *P*: What would I consider/sensi-
>
> *C*: /you said yourself that you'd been strong enough to think about AIDS sensibly rather than as a depression what would sensibly be?
>
> *P*: hhh in an analytical way
>
> *C*: Mm

The patient here is an HIV seropositive haemophiliac man. Notice two things: he refers to being 'at the stage I could sensibly start thinking about AIDS'; and later, when he is asked the question, he asks, 'in an analytical way'. This is interesting because it shows graphically how counselling constructs a particular subject, one who examines himself. What it suggests, if pushed to extremes, is that counsellors face subjects whom they themselves have constructed.

But this patient has HIV infection. What about those who do not? Think of the prevalence of counselling one form or another in the problem pages of magazines. Think about counselling as it is used in a whole variety of therapeutic contexts. As noted above, Taylor (1986) has treated counselling as an emblem of post-modern society. This parallels Rose's (1989) book on counselling in which he asks, 'How has personal meaning become definitive of our existence? How have questions of truth become more important than questions of wisdom or faith and tradition? How have questions of efficacy, scientific solutions, become more important than ethics?'

What seems to be at stake here is the nature of normality itself. Hence counselling is not just about techniques of the control or regulation of problematic behaviour. It is also about encouraging or inciting us to speak (Foucault, 1979). It is about the problems of living, choosing a lifestyle and finding a meaning in the choices we have made. So we have developed what Rose calls 'professions of the self', and these professions have what he calls 'an expertise of subjectivity'. They provide us with a grammar for speaking about personal troubles and with techniques for dealing with them. In considering counselling, then, we are looking at a phenomenon that just might be a nodal point of contemporary cultural life. To view HIV counselling as part of a progressive programme of 'enablement' or 'empowerment' must, therefore, not blind us to a broader cultural agenda of which it is inescapably a part.[8]

Notes

1   While I was present recently at one clinic, the London tabloid newspaper, *The Sun*, ran a story that it was 'impossible' to contract AIDS (as it calls HIV) heterosexually. During that day and two days afterwards, nobody came for an HIV test.
2   Contact-tracers are used in STD clinics to identify the sexual partners of people with sexually transmitted diseases and to request their attendance for diagnosis and, if necessary, treatment. The source of information (the 'index case') is not identified to the partner.
3   This was personally asserted to me by consultants in genito-urinary medicine and by some health advisors working in their department.
4   This was a comment made to me by a worker at a leading community support agency.
5   This was a comment made to me by a health advisor in a regional centre.
6   Comment taken from field notes.
7   It may well be that outreach programmes like that run in Plymouth by a senior health advisor and a drugs worker may be more effective for injecting drug users than conventional hospital-based clinics.
8   Transcription symbols used throughout this chapter:
    C   Counsellor
    P   Patient
    (0.5) pause in seconds
    (?)   untranscribable utterance
    test emphasized word
    /   overlapping utterances.

References

AGGLETON, P. (1989) 'Evaluating Health Education about AIDS', in P. AGGLETON, G. HART, and P. DAVIES (eds), *AIDS: Social Representations, Social Practices*. Lewes, Falmer Press.

AGGLETON, P., HART, G. and DAVIES, P. (eds) (1989) *AIDS: Social Representations, Social Practices*. Lewes, Falmer Press.

BIGGAR, R., *et al.* (1988) 'Effect of Knowledge of HIV Status upon Sexual Activity among Homosexual Men'. Paper given at the Fourth International Conference on AIDS, Stockholm.

BOR, R. and MILLER, R. (1988a) 'The Essentials of AIDS Counselling for the Clinician'. Paper given at the Fourth International Conference on AIDS, Stockholm.

BOR, R. and MILLER, R. (1988b) 'Managing Staff Stress from Working with Patients with AIDS/HIV'. Paper given at the Fourth International Conference on AIDS, Stockholm

BOWEN, G. S., *et al.* (1988) 'AIDS Risk Behaviour in Family Planning Clinics'. Paper given at the Fourth International Conference on AIDS, Stockholm.

CHESTER, R. (1987) *Advice, Support and Counselling for the HIV Positive*. A Report for the DHSS, University of Hull, Institute for Health Studies.

D'ERAMO, J. E., *et al.* (1988) 'The '800 Men' Project: A Systematic Evaluation of AIDS Prevention Programs Demonstrating the Efficacy of Erotic, Sexually Explicit Safer Sex Education on Gay and Bisexual Men at Risk for AIDS'. Paper given at the Fourth International Conference on AIDS, Stockholm.

DE RON, C., *et al.* (1988) 'Swedish HIV Legislation: Two Year's Experience'. Paper given at the Fourth International Conference on AIDS, Stockholm.

EUROPEAN STUDY GROUP (1989) 'Risk Factors for Male to Female Transmission of HIV', *British Medical Journal* 298, pp. 411–15.

EVANS, P. E., *et al.* (1988) 'Trends in HIV Testing and Counselling Programs in San Francisco'. Paper given at the Fourth International Conference on AIDS, Stockholm.

FOUCAULT, M. (1979) *The History of Sexuality*, Volume 1, London, Allen Lane.

David Silverman

FREUDENBERG, N., et al. (1988) 'An Evaluation of a Training Program for AIDS Counsellors'. Paper given at the Fourth International Confrence on AIDS, Stockholm.

GRABAU, J. C. and MORSE, D. L. (1988) 'Changing Patterns of Client Characteristics and Seropositivity at Upstate New York HIV Alternate Test Sites'. Paper given at the Fourth International Conference on AIDS, Stockholm.

GREEN, J. (1988) 'Projecting the Impact of AIDS on Health Services in Western Europe'. Paper given at the Fourth International Conference on AIDS, Stockholm.

HEARST, N. and HULLEY, S. (1988) 'Preventing the Heterosexual Spread of AIDS: Are We Giving Our Patients the Best Advice', Journal of the American Medical Association, 259, 16, pp. 2428–32.

HENRIKSSON, B. (1988) 'Prevention Policies in Sweden'. Paper given at the Fourth International Conference on AIDS, Stockholm.

HERLITZ, C. and BRORSSON, B. (1988) 'The AIDS Epidemic in Sweden: Estimates of Costs, 1986, 1987, 1990'. Paper given at the Fourth International Conference on AIDS, Stockholm.

HULL, H. F., et al. (1988) 'Comparison of Antibody Prevalence in Patients Consenting to and Declining HIV Antibody Testing', Journal of the American Medical Association, 260, pp. 935–8.

JOHNSON, W. D. (1988) 'The Impact of Mandatory Reporting on HIV Seropositive Persons in South Carolina'. Paper given at the Fourth International Conference on AIDS, Stockholm.

KAGELES, S. M., et al. (1988) 'A Comparison of Current and Early Utilization of Alternative Test Sites for HIV Antibody Testing'. Paper given at the Fourth International Conference on AIDS, Stockholm.

LIDMAN, K., et al. (1988) 'Contact Tracing in a Country with Low HIV Prevalence'. Paper given at the Fourth International Conference on AIDS, Stockholm.

LOVEDAY, C., et al. (1989) 'Human Immunodeficiency Viruses in Patients Attending a Sexually Transmitted Disease Clinic in London, 1982–7' British Medical Journal, 298, pp. 419–22.

MASSARELLI, V. B. (1988) 'Council of Europe Recommendations on a Common European Public Health Policy to Fight AIDS'. Paper given at the Fourth International Conference on AIDS, Stockholm.

MILLER, D. (1987) 'HIV Counselling, Some Practical Problems and Issues'. Journal of Royal Society of Medicine, 80, 278–88.

MILLER, R. and BOR, R. (1988) AIDS: A Guide to Clinical Counselling. London, Science Press.

MULLEADY, G., et al. (1989) 'Injecting Drug Use and HIV Infection: Intervention Strategies for Harm Minimization', in P. AGGLETON, G. HART, and P. DAVIES (eds), AIDS: Social Representations, Social Practices. Lewes, Falmer Press.

NELKIN, D. (1987) 'AIDS and the Social Sciences: Review of Useful Knowledge and Research Needs', Reviews of Infectious Diseases. 9, 5, pp. 5–21.

PACHARZINA, K., et al. (1988) 'AIDS Counselling Skills for Health Professionals in Public Health Centres and Private AIDS Organizations'. Paper given at the Fourth International Conference on AIDS, Stockholm.

PADIAN, N. (1987) 'Heterosexual Transmission of AIDS: International Perspectives and National Projections', Reviews of Infectious Diseases, 9, 5, pp. 947–60.

PUBLIC HEALTH LABORATORY SERVICE (1989) 'HIV Infection in Patients Attending Clinics for Sexually Transmitted Disease in England and Wales', British Medical Journal. 298, pp. 415–18.

REES, M., et al. (1988) 'The Impact of AIDS/HIV on the Activities and Costs of St. Stephen's Hospital, London'. Paper given at the Fourth International Conference on AIDS, Stockholm.

ROBERTS, T. (1989) 'A Street Counselling Service for Prostitutes'. Paper given at Forum on Communication Issues in HIV Infection and AIDS, Royal Society of Medicine, London.

ROSE, N. (1989) Governing the Soul: Technologies of Human Subjectivity. London, Routledge.

SADLER, C. (1988) 'Sexually Transmitted Disease, More Than Tea and Sympathy', Nursing Times, 84, 49, pp. 30–4.

SANKARY, T. M. (1988) 'Diversity in Risk Factors, Seroprevalence, Urgency, and Utility of HIV-Antibody Testing'. Paper given at the Fourth International Conference on AIDS, Stockholm

SHERNOFF, M. (1988) 'Integrating Safer-Sex Counseling into Social Work Practice', Social Casework, The Journal of Contemporary Social Work. pp. 334–39.

SILVERMAN, D. (1987) Communication and Medical practice: Social Relations in the Clinic. London and Beverley Hills, Sage.

SILVERMAN, D. (1989) 'Making Sense of a Precipice, Constituting Identity in an HIV Clinic', in P. AGGLETON, G. HART, and P. DAVIES (eds), *AIDS: Social Representations, Social Practices*. Lewes, Falmer Press.

STALL, R. nad McKUSICK, L. (1988) 'The Prevalence of High Risk Sexual Behaviour among Heterosexual and Homosexual 'Pick Up' Bar Patrons in San Francisco'. Paper given at the Fourth International Conference on AIDS, Stockholm.

STIMSON, G. V., *et al.* (1989) 'Syringe-Exchange Schemes in England and Scotland: Evaluating a New Service for Drug Users', in P. AGGLETON, G. HART, and P. DAVIES (eds), *AIDS: Social Representations, Social Practices*. Lewes, Falmer Press.

TAYLOR, C. (1986) 'Foucault on Freedom and Truth', in D. HOY, (ed.), *Foucault, A Critical Reader*. London, Basil Blackwell.

US NATIONAL CENTER FOR HEALTHSTATISTICS, D. A. DAWSON (1989) 'AIDS Knowledge and Attitudes for September 1988: Provisional Data from the National Health Interview Survey'. *Advance Data from Vital and Health Statistics*, No. 164, DHHS Pub. No. (DHS) 89–13250, Public Health Service, Hyattsville, MD., USA.

WARWICK, I., *et al.* (1988) 'Constructing Commonsense: Young People's Beliefs about AIDS', *Sociology of Health and Illness*, 10, pp. 213–33.

WATNEY, S. (1987) *Policing Desire*. London, Comedia/Methuen.

WATNEY, S. (1988) 'AIDS, Moral Panic Theory and Homophobia', in P. AGGLETON, and H. HOMANS (eds), *Social Aspects of AIDS*. Lewes, Falmer Press.

WATNEY, S. (1989) 'The Subject of AIDS', in P. AGGLETON, G. HART, and P. DAVIES (eds), *AIDS: Social Representations, Social Practices*. Lewes, Falmer Press.

WEEKS, J. (1989) 'AIDS: The Intellectual Agenda', in P. AGGLETON, G. HART, and P. DAVIES (eds), *AIDS: Social Representations, Social Practices*. Lewes, Falmer Press.

WINKELSTEIN, W., *et al.* (1987) 'The San Francisco Men's Health Study III: Reduction in HIV Transmission among Homosexual/Bisexual Men, 1982–1986'. *American Journal of Public Health*, 9, pp. 685–9.

Chapter 15

Local Authorities and HIV-Related Illness

Terry Cotton with Vijay Kumari

AIDS is perhaps the single greatest challenge ever faced by local authorities. But, although HIV and AIDS are new medical problems, it does not necessarily follow that all the issues surrounding them are new or that we require novel methods and systems to cope with them effectively and efficiently (Foy, 1988). Issues such as confidentiality in relation to personal information, staff training and support, anti-discriminatory functioning, health and safety, staff and client consultation in decision-making, and policy and guidelines are all matters which are familiar to local authorities. In effect, AIDS has exposed the inadequacies of local authority policy and practices, and has brought about an urgency to examine each of these concerns afresh. The challenge of AIDS means that local authorities, as providers of health and social services, must confront these issues and tackle the very questions which until now have been so easily brushed aside.

For some time now, Hammersmith and Fulham Council in London have been at the forefront of local authority work with HIV-related illness. In July 1989 there were over eighty people with AIDS living in the area for which the authority has responsibility, and support services are provided to over fifty people. Over 280 people were HIV antibody positive and unwell, and there were an estimated 3,000–5,000 people with the virus in the borough.

This chapter offers a brief case study of the Council's experience in facing the challenge of AIDS, and developing community support services that are sensitive and appropriate for people with HIV-related illnesses. Three main areas of interest are covered: first, how the authority was forced to confront issues such as staff training and discrimination, and some of the problems that were faced in tackling these issues; second, the range of services made available to people with HIV-related illnesses; and finally, the planning mechanisms which were developed within both the local authority and the health authority.

Issues and Problems

Since 1983, Hammersmith and Fulham Council has provided a comprehensive range of services to people with HIV-related illnesses. However, until 1985 the number of cases had been few, and the authority had worked from the assumption that the situation would remain unchanged—that AIDS would not become 'a problem'. In early 1985 two incidents dramatically illustrated how misguided this assumption had been. The first concerned a client with AIDS who had died in hospital. His name and cause of death appeared on the front page of a local newspaper, along with reports that his hospital room had been fumigated and that the hospital porters had refused to take his body to the mortuary. The client had been supported by six different home helps while at home. Predictably, the reaction of the home helps and their union was one of fear and anxiety, and the whole situation rapidly turned into an industrial relations problem, with many home helps and 'Meals-on-Wheels' staff refusing to work with people with AIDS (PWAs). Hammersmith and Fulham Council responded by organizing a study day for its 350 home helps. On the study day, the Home Care staff managed to raise 130 questions of the following nature:

Will I be forced to work with PWAs?
Can I refuse to go in?
Will I be told a client has AIDS?
Do they really know how you can catch AIDS?
Can I catch AIDS from client's money?
Can I tell my family I'm working with PWAs?
What training do I get
Why should I work with homosexuals?

Many home helps who were working with AIDS did not wish to be identified on the study day for fear of rejection by their colleagues and friends. This fact, coupled with the type of questions raised by the Home Care staff, highlighted the scale of the problem facing the Council.

The second incident concerned an employee who informed the Council that he had been diagnosed with AIDS and wished to be re-deployed. While much attention had been placed on clients, little consideration had been given to employees with HIV-related illnesses. Questions surrounding confidentiality and reactions of colleagues required urgent attention. The Council's response to the two events was twofold: a corporate group was established who produced a policy guidance booklet for managers and staff; and the Council embarked on a large training initiative.

In terms of developing service provision, AIDS forced the authority to examine issues which had previously been ignored: issues such as health and safety, confidentiality, discrimination, attitudes towards gay men and injecting drug users, and staff support. AIDS highlighted a range of deficiencies in existing work practices, particularly those to do with good standards of hygiene, regardless of the HIV status of the client. The involvement of the trade unions in this process was vital, since they can ensure that discriminatory practices do not occur and that members do not place themselves at occupational risk from HIV. The leadership of local trade unions also played an important role in assisting management to take into account the possible industrial relations problems which might arise, while trade union forums provided an appropriate platform for discussion on AIDS. The corporate group found that staff supervisors and managers were also voicing the same fears and prejudices as the staff. Setting up training sessions for shop stewards and joint staff committees has been important, since many members have initially turned to their shop stewards for advice rather than approach management.

The Council's guidelines were drawn up with the trade unions and were approved by full Council in January 1987. The guidelines sought to ensure that appropriate and sensitive services were provided to people with HIV-related illnesses, and to ensure that they did not experience discrimination in service provision. Additionally, policies, practices and procedures were to be regularly reviewed and updated. Policy and guidelines are crucial aspects of developing services for people with HIV-related illness. Hammersmith and Fulham's guidelines, for example, state that a breach of confidential information about their clients and their diagnoses can lead to disciplinary action being taken. With AIDS, confidentiality and the need to know has always been a contentious issue. AIDS has led us to examine our general practices regarding confidentiality. We have often worked in a climate where we have been extremely liberal in passing information from one person to another, without considering the implications of our actions. It is important to re-assess present practices, while bearing in mind the following points. First, the 'need to know' is not based on infection control concerns, but on the need to provide appropriate care. For example, home helps are told with client consent. Second, the client may need to be assured that giving information is about providing appropriate care and that the information will be kept confidential. Third, in order to avoid an accidental disclosure of information, there is a need to ascertain exactly who is, and who is not, aware of the person's diagnosis.

The refusal of some staff to work with people with AIDS was another area of much concern. All new staff recruited to the authority are informed at an interview of the Council's policy on HIV infection and of the Council's expectations. For existing staff, the guidelines state that they should not be instructed to work with people with AIDS if they refuse. We have found that if staff members refuse to work with people with HIV-related illnesses, then talking about their concerns with an informed person has often helped. Training is obviously an important area. There is a compulsory initial training course for all home care staff, with optional further training, including a three-day counselling skills course. Home care staff are given priority for places on these courses as they usually have more client contact than any other professionals. As a rule, we do not force a member of staff who has refused or is clearly homophobic to care for a gay man with AIDS. We have found that good training greatly reduces staff anxiety and fear. The Social Services Department always includes people with HIV infection on all its training courses. For staff to hear someone with HIV/ARC/AIDS talk about their experiences is often the most powerful part of a training course. Staff can hear first-hand what it is like to live with a HIV-related illness, and can also empathize and begin to consider how this person could easily be a member of their family, a close friend or indeed themselves.

The specific need for personal support for social workers has been discussed in more detail elsewhere (Davison, 1988). In Hammersmith and Fulham, many social workers and home carers working with people with AIDS frequently inform us of their feelings of isolation and stress. Working with people with AIDS can be a very stressful and sad experience, and for staff to function well when working with people with AIDS, they themselves need strong support. Peer group support is encouraged within the authority, and we now have four staff support groups which carers are able to attend during work time. The staff consider it an important opportunity to exchange information, experiences and feelings.

Discrimination is probably the largest single issue in AIDS, and the illness has become inextricably linked with male homosexuality. Particularly in the early days, staff anxieties about working with people with AIDS included not only fear of infection but also hostility and prejudice towards gay men and injecting drug users. These two groups were seen as the 'guilty perpetrators' of HIV infection, while children and people with haemophilia were considered the 'innocent victims'. Given that gay men and injecting drug users have been the main groups affected by HIV in Britain, they will form a majority of the people seeking local authority support (Bebbington and Warren, 1988). The majority of people we have supported have been gay men, and it is has been important for our staff to examine their own attitudes and feelings towards gay men. Indeed, the general training of health and social workers needs closer examination, for it has traditionally focused on the conventional heterosexual family to the detriment of other units (Harvey, 1988). Clients are often concerned about how staff may react to them, so it may be helpful if they can be introduced while the client is still in hospital. It is important for health and social workers to express their anxieties and concerns to the client. Indeed, not only clients but also their families, friends and lovers may have anxieties, and they will need to be assured that they can talk to someone who is 'safe', someone who does not make moral judgments, and someone who can offer assistance in decision-making (Vernon, 1987). Honesty is fundamental in supporting clients and maintaining a quality relationship between staff and client.

Another important issue is consultation and partnership. People with HIV-related illnesses are, generally speaking, young, often articulate, and frequently knowledgable about their illness. Consulting and involving the person in any decision affecting them are vital. It is essentially a matter of partnership not one of assuming that we, as service providers, know what is best for 'them'. Hammersmith and Fulham Council includes many people with HIV-related illnesses on various planning forums on AIDS established within the Council and the health authority.

Service Provision

The greatest impact on demand for services has been placed on the Social Services Department. Through the provision of home help services, the role of domiciliary care has been very important. A range of services has been involved in the care of people with HIV-related illnesses: the Hospital Discharge Team who provide intensive support for up to eight weeks after discharge, the Area Home Help Service who provide practical tasks to assist daily living, the Home Care Team who work particularly with people facing terminal illness, and who can provide respite and overnight care, and finally, the specialist home helps who work with children and families at risk. It has been found that in the three to six months before death, the equivalent of a full-time home help is often required. Good liaison between the Home Care Manager and hospital services no doubt facilitates planned discharge and an early assessment of the client's needs in the community. Indeed, the very process of liaison builds trust and confidence between the client and available community services.

The issue of respite care is one which we have recently been considering. Respite care has been provided to give the carers of people with AIDS a much deserved and needed break, particularly in case of AIDS Dementia Complex (ADC). Our respite care facilities need to be developed and possibly examined with certain questions in mind. For example, should respite care be placed in the client's home?

Another service which is being examined is 'Meals-on-Wheels' which we have been providing to people with HIV-related illness. A recent review of this service with the Meals Service Manager, Community Dietician and Clinical Nurse has highlighted the specialist dietary needs of people with HIV-related illnesses, and we are currently working to ensure that healthier and more varied diets are provided.

The role of the Area Social Worker is important in many ways: in undertaking an early and wide ranging assessment of the client's physical, financial, social and emotional needs; in co-ordinating health district and local authority community services; in acting as an advocate in relation to welfare benefit and housing problems; and in providing longer-term counselling support to people with HIV-related illnesses and their carers. Social workers need to ensure that a care plan is drawn up to meet the needs of the client and that this is regularly reviewed as the client's physical, social and emotional needs change.

Visual handicap specialist social workers are important in cases of cytomegalovirus retinitis as they can assist in rehabilitation at home and can loan various pieces of visual handicap equipment. Specialist workers have also been involved in cases where clients fear they may develop CMV retinitis. Occupational therapists can take a full assessment of the client's physical needs in order that the loaned equipment and adaptations can be provided. They can also offer advice about the physical care needs of the client, particularly if the client becomes increasingly disabled as a result of AIDS-related illness. Under the Chronically Sick and Disabled Persons Act, social services can also provide clients with telephones and travel permits.

The Housing Services Department's role has been to provide general advice on housing problems, for example, where rent arrears occur because of inability to pay. The department has rehoused people because of homelessness, harassment, or where ill health constitutes a need to be rehoused to more suitable accommodation. It has also provided adaptations and improved heating. The importance of good housing cannot be overstated. A safe, secure, warm and accessible living environment offering people control over their lives is a key component of the support systems that enable people with HIV-related illness to continue to live in the community.

Other council departments have also been involved in AIDS-related work. We have, for example, been running an AIDS awareness week through the Advice and Law Centres, and the Libraries Division. This campaign has been particularly aimed at women, and a health education and advice campaign targeting the various ethnic minority groups in the Borough is being developed.

Planning Mechanisms

A task-orientated planning team for HIV infection has been established with Riverside Health Authority. It consists of representatives from the Health Authority, local authority, Community Health Council, Family Practitioner Committee, housing associations, local voluntary organizations and AIDS organizations. It aims to develop policies and practices in the provision of services, and is considering issues such as information, models of care, service development, the provision of resources, and the balance of care to ensure that different bodies provide their services in a complementary rather than competitive manner.

Within the Council, two planning teams have been established. In the Social Services Department, the HIV Policy and Practice Group is considering policy, practice and resource issues in the provision of social services to people with HIV-related illnesses. The membership of the group includes frontline staff such as home helps and social workers as well as the Director of Social Services. It also includes representatives from the local AIDS Housing Needs Planning Team who are considering the development of policy and practice regarding housing services for people with HIV-related illness, and are also responsible for the training and support of housing staff.

Since 1983, Hammersmith and Fulham Council has provided services to over 200 people with HIV-related illnesses at a cost in 1988/89 of £910,000. Every ten months there has been a twofold increase in the number of referrals for Council services, and this chapter has highlighted the important role of local authorities in the care of people with HIV and AIDS. Existing local authority services can readily be tailored to meet the needs of people living with HIV-related illnesses, and it has been our experience that specialist teams do not necessarily need to be created. Indeed, a combination of specialist and generic services appears to be the way forward to developing practice within the existing service provision system. The Council is committed to providing appropriate and sensitive services to people living with HIV-related illnesses and ensuring that they do not experience discrimination. This has meant addressing many issues. In particular, it has meant examining how we, as service providers, work with our clients. Training for our staff has been vital, and all local authorities must ensure that their staff are adequately trained for future HIV-related work.

In 1985 a borough resident diagnosed with AIDS said that his diagnosis presented him with a choice, ' . . . to give up and die as a victim of AIDS or the chance to make my life right now what it always ought to have been . . . ' There is much uncertainty regarding AIDS, but while the quantity of life for people with AIDS is uncertain, our role as service providers is to ensure that their quality of life is maintained. Over the next decade all local authorities will be involved in the care of people living with AIDS. It is crucial to plan now and not wait for the first person needing support to come forward. AIDS is clearly a community care issue, and, on the whole, British community care is in need of urgent updating. AIDS highlights a multitude of community care issues and the inadequacies of our system, but it also offers the chance to put present systems in order. In many ways, therefore, AIDS challenges local authorities to make the community care system into what it always should have been.

References

BEBBINGTON, A. and WARREN, P. (1988). *AIDS: The Local Authority Response.* Personal Social Services Research Unit (PSSRU), University of Kent at Canterbury.

DAVISON, H. (1988) 'Impact of AIDS on Social Work and Social Workers', *Social Work Today*, 20, p. 5.

FOY, F. (1988) 'HIV Infection and AIDS — What's New?', *Social Work Today*, 19, p. 51.

HARVEY, N. (1988) 'AIDS: A Terminal Disease Becomes a Family Affair', *Social Work Today*, 19, p. 28.

VERNON, R. (1987) 'Responding to AIDS: Practice and Policy', in J. KINGSLEY, *Sex, Gender and Care Work.* London, Research Highlights in Social Work, 15, pp. 0–00.

Chapter 16

Responses to AIDS: 1986–1987

Zoe Schramm-Evans

The period from 1981 to 1989 has seen a variety of responses to a medical condition which has attracted the most intense simultaneous analyses ever. Such analyses have revealed that the history of AIDS, although short, has it own eras and timescales, divisions, boundaries, assertions and refutations. It is a history chequered by the untimely deaths of young people, by the responses of their friends and supporters, by the medical profession, by the media, by the public and by government. From this chronicle has emerged a distinct period, during which many of the forces engaged in the historical process met, clashed, parleyed and agreed a truce before going their own ways. This period, from spring 1986 to summer 1987, saw unparalleled media and public interest in AIDS, shifts in government attitudes and the growth and subsequent decline in the power of the voluntary, now often referred to as the non-statutory, sector.

In the autumn of 1986 I began research into social policy and AIDS and this was facilitated through my work with the Terrence Higgins Trust, the National AIDS Helpline, television and radio and, perhaps most revealingly, through my own friends. The analysis which follows results from three methods: participant observation, interviewing and secondary analysis. Three main subjects which the research addresses are the development and function of the Terrence Higgins Trust, the response of the public domain — which includes the media, the population in general and helplines, and the role of government.

Each of these three subjects has its own history. In telling it, choices had to be made: what were the most important features of those histories, how were they important, to whom and what was their provenance? This is work still in progress and, for the purposes of this chapter, I have chosen to consider the main tensions at work between all three subjects; the contradictions and ironies which bound them together and simultaneously forced them apart. By an examination of the tensions, both internal and external, separate and collective of each subject area, I hope to show the cause of such tensions and their effects on the story of an illness.

In 1982 AIDS first came to the notice of gay people in Britain with the death of several men from the disease. In 1983 friends of Terrence Higgins, one of the first people to have died with AIDS in Britain, organized a group of concerned people and, with the assistance of the Greater London Council (GLC) and the Health Education Council (HEC), held a conference at London's Conway Hall; this included a speaker from the Boston AIDS group. From this community event grew an organization producing AIDS education leaflets, initially for gay men but very quickly for a wide and varied audience, and general medical information. In the early years, Terrence Higgins Trust funding came entirely from the gay community; from legacies, donations, gay businesses, raffles in pubs and rattling buckets. During the years prior to 1986, the Terrence Higgins Trust lobbied for government recognition of AIDS as an issue of national and international importance. Not until September 1985 was the first government grant of £35,000 received, intended for producing more leaflets and funding the helpline which had been in service since St Valentine's Day 1984. In the years prior to 1986 there was no one else to turn to. If you wanted advice, help or comfort, you rang the number of the Terrence Higgins Trust.

Meanwhile, in the statutory sphere, the Medical Research Council established its own working party on AIDS in 1983. In the political arena, the government set up EAGA — the Expert Advisory Group on AIDS — in the last days of January 1985. This was a move which coincided with the death of Chelmsford prison chaplain, Gregory Richards, an event which caused unprecedented public concern, as Vass has suggested: ' . . . alarming forecasts brought to the forefront of debates the growing realisation that "the homosexual plague" was about to endanger the existing "order" of society and put the heterosexual community at risk . . . ' (Vass, 1986:30). This 'growing realization' that AIDS was not confined to peripheral groups was an indicator of how government policy might be expected to deal with the problem. In keeping with such indications, the first significant government action in relation to AIDS was the implementation in March 1985 of the Public Health and Control of Diseases Act 1984. This allowed for the detention and enforced hospitalization of people with AIDS. Within weeks, Barney Hayhoe, then Minister of Health, announced a £4 million blood screening programme to be operational by the autumn. However, since the cost of this was to be met from existing local health authority funds, it was a tardy and partial solution. Also in March the Government faced widespread public concern about its intentions to close the Public Health Laboratory Service (PHLS) and in August it censored a report critical of its plans for the PHLS. In the same month the Department of Health asked local Health Authorities to provide estimates of projected AIDS-related costs and announced its health education campaign to be launched the following spring in the national press. In September 1985 the Government promised £900,000 to AIDS work, one-ninth of which was allocated to the Terrence Higgins Trust. By November 1985, £6.3 million had been set aside for AIDS funding, with a further £1 million agreed in December.

What of the public domain during this period? What little people in general knew about AIDS prior to 1986 was chiefly the result of media attention, and most would agree that much early reportage aimed to produce scandal, scapegoats and shock headlines as a means of selling papers. The 'quality' press was equally capable of a moralizing bias as and when it saw fit. Television and radio reports tended to be less dramatic and generally better researched; in 1983 Horizon's 'Killer in the Village' documentary began a long chain of AIDS programmes. By 1984 the press had all but convinced a willing public that AIDS was the 'gay plague'. The coverage of the death of Gregory Richards aggravated a rising wave of panic and initiated an increase in the publication of official and ministerial comment in the press; as Vass again reminds us:

> ... the health Minister was quoted ... making predictions that there would be thousands of AIDS casualties in the near future. The Chief Medical Officer ... also predicted that there would be over 2,000 victims by 1988, and possibly up to 5,000 by 1991. Similarly, these predictions coincided with forecasts made by the Royal College of Nursing that there could be not just thousands, but one million AIDS sufferers by 1991 ... (Vass, 1986:30)

Thereafter, media disease — panic — was no longer confined to the 'masses'.

The Terrence Higgins Trust

What conclusions, if any, may be drawn from this highly compressed history? With regard to the gay community initiatives, it could be suggested that in the absence of any integrated government strategy the Terrence Higgins Trust took up arms and created the only viable information base. However, it was argued within the House of Commons by the then Conservative MP for Renfrewshire that ' . . . the Trust may be expiating some sort of guilt, but ... its view of life is distorted . . . .'[1] Even the most superficial of accounts provides a rich contrast of opinions and thus opportunities for conflicting ideas to find support. Below the visible, public activity of the Trust, many tensions and contradictions existed within the *internal* structure, which materially and fundamentally affected its objectives and the pursuit of those objectives in the public arena. If we accept that such tensions *did* exist within the Trust, a relatively small voluntary organization, what kind of tensions might be expected within government over a matter as controversial as AIDS; within the media interpreting that controversy; and within a public left to assimilate and act upon information from these three often diverging and opposing sources? Such tensions are the result of individual and collective contradictions and ironies which may manifest themselves in the public sphere as dilemmas.

In spring 1986 the Terrence Higgins Trust was still the only central source of education, comfort and indeed hope for many either suffering with or concerned about AIDS. This uniqueness was powerful. It is not easy to describe the sense of authority which some gay men, and women too, felt at that time through their work at the Trust. It came from the knowledge of being able to *do* when others could not, from the sense of being valuable, if not yet valued. But the price of that power was a high one — the public and sometimes private denial of the gay essence of the Trust.

A gay lifestyle is often associated in the minds of onlookers with extremism and anarchy, deviation from one 'norm' being necessarily associated with deviation from all. This was certainly not the case within the Terrence Higgins Trust. Between 1986 and 1987 many of those in positions of authority on committees and subcommittees — almost entirely non-elected — were highly conservative. The organization was administered, with a few exceptions, by white, middle-aged, middle-class men whose own political and social affiliations powerfully influenced its internal structure and management. Those who carried out the day-to-day functions within the organizations either had no stomach for authority, or were women.

By spring 1986 there were two members of staff and a fast rising number of volunteers. Some were highly trained and skilled in counselling, information provision and fund raising. However, few had experience in or wished to be involved in management. To them, service provision was more personally rewarding than developing a management structure.[2] As a result of this attitude, very few people were skilled in administration or management, and so the members of the cumbersome committees jostled and fought over the cover of the next leaflet quite unaware of any political considerations outside the room, as the minutes of such committees demonstrate. Yet at this time of inadequate funding, low staffing levels, poor working conditions and apparently almost non-existent political awareness, the Terrence Higgins Trust was at the peak of its power. Despite the biased nature of media reporting and the image of 'AIDS carriers' that it portrayed, the reality for some gay men was that they were steadily becoming not only visible but more acceptable. What was the reason for this? The Trust hierarchy — again committee minutes demonstrate this clearly — was aware that the same reactionary, apolitical stance that so stultified the internal workings of the organization was the very thing that made it palatable to a wide audience.

The root of the Terrence Higgins Trust's power lay, of course, in the ignorance and fear of the wider population, and the cause of that fear was not in reality AIDS, but sex and sexual guilt. Members of the Trust itself were not entirely free of such guilt. The type of internal damage caused by those not entirely 'glad to be gay' has been persuasively exposed by Randy Shilts (1987: 406).

> . . . It was a truism to people active in the gay movement that the greatest impediment to homosexuals' progress often were not heterosexual bigots

but closeted homosexuals. By definition the homosexual in the closet has surrendered his integrity. This makes closeted people very useful to the establishment. Once empowered such [a person is] guaranteed to support the most subtle nuances of anti-gay prejudice . . . is far less likely to demand fair or just treatment for his kind, because to do so would call attention to himself . . . Again and again this sad sequence of self-hatred and policy paralysis played out in the AIDS epidemic . . . .

By mid-1986 a further £100,000 had been received from the government to enable an expansion of the Terrence Higgins Trust's health education activities. Accepting central funding created a dependence which in turn led to lack of autonomy. But so great was the desire within the Trust to *do*, that it wanted the money in order to do *more*.

Internal problems reached their climax in the summer of 1987, with the collapse of the accounting system, the fiasco of the annual report and a spate of resignations. The desire to 'do' had become self-defeating, and the organization was on the brink of imploding under a workload both externally and internally imposed; shaken by poor administration, but also by its growing dependence on central funding. Because of the general election in June 1987, promised monies were delayed by months. The sum finally received, £330,000, fell a quarter of a million pounds short of the budget that had been requested. No more money was granted for leaflet production — the Department of Health and Social Security (DHSS) had perhaps been satisfied by its own leaflet drop six months earlier. Though not a large percentage of its budget, the acceptance of government funding allowed the Trust to do many things, to employ more staff, to consider moving to larger premises, to make leaflets for a wider public and to assist other local AIDS groups to organize and establish themselves. The Trust did all of these things and more between 1986 and 1987; in so doing, it effectively created a deeper and more crucial dependency, while simultaneously reducing the uniqueness that was the source of its power. One possible interpretation of the results of such activity is that the Terrence Higgins Trust marginalized itself out of the future politics of AIDS, thereby reducing the extent of its power to enable and assist either people with AIDS or gay men. We should not forget that between 1986 and 1987, as now most people with AIDS were gay men.

Despite its internal wranglings, the Terrence Higgins Trust's successes were undeniably impressive, a tribute to all those who gave their time and effort to others. Ironically, it was this very 'British' public spiritedness which the government managed so effectively to manipulate. In return for a comparatively small sum of money, the government achieved a great deal in terms of public health education, information and training — all without becoming too visibly involved in the seamier side of AIDS itself. Restrictions placed on advertising condoms and the use of terms like anal sex were counterbalanced by the work of the Trust and, increasingly by mid-1987, other non-statutory agencies and regional AIDS organizations. Trust spokesman Nick Partridge summed up the political issues surrounding its policy very succinctly when he pointed out that a desire to have sex has little to do with political bonds.[2]

Government Responses

The leaflet 'Don't Die of Ignorance' was reportedly dropped into 23 million homes across Britain in January 1987, causing a near panic in many thousands of people. What was the background to this event? Prompted perhaps by the US Surgeon General's report published in the previous October, by continued pressure from medical experts, from lobbyists within the non-statutory sector, by media hype, growing public concern or indeed the imminent general election, the government rushed into action in November 1986 with the first parliamentary debate on AIDS. The fact that parliament thus publicly acknowledged the existence of AIDS, and stated its intentions of doing something about it, changed the complexion of AIDS policy in this country irrevocably. The release of £20 million pounds surprised even the opposition; less surprising was the fact that very little of that money would ever be seen by those doing most of the educational work — the non-statutory agencies. A further indication of government intent was the announcement of the restructuring of the Health Education Council (HEC), which had been one of the few statutory bodies outside teaching hospitals to challenge government negligence over AIDS. As the re-formed Health Education Authority (HEA), its reward was to be given a larger budget and greater responsibility for AIDS; its punishment was to lose most of its autonomy through what Norman Fowler, then Minister of Health, described as its 'accountability to Ministers and Parliament'.[3] As a result of this policy, many of those staff who had worked on AIDS for the HEC left the organization. As with the Terrence Higgins Trust, the HEC found the results of zeal to be more cash but less authority.

In January 1987 the all-party Social Services Committee began its government commissioned investigation into the state of AIDS and AIDS care in the nation. The results, when published the following May, were highly critical of the government record on AIDS: ' . . . in all the areas we have covered in this report we have identified a need for more money, more manpower, more facilities, more resources of all kinds. It is not good enough for the Government to say "We have given something"; effective . . . care will require a continuing financial commitment.'[4] The government response to this report was not published until mid-1988 and, despite the fact that it had ordered the investigation, it conspicuously ignored the above recommendations and many others. These included recommendations regarding the monitoring of drug use and homosexual behaviour in prisons, still to receive the attention they deserve.

The government paid large sums of money to the advertising company TBWA, to conduct its campaigns, rather than those organizations already involved in education work; but, in a typically ironic gesture, it acknowledged the role of the Trust and organizations like the London Lesbian and Gay Switchboard by including their telephone numbers on the leaflet, but without giving such agencies the financial means to counter the national panic the leaflet engendered. The DHSS forcibly introduced the concept of male homosexual behaviour into 23 million homes, but condoms could still not be advertised.

The funding allocated prior to 1987 had not been 'new' money but had come out of the budgets of already struggling local health authorities. More cash was released in 1987, but for political reasons this could not be distributed with any real sense of equity. It has been argued that, in allocating funds, the government had to consider the various shades and dimensions of its party, particularly the New Right vote which would have been seriously affected in 1986–87 by any softening towards those supposedly reaping the wages of sin; needle exchange programmes and free condoms for gay men being particularly offensive to moral re-armers. By the autumn of 1987 the Terrence Higgins Trust had received a total of £466,000 from central funding. On 16 November 1987 the press widely reported an ex gratia government payment of £10 million to the Haemophilia Society to assist them in the setting up of a trust fund. No one would question the needs and rights of haemophiliacs. What perhaps should be questioned is the political and ethical processes at work behind such financial decisions within the government.

The Public Domain

By 1986 the public were being subjected to almost daily doses of AIDS 'news' in the tabloid press. The 'quality' press examined AIDS through a more heavily disguised moral diatribe; even those attempting a rational and humane approach did so within the limits and restrictions of journalese. Examining the period with hindsight, it is possible to distinguish a pattern, a process, beginning with newspaper stories which passed via the reader to the AIDS helplines which in turn became a kind of metaphor of disgorgement, where all the poison and inanity could be spat out.

The Terrence Higgins Trust helplines and, since December 1986 what later became the National AIDS Helpline, were antennae listening in on the moral heartbeat of the nation — a heart made to beat faster according to one's newspaper of choice. The nature of calls altered rapidly with the onset of government involvement; instead of taking calls from mainly gay men needing specific advice and information, the 'phone counsellors found themselves facing a panic of national proportions. The closets of the nation had suddenly become a Pandora's box. Callers were evidently at once terrified and fascinated by the tales they read, like *The News of the World's* 'I've

Given My Bride AIDS Says Deathbed Groom': 'Tragic superstud Andy Filby wed his sweetheart in a bizarre deathbed ceremony haunted by the knowledge that he had given her AIDS.... Doctors told guilt-ridden Andy, who had slept with 50 other women, that he had only 24 hours to live'.[5]

Most callers hoped to have their fears allayed, but records kept during calls would seem to indicate that some callers dreaded the emptiness such assurances might create. The pseudo-medical information sold by the tabloid press, and on occasions by 'quality' newspapers too, pandered to that guilt and created serious problems for those trying to dispense accurate information. The DHSS material published in the press in March 1986, and in the leaflets of January 1987, conflicted with much that the public had absorbed years before. Helpline statistics suggest that, in those early days of government activity, the public chose to believe the press rather than the DHSS, which left the helplines to distinguish fact from fiction for those unempowered to do so for themselves. Our culture ensures that our personal development is estranged from the concept of sex, if not the reality, and the gulf between those two points allowed those so estranged to seize on reasons and causes, to expiate their consciousness of sin. In this sense, the helplines provided the new confessionals.

Helpline data collected at this time reinforce the notion that guilt precedes blame in both personal and public contexts. Ironically, that blame did not land quite where it was expected. The backlash against gay men did not fully materialize, though some might dispute that. Increased TV and radio coverage of gay issues, both with and without AIDS, apparently produced the interesting effect of increased public tolerance of homosexuality — or at least of gay men — and a decreased tolerance of sex in general. Polls indicated that young people surveyed were favouring a return to so-called Victorian values; many blamed their parents' excesses in the 1960s and 1970s — a particularly New Right stance — though whether the blame was for causing AIDS or for spoiling their own fun was unclear.

Patterns of Response

How did the three main pieces of the puzzle relate to each other throughout the year? At its heart lay an unmanageable collective of guilt which all three were forced by circumstances to confront. Weeks has eloquently expressed the deepseated nature of the conflicts which lie at the core of cultural guilt and which generate the contradictions which appear as usually unsolvable dilemmas: ' ... The erotic acts as a crossover point for a number of tensions whose origins are elsewhere: of class, gender and racial location, of intergenerational conflict, moral acceptability and medical definition. This is what makes sex a particular site of ethical and political concern and of fear and loathing ... ' (Weeks, 1985: 44).

As the Terrence Higgins Trust, the HEC, the College of Health and medical experts lobbied throughout 1986 for increased government attention and concern, some in parliament were considering the re-criminalization of homosexuality. This leads to the question: was the fervour with which the Trust sought to educate and inform others a means of protecting not only itself as an organization, but also the rights of lesbians and gay men in general, although, as mentioned earlier, the organization denied its own gay essence? In 1986 few people in the Trust who had any knowledge of the political epidemiology of AIDS believed that it would ever spread significantly into the heterosexual population. It eventually became clear that an idea was being created, an idea accepted not only by panic stricken heterosexuals but by most of the gay people who helped them.

The idea of 'everyone' being at risk was a powerful weapon against anti-gay prejudice in 1986, and it was the only one that the gay community, such as that was, had with which to protect itself at a time of brutal public attack. Risking the opprobrium of the general public, the Terrence Higgins Trust hierarchy sought to persuade the government that the nation itself was endangered, while not entirely believing that fact itself. What was in 1986 an unproven epidemiological projection is, in 1989, a matter of heated political debate. Perhaps the most punitive effect of this for gay men was that the agony of AIDS, compounded by the press, brought them into a kind of community that would have been unlikely before 1982. In saving itself, the gay community, in the persona of the Terrence Higgins Trust, educated and informed, and thus 'saved', countless others.

The government proceeded to take up the Trust line of 'everyone', and perhaps still mindful of the public response to Gregory Richards's death two years previously, sought to pre-empt media criticism by flooding the nation with panic striking material, leaving the Trust and other gay organizations such as the London Lesbian and Gay Switchboard to manage the resulting commotion without adequate support. Perhaps the government did not entirely believe in the potential for massive heterosexual spread but were taking out political insurance. The only people who, it seems, *did* believe it were those terrified into calling the helplines; as counselling records from the time testify, as many calls opened with 'I read in *The Sun* this morning . . . ' as with 'I read in the leaflet that came through my door . . . .'

Those working on the DHSS funded National AIDS Helpline created in December 1986 were almost entirely drawn from the Trust, or from Gay Switchboard telephone counsellors. Within three months of setting up the lines, however, such people found it increasingly hard to book shifts, as new counsellors — many untrained in the specifics of AIDS — were drafted in from non-gay agencies like the Samaritans, the Pregnancy Advisory Service and Drug Dependency Units. The DHSS had, it appears, pressurized the management of the national helpline to broaden its counselling base, fearing that the public, through the media, might discover that it was being advised by a 'bunch of queers'. The fact that no-one was better qualified at that time to advise and inform, refer and support if necessary, was clearly not an issue for the DHSS. Customer service came a rather poor second behind party policy.

Reading an AIDS debate in *Hansard* is like opening a window onto a fantasy world where the inhabitants live quite independent of reality. As Sir Ian Percival, MP for Southport, declared:

> ... Among the guilty are those who since the early 1960s have actively promoted what they choose to call the 'permissive society'. In this Chamber I have even heard it called 'the civilized society'. They have actively promoted every form of deviation from those normal values until the mystery and the beauty of sex have been dragged down to levels of what we have to talk about in this debate . . . . [6]

The present government as mentioned earlier, is in a stultifying position with regard to AIDS. It walks the line between its liberal 'wets'; the New Right who clamour for a return to family values, monogamy and/or chastity; and the demands of the public and media. If one listens to that first debate in November 1986, it becomes clear that what was being offered then was death before dishonour. The rhetoric of both parties, but the right in particular, created a stance of good versus bad, morality versus AIDS, Christian heterosexual marriage versus pagan homosexual promiscuity. In one brief paragraph, the MP for Stafford succeeded in speaking volumes: ' . . . is it not extremely difficult to justify a position in which one would condone sexual behaviour by avoiding the fact that many of the figures show that AIDS has been generated because of sexual behaviour of one sort? Surely we should not only try to prevent it from happening, but should try to prevent it from spreading? . . . '[7]

The work of the government, however, when it began, was made much more difficult because of the freedoms accorded to the press over the preceding years; yet in May 1987 it joined Robert Maxwell — whose Mirror Group had been to the forefront of inaccurate and homophobic reporting — in establishing the National AIDS Trust. Members of Parliament were clearly aware of the effects of 'gutter' reporting and the costs of such, as MP Archie Kirkwood reminded the House: 'The popular press has dealt with this matter in a sensational way and has done itself no credit. It will take us many months to try and redress some of the damage it may have done.'[8]

As a result of its own laxity in relation to the press coverage of AIDS, the government was obliged to give larger budgets to gay-based organizations like the Terrence Higgins Trust, who, in return for that money, gave their cooperation and collaboration in educating those who still believed and hoped that AIDS was a disease as prejudiced as themselves. But the effect of all these seeming contradictions was to create a collective effort between 1986 and 1987 which would have been inconceivable half a decade earlier, and which since 1987 may in some respects have become increasingly unnecessary with the statutorization of health care provision and counselling.

Conclusion

Collective effort made guilt manageable. The work was subdivided and with it the power to influence policy. The results of this were to permit a sense of achievement, of control. The government succeeded in moving into the general election with an agenda on AIDS which, while it did not please many, did not offend anyone perceived as worth offending. The Trust continued its work with the public but became merely the first and still largest of a growing number of voluntary-based AIDS charities throughout the country. Within six months of concluding my fieldwork, a heterosexual man held the post of chief executive of the Trust. The media balanced the outrages of the press with the usually more humane approach of TV and radio. The public continued to be deeply influenced by the media, as statistics of helplines calls verify. As the immediate issue of AIDS passed to the back rather than the front of the public mind, the helplines increasingly became an agony service for all kinds of sexual/guilt-related problems, most of which used AIDS merely as an introduction to the deeper issue beneath; some calls never even mentioned the syndrome.

The comfortable notion that knowledge dispels fear was itself dispelled by AIDS. The government leaflet issued in January 1987 created more panic than it allayed; fears and anxieties born of guilt cannot simply be removed by the provision of scientific and medical information. AIDS is old news in 1989, and it may take the deaths of many numbers of heterosexual people to revive the public concern that we saw between 1986 and 1987. But the guilt is still there, perhaps just a little less deeply buried than it was then. The particular dilemma of AIDS is that it is at once terminal illness, a social problem and a moral question. The glove laid down in 1982 has only been partially taken up in 1989. There is a very long way to go before we can look over our shoulder at AIDS and its wider meanings and not then turn round and find them all in front of us still.

Notes

1 Anna McCurly MP, reported in *Hansard*, 21 November 1986, p. 844.
2 Interview with Nick Partridge, then External Liaison Officer for the Terrence Higgins Trust, 15 March 1988.
3 Norman Fowler, Minister of Health, reported in *Hansard*, 21 November 1986, p. 2.
4 Third Report of Social Services Committee, *Problems Associated with AIDS*, 13 May, 1987, Recommendation 69.
5 Reported in *The News of the World*, 6 December 1987.
6 Sir Ian Percival MP, reported in *Hansard*, 21 November 1986, p. 836.
7 William Cash MP, reported in *Hansard*, 21 November 1986, p. 820.
8 Archie Kirkwood MP, reported in *Hansard*, 21 November 1986, p. 849.

Zoe Schramm-Evans

References

SHILTS, R. (1987) *And the Band Played On*. New York, St Martin's Press.
VASS, A. (1986) *A Plague in Us*. Cambridge, Venus Academica.
WEEKS, J. (1985) *Sexuality and Its Discontents*. London, Routledge and Kegan Paul.

Chapter 17

No One Knew Anything: Some Issues in British AIDS Policy

Philip Strong and Virginia Berridge

Large-scale, lethal epidemics reveal something of the strengths, weaknesses and dispositions of the societies with which they interact. Studying the social impact of AIDS sheds light on our ethical, industrial, political and scientific capacity; on our health and social services; and on the wider world in which we live, both human and natural. Systematic enquiry into such matters has only recently begun, but in Britain, in one central area of work — the policy response — there have already been articles from an historian (Weeks, 1989), from management scientists (Ferlie and Pettigrew, forthcoming), from a political scientist (Street, 1988, forthcoming) and from an historian and two political scientists (Fox, Day and Klein, forthcoming).

One core question runs through much of this enquiry: how did governments respond to AIDS, given its initial identification with gay men? Reflecting on this issue invites us to consider a common set of political and scientific concerns: the nature of deviance, élites, expertise, morality, the masses, minorities, the media, policy, sexuality, the state, science and stigma. Yet, if the key questions and topics are often the same, the analyses can be very different. Some see in key parts of the British response to AIDS a disturbing reminder of the witch-hunts and pogroms historically associated with great epidemics. For others, its most striking feature has been the weakness of such reaction, policy being dominated instead by the scientific, medical and bureaucratic élites which have shaped the government of health for most of this century.

This chapter aims to cast fresh light on these matters through preliminary interviews with some key participants in the AIDS policy story. Our analysis seeks to identify the beginnings of what may be described as a sociological perspective on these issues. Another preliminary paper, written mainly from the viewpoint of social history, considers chronology, periodization and some policy themes (Berridge and Strong, forthcoming). Both essays stem from the pilot phase of a long-term research and archival project, funded by the Nuffield Provincial Hospitals Trust, into the history of the social impact of AIDS in Britain.

Background and Context

There is general agreement in the literature to date that there have been two main phases in the social and political trajectory of AIDS in the UK. In the first period, the emergency gradually became visible, slowly to begin with, then rising to an intense feeling of national crisis. This was succeeded by a second phase whose key characteristic has been major, though possibly selective, intervention by central government. However, if there is a broad agreement over the existence of two main stages, there are important differences in matters of emphasis. We shall focus here on the work of Weeks (1989) and on that of Fox, Day and Klein (forthcoming). Both papers address the question noted earlier: how, when and why did governments respond to AIDS, given its initial location in a highly stigmatized minority? The answers they provide, however, stem from two very different traditions in policy analysis. The aim here is to add a further voice to the debate.

Both sets of authors start from an historical perspective. Weeks approaches AIDS as yet another instance of the way in which both epidemics and deviant minorities are reacted to by the wider society. He focuses with particular force on the crisis phase and on the dangers of collective social hysteria that large-scale fatal epidemics still seem to pose; dangers that were dramatically increased by the social marginality of the group that AIDS first affected in the West. The identification of AIDS as a 'gay plague' in the popular press in both Britain and the United States led, so he argues, to a rapid escalation of media and popular hysteria and to an upsurge of moralizing about the 'innocent' and the 'guilty' victims of the disease. The scale of the moral panic was only strengthened by the appearance of the virus in a second, even more marginal group, injecting illegal drug users.

In both Britain and America, so Weeks argues, state policy reflected and fed off this moral panic, for the 1980s were an era in which New Right governments engaged in a symbolic crusade against the moral excesses of the 1960s and 1970s, at least as they saw them. Aside from haemophiliacs, serious government intervention against AIDS occurred only when it became clear that the heterosexual population was also in danger. Moreover, although major government action — when it did come — obviously had its beneficial side, the advent of massive medical and scientific resources has also produced major tensions. The gay self-help movement which had achieved such marked success in health education and social support has been displaced as professional experts moved in. Important conflicts have developed both between clients and services and within the gay community itself. These tensions have been mirrored by major internal conflicts within government policy. Detailed public education about the transmission of the virus has clashed with the new doctrines on sex education in school. The strategy of harm minimization has contradicted the previous tough policies aimed at illegal drug users. Thus, while action has come at last, fundamental contradictions within it exist and future policy remains uncertain.

Fox, Day and Klein present an equally sceptical picture of events, but their cynicism is of a different kind. Their focus is also slightly different. They compare not just Britain and the United States but Sweden too. Their main interest, moreover, is in state intervention, not in the initial crisis period. For them, the most striking feature about AIDS has been just how little impact populist moralities have had upon government policy, despite the great potential for popular hysteria. By and large, tabloid journalists, fundamentalist preachers and neo-conservative politicians have been excluded from inner policy-making circles. For the most part, whatever public fuss they made, their effect has been negligible. Instead, the main political response to AIDS has been shaped by the technical doctrines and liberal values of the traditional bio-medical élite; or, as they term it, by 'the power of professionalism'. AIDS might be novel and threatening, but it has been firmly defined as a medical not a moral issue and doctors have stayed firmly in control of the medical sphere. The emphasis of their paper is, thus, not upon conflict but upon continuing consensus:

> . . . In late 1988, the health policies of all three countries (Sweden, the UK and the USA) defined AIDS primarily as a professional issue . . . [as such], the epidemic was mainly a problem for experts in clinical medicine, research and public health and was, by and large, an unseemly topic for partisan debate. In each country some people emphasised moral and emotional issues in the epidemic. But even in the United States, where these groups have been loudest and occasionally effective, policies have been made mainly in response to the customary actors in health affairs . . . Policy in the three countries has, in the main, been based on consensus, both professional and political: a consensus that has ruled out certain options (like widespread mandated screening for infection) . . . [and] on agreement that the epidemic, whatever its unique features and however menacing it might appear, is a disease like any other as far as research and treatment is concerned. (Fox, Day and Klein, forthcoming: 1–2)

Our own focus is solely on the UK, for we have yet to examine any comparative data. Our starting point is the extraordinary shock and novelty of AIDS — something that both sets of authors acknowledge but make relatively little of, save for Weeks's emphasis on scapegoating. For us, however, the initial shock is worth exploring in depth, because, though obvious enough, it seems closely linked to key aspects of the wider impact of AIDS and the ensuing policy response; aspects which are less than adequately characterized in the accounts that we have so far considered.

Methods

The pilot phase of our research was conducted by analysis of the secondary literature, by a brief examination of some primary sources and by informal interviews with some policy-makers and observers. Since this was the pilot phase, only a small number of key actors were interviewed and some important areas and institutions were underrepresented. However, though access was difficult at times, we spread our net widely, talking to some of the staff of voluntary organizations, professional bodies and pharmaceutical companies, and with a few civil servants, health service managers, clinicians, scientists, journalists, research funders and a variety of other informants. These interviews, which took place at the end of 1988 and the beginning of 1989, were highly informal and were recorded by hand, not by tape. (Names and identifying details have been changed in the quotations which follow.) We described the long-term nature of the project, stressed that this was merely a first, exploratory interview, then asked our respondents to fill us in on the salient background, history and issues as they saw them. For many of them, the most obvious and immediate topic was the jolt that AIDS had initially caused.

A Shocking Novelty

AIDS came — and still comes — as a terrible shock to those diagnosed with it. What sets it apart from other fatal conditions is the way in which so many others were shaken too: even those whose daily work it is to deal with disease and suffering. The following quotations, which illustrate this, come in turn from a gay community health worker, a senior civil servant and a general practitioner:

> ... I got into AIDS via a student gay-group help-line which was set up in '83 .... We were all groping in the dark. There was no sense of anyone to turn to.

> ... AIDS really hit us in '85 .... It came through the media as much as anywhere. It didn't come to the politicians and civil servants via experts as opposed to any other source .... It just gradually bubbled up .... It was a phenomenon with which we were totally unfamiliar .... Nothing like this had happened in the living memory of anyone. With everything else you knew something of what could and could not be done — cancer and things like that — but here, no one knew anything.

> ... I've had to break bad news to lots of patients and you get used to it; it's part of the job .... What surprised me when I saw my first AIDS patient ... I suddenly realised, this must be AIDS ... I felt my heart

pounding away and found myself wondering whether I could cope . . . I was in a real state.

Given the novelty and gravity of AIDS, some of those to whom we spoke could remember the precise circumstances when the news about the disease first really hit them:

> . . . It's a bit like when Kennedy was shot! I didn't hear about it until the summer of '83 which is amazingly late for someone in Community Medicine. I heard through a friend in the Gay Medical Association. I had vaguely noticed an article about it in the BMJ [*British Medical Journal*] but I hadn't paid any attention. Then in Christmas '84, I was pinning up the mistletoe for the office-party and Jim [clinician] came up to talk to Bob [medical officer]. It was the first time it hit the [regional] health authority agenda. (community physician)

What can be made of such remarks? Of course, those involved in AIDS may often have powerful reasons to stress its importance and novelty. but there may also be powerful reasons to play down some aspects of it. Weeks emphasizes the disequilibrium that AIDS initially caused among gay men. How far does his commitment to that community prevent him from giving equal weight to the potentially similar disorientation it seems to have produced in those who were less corporeally affected — those in medicine, natural science, Whitehall, the mass media and the rest of the population?

Likewise, how far may a narrow, disciplinary perspective downgrade the initial impact of AIDS? In Fox, Day and Klein's analysis, the new disease turns out to be just another health policy issue for which traditional medical solutions were found. Their tale, in essence, is the reiteration of the jaundiced view, common to many political scientists, that most of the time nothing much changes, whatever the surface appearance of things. The élite machinery through which state policy is made is sufficiently powerful to ride out almost all public storms, however alarming the tempest may appear to the many politically inexperienced actors caught up with the sound and fury of a particular issue. Like Weeks's radicalism, such scepticism is salutary. However, one may still wonder how far the professional cynicism of political scientists leads them to underestimate the great ravages that AIDS seems to have caused, at least initially, to the small world in which policy is normally formed?

Bio-medical Expertise

AIDS was indeed novel. Not only had no large-scale, fatal epidemic happened in the West for many years, but the possibility of such epidemics had largely vanished from both popular and medical consciousness. Moreover, not only was the condition new to medical science, but it was also enormously complicated and of an obscure and largely unknown type. All this, as we shall see, seems to have created both a scientific and a policy vacuum, with several striking consequences. On the policy side, at least to begin with, some bio-medical experts in key advisory positions to government found it hard to appreciate the significance of what was happening, while others, though better informed, were often at a loss as to what to do next and how to persuade others of the very real danger. As a result, in the early period, some outsiders had a distinct comparative advantage in relevant expertise. These newcomers to conventional policy-making — gay men, journalists, young doctors from Cinderella specialities, social historians — either fought their way in, or were invited, to fill the resulting policy vacuum.

The main trends in post-war bio-medicine had led in quite the opposite direction from that taken by AIDS. Many of the doctors in closest initial contact with the condition were on the bottom rungs of the medical ladder. It is hard to think of a segment of the medical profession with less prestige than community medicine — except perhaps for genito-urinary medicine (GUM) and those involved in the provision of services for injecting drug users. Moreover, the UK, unlike the USA, had no tradition of infectious disease specialists:

> . . . The infectious disease area is where UK capacity has lagged behind the States and probably several European countries . . . . I don't know why the UK lost interest post-antibiotics . . . for medical graduates who want to do good basic infectious disease science and go on to become a consultant, the posts just don't exist here as they do in the States. (Medical Research Council manager)

Weeks mentions the Cinderella status of the relevant disciplines, but he fails to emphasize sufficiently that, as a result, they were mostly removed from positions of immediate power and influence within wider medical and scientific circles. Experts from these ranks still made it into the first MRC committee on AIDS established in 1983, but from the accounts we have elicited, that committee seems to have had little or no power:

> . . . It was just a political expedient. It was not given the wherewithal to do anything. There is a genuine sense in which AIDS was not seen as important by MRC . . . . The story has a number of echoes with Randy Shilts' book . . . . In a sense, NIH [the American equivalent to MRC] was the same story . . . . MRC is full of the same human failings as everywhere else. People just made the wrong judgments. (clinician)

> . . . It wasn't just MRC that was slow . . . [just why they were slow] is terribly complex — partly the belief that it will go away; partly because it

was STDs; partly because it was gay men. And the sort of people who were involved than were not establishment — whereas the people in the Directed Programme [MRC's main AIDS programme post-1987] are very much establishment people. Oxford had to be diverted from other things! And then, it was a much younger group of people with no reputations . . . . If you look at the product champions of AIDS, to be fair, there were no senior people in the area. Part of the reason was that there were very few people who could see what was happening — patients were being seen in GU medicine which is very low down the pecking order. The people who were making the fuss were those who'd been to the States and seen the cases. (clinician)

Thus, according to some accounts, it was not only gay men who were outsiders; so also were the relevant clinicians. Their sort of professionalism was still some way from power. They lacked many of the establishment contacts, the links to the media, the experience of political lobbying. In consequence, in the early crisis period, the gay voluntary movement seems to have been matched by an equivalent network of clinicians and natural scientists also trying, in their own way, to bring AIDS to serious public and governmental attention — as well as the attention of their older and more prestigious colleagues: '. . . We just tried everything. It was only later that you realized what made the difference. It wasn't sophisticated lobbying. We just did a lot of it' (clinician).

Just as the initial AIDS experts in bio-medicine were some considerable way from real power in medical circles, so some of them also had links with groups external to medicine. Social scientists, as a whole, have had little direct effect upon the formation of AIDS policy, but one branch of that science — social history — may well have exerted a powerful, if surrogate, influence. The AIDS policy memoranda submitted to the House of Commons Social Services Committee by the DHSS and BMA (HMSO, 1987a, 1987b) leant heavily on an informal but forceful theory about the conditions for compliance with public health measures. Consider, for example, the discussion of compulsory notification in the DHSS memorandum to the Social Services Committee:

It has been suggested, however, that the Government should go further and make AIDS a notifiable disease under the Public Health (Control of Disease) Act 1984. The main purpose of statutory notification is to enable fever contacts to be traced and isolated in aerosol spread conditions like African haemorrhagic fever; and to enable infected food or water sources to be traced (for example with typhoid) by establishing an infected person's movements. There are clear public health arguments for applying statutory notification procedures to such diseases. This is recognised by the medical profession and the public who generally cooperate well as a result. With HIV infection and AIDS, public health arguments for making the infection

> notifiable are not so clear-cut. As HIV is not transmitted except in very limited ways, and the incubation period is so long, notification would not assist in containing the spread of infection. Because of the length of incubation, compulsory contact-tracing would not be practicable either. It could be argued too that compulsory notification might be counter-productive and lead to fewer people coming forward for advice and testing. (HMSO, 1987a: 10)

How did this theory originate? As the quotation indicates, public health medicine does have contemporary experience of fatal infectious disease. But African haemorrhagic fever is a rarity, and so too is typhoid. The last major, fatal epidemics in the Western world are remote from the personal experience of all practising doctors. Historians are thus the main experts both on the social and political aspects of large-scale, fatal epidemics and on the lessons for control which may be drawn from them (see, for example, Brandt, 1988; Porter, 1986).

Of course, it is one thing to possess a body of expertise, and quite another for it to be used in policy formation. While many doctors have an antiquarian interest in the past, medical history is rarely an object for systematic enquiry, more a totem to be ritually invoked. What made AIDS different? One factor was the particular consciousness of some of the most affected medical disciplines. The inaugural lecture of the UK's only professor of GU medicine (an important figure in the UK AIDS story) had focused on the history of STDs (Adler, 1980), while community physicians are some of the most historically and socially conscious of all the branches of medicine. But more important, perhaps, was the sheer novelty of the situation. In other areas — drugs policy, for example — historical scholarship, however salient, has made little headway against long-held and deeply entrenched positions. With AIDS, however, almost everything was up for grabs.

There is one final point on professional dominance. Not only was bio-medical expertise more open to external influence than current analyses have suggested (a point which will be returned to in the next section) but the location of expertise within bio-medicine has changed over time. Street (forthcoming) has argued that medical influence peaked in 1986; that once a national crisis had been declared and the main lines of policy established, the politicians and civil servants pushed the doctors firmly to the sidelines. There is a good deal to this argument, but it is also the case that with decisive government intervention new and more traditional cadres of experts were brought in as well. The MRC AIDS Committee was reformed and so too was the membership of the Expert Advisory Group on AIDS at the DHSS. As one scientist commented: ' ... The mandarins moved in ... It's symptomatic of the old-boy network of British science ... [the new members] were no longer the 'experts' — though they're regaining that expertise now. X is now very expert on AIDS; but he wasn't then. He had to ring me up before meetings.'

Thus, as AIDS became Big Science (de Solla Price, 1963), so Big Scientists moved into the arena in force — so too did fresh cadres from all kinds of other trades, health counsellors, health educationalists, social scientists and so forth. The influx caused tricky problems of adjustment for all those who had been involved from the early days — for doctors quite as much as gay activists: '... We have to learn that AIDS is everybody's business.... No one can be Mr AIDS. No one can hang onto AIDS as their own. A lot of us find that difficult if we were involved from the beginning. It's very hard to let other people get in on the turf' (clinician).

Gay Expertise

To begin with at least, the novelty of AIDS meant that less established doctors and scientists could move into the policy vacuum. So too could people from quite outside the circles in which state matters are conventionally decided. However, Weeks's particular version of professional dominance does violence to the important links between some clinicians and clients. Well in advance of AIDS, a small number of clinicians had been trying to offer a better service to injecting drug users and gay men with sexually transmitted disease. Moreover, just as some diabetic doctors become diabetologists, so some gay doctors had taken an active interest in gay medical matters and, eventually, in AIDS; a point duly noted by others: '... *The Times* reviewer commented about a TV programme I was on, about "The usual collection of moustachio'd doctors talking about AIDS!"' (gay clinician).

Clients too had the capacity to shape events. Consider the concentration and location of medical expertise. Fox, Day and Klein note that AIDS so far has been a fundamentally local phenomenon. Within London itself, just three district health authorities have treated most of those affected. What might explain this? Weeks rightly points to the striking display of client power among gay men, but other clients have exerted their own influence. On one hypothesis, there has been a process of dynamic interaction over time between clinics, friendly and unfriendly, and a young, mobile and well informed clientele:

> ... There's nothing as rapid as the AIDS grapevine (amongst gays)! .... Think of what happened to the reputation of X [hospital]. Terrence Higgins died there in abject misery and for four years no one went there! It was only by the huge efforts of Dr. Z that they got people back. (nursing manager)

> ... A lot of the referrals have been patient-led. The districts are now happier [to take AIDS cases] but the patients are only changing a bit. It probably needs a critical mass. (London Regional Health Authority manager)

Early reputations may have had striking consequences for different hospitals and health authorities as big money became available for both services and research. Moreover, though injecting drugs users could only vote with their feet, gay men, largely through their contact with events in the United States, undertook an active educational, medical and political campaign well ahead of the rest of the field:

> ... You hear physicians saying now that the government wouldn't do anything — but, in fact, doctors then [at the beginning] were very reluctant to do anything. I said, 'Who'll take the handle off the Broad Street pump?' [John Snow's action in the London cholera epidemic of 1854] ... The term public health wasn't introduced 'till '86 in the AIDS area at the Paris conference. [Many of] the clinicians here had a very non-judgemental attitude to STDs. That was the tradition. So it was very hard to switch to a health education approach. It was the Terrence Higgins Trust that raised public consciousness, not the physicians. (Community physician)

The influence of the Terrence Higgins Trust in the early crisis years seems to have been far-reaching indeed, though that influence was primarily exerted through informal mechanisms. However, just like the first wave of medical experts, that influence seems to have waned once politicians began decisive state action:

> ... The Terrence Higgins Trust were very involved early on ... [For example] it had actually been proposed to circulate them [explicit THT leaflets on safer sex] to all schools ... Civil servants had convinced themselves that we were in a crisis and in a crisis you'll do anything. (civil servant)

> ... The relation of Ministers and the CMO to the Trust was much more informal then ... Tony Whitehead would pick up a phone and ring Acheson. But once the government itself started intervening in AIDS, the Trust gradually lost influence and relations became more formal. (voluntary worker)

Scientific Research and AIDS Policy

If the autonomous power of the medical profession has been overrated in some versions, there has also been a corresponding tendency to underrate the independent role played by science in the trajectory of AIDS policy. Of course, the discovery of the virus is mentioned, as is the initial scientific uncertainty. However, policy accounts so far concentrate primarily on gay men, on doctors and on politicians and ignore the central roles — both technical and metaphysical — that research has played in the story. We shall argue that scientific enquiry was crucial to the establishment of a public consensus and to the dramatic pace and character of many of the key policy issues.

For all his stress on conflict and contradictions, Weeks argues that no major backlash has yet occurred against gay men. How has this come about? Fox, Day and Klein produce an essentially élite account. Policy, so they argue, has been 'based on consensus, both professional and political' (forthcoming). This seems too narrow an analysis. The general acceptance of medical rather than moral interpretations of AIDS has depended not just on their plausibility to élites but on their credibility among the general public. The modern power of medical professionalism has rested on a strong popular confidence in its technical authority. A vital part of the AIDS story, therefore, lies in the massive, initial challenge made to public faith by this frightening and hitherto unknown condition. Here Weeks's focus on panic is surely correct. Yet, despite his interest in popular attitudes and belief, Weeks does not systematically consider the nature of that faith or the assault upon it that AIDS represented.

Questions of sickness and disease are always and in every society shot through with powerful notions of morality (see, for example, Strong, 1979). Likewise, magic retains a powerful, if inchoate grip on us all (Miner, 1956). Nonetheless, the scientific revolution has wrought fundamental change. There is systematic evidence from anthropology (Murdoch, 1980) that elaborate and essentially supernatural theories of illness were of overwhelming importance in pre-literate societies. Bio-medical science has, however, placed a great gulf between the Gods and ourselves. We now live in the natural realm and the Gods (if we believe in them) in quite another. Naturalism has become the dominant, organized mode of explanation, while supernatural theories exist, for the most part, only in fragments — the mere wreckage of what once were powerful intellectual traditions.

But when the cause of AIDS was unknown, and its modes of spread uncertain, the easy flow of scientific answers to human questions about the natural world was, for a time, dramatically halted. There was much greater potential scope — as there was in pre-scientific societies — for moral rather than medical explanations, for aetiological theories which emphasized taboo, pollution, witchcraft and divine retribution. The novelty and shock of AIDS set the preconditions for the moral panic on which Weeks himself focuses.

For some of those with the virus, scientific authority has never been fully re-established. In the absence of viable, bio-medical alternatives, alternative medicine has achieved a powerful grasp on some of those affected. For many others, however, the moment soon passed. Though much about the virus remains uncertain, the pace of discovery has been such that, for the most part, conventional scientific and medical authority seems to have been quickly re-affirmed rather than seriously questioned. Rapid technical advance — and not just governmental action — closed the potential gap in the metaphysical firmament that AIDS had ripped open; or so one may hypothesize.

The transition from crisis to response is not just a shift from amateur to governmental and professional intervention, but seems also to have been — and just as importantly — a transition from uncertainty to certainty, from ignorance to knowledge, from popular scientific argument to popular and scientific consensus. The vast campaign both of self-help and of public education, the wave of textbooks, the educational programmes for health and social service workers, the extraordinarily rapid shift in public knowledge about the virus and its means of transmission: none of these would have been possible without speedy biological, clinical, epidemiological and social scientific advance. Experts retained their authority because, though sorely tested at first, they did, eventually, prove to have expertise. Popular consensus was dependent on scientific advance and without such development both gay and populist activists would have continued to threaten the traditional health policy-making élites.

A second aspect of scientific discovery that deserves more consideration is the unusually dramatic and often conflicting influence that research seems to have exerted upon the details of policy debate during the crisis period. With other, more established conditions, scientific advance has occurred over many decades, often centuries. With AIDS, however, a huge amount had to be filled in very quickly — nosology, aetiology, epidemiology, natural history, therapy. In all these basic areas, everything had to be done from scratch. In the early days of research, therefore, huge policy consequences followed rapidly from relatively simple scientific advances. Breakthrough followed breakthrough, particularly with respect to the aetiology of the syndrome, each producing major media headlines and stirring the policy pot still further.

Some of these advances had fundamental but conflicting effects. On the one hand, they might help reinforce the traditional authority of science. Some scientific answers could at last be given. Equally positively, they might also provide potentially new ways of handling the crisis. But on the other hand, since there was no news of any cure, much of the new knowledge only added to the growing fear, at least initially.

Consider the discovery of the virus. This innovation had striking consequences for the development of the public crisis over AIDS. On the one hand, it provided a cause for the disease and raised hopes for a potential vaccine or cure. The new virological knowledge, when coupled with epidemiology, established with some certainty just what, and what were not, the principal means of transmission — and thus laid the basis for huge schemes of public health propaganda. Such knowledge also led rapidly to a much safer blood supply; thus cutting off a key route of transmission. On the other hand, the development of reasonably reliable diagnostic tests (which followed on immediately from the identification of the virus) also gave grounds for much greater public panic. Testing revealed the startling size of the epidemic among haemophiliacs, among gay men attending GU clinics in London, among Edinburgh drug injectors and among a whole age cohort in the urban population of some central African cities. Moreover, the very existence of tests created demands to test everyone, for quarantine, for 'green cards', for insurance tests and so forth. Thus, to understand the peculiar policy history and social impact of AIDS, close examination is needed, not just of its politics, but of its science and technology also.

Moral Panic

As we have seen, Fox, Day and Klein tend to discount the influence of popular attitudes, while Weeks shows little interest in the ups and downs of popular faith in scientific authority. Weeks does, however, place great emphasis upon some important aspects of the widespread shock that AIDS first created — the witch-hunting, the various signs of mass panic and the ugly moral positions that were taken by some key actors in the early years of the epidemic. What can be made of such events? The concept of 'moral panic' has been regularly used by many socialist observers of popular morality since it was first introduced by Cohen (1972) in a study of the media reaction to mods and rockers. However, though there do seem clear instances of moral panic in the British AIDS story, there are several problems in its general use as proposed by Weeks.

For a start, 'moral panic' is very often not an external detached theory with which to analyze moral debate but a move within a particular debate. Cohen, when he introduced the phrase, was taking an active part in the moral and political debate over mods and rockers. The claim that a moral panic has occurred thus serves to discredit one moral position and assert another. Watney (1988) has already criticized the blanket application of this kind of theory to AIDS. Tied to one particular side in the argument, it is unable, so he argues, to capture the sheer range and diversity of the debate over AIDS and the way that many different interest groups have invoked AIDS in their own cause. This argument is important and may be extended. We shall argue that to characterize the whole crisis period in this fashion conflates four potentially separate phenomena — stigmatization, moral debate, panic and fear — each of which needs its own analysis.

Take stigmatization first. Analysis of key segments of the mass media in the early crisis phase (Vass, 1986; Wellings, 1988) reveals a very striking invocation of a popular morality, with a clear division of those with AIDS into those who were supposedly 'innocent' and those who were supposedly 'guilty'. Correspondingly, many of those with AIDS in the early period — and some of those working on AIDS or with people with AIDS — seem to have experienced massive discrimination and personal abuse from, variously, colleagues, relatives, neighbours, employers, landlords, classmates, lovers, doctors, ambulancemen, pathologists and undertakers (instances are cited in McKie, 1986; Vass, 1986; Costick, 1987). To give yet another example:

... The response from some nurses (to the Royal College of Nursing's

> guidelines for nursing people with AIDS) was really quite horrendous. We got anonymous hate mail from all over the country — claims that we were putting nurses' lives at risk; that if we were so fond of these pooftahs, we should look after them ourselves. For about a month or so, we got three, four, five anonymous messages left on the RCN phone every night. (nursing manager)

There is also possible evidence from this period of government panic. In legislation extending the 1984 Public Health (Control of Disease) Act, the bodies of those who had died of AIDS had to be placed in body-bags and leak-proof coffins; a measure which does not seen to have found much favour elsewhere. Yet, if there is plenty of evidence of stigma, there is still a need to distinguish the different elements in what occurred. The crisis phase was marked not just by aggressive moralizing but by intense moral debate; a debate that took many different and conflicting forms. The churches, for example, were riven by disputes between the varying weight to be put on chastity and charity (see, for example, the debates in the collection of Christian essays edited by Costick, 1987). The gay community also was torn by moral conflicts, as Weeks notes in his discussion of the contradictions within it. All these debates took complex, subtle and changing forms that cannot be reduced to simplistic notions of moral panic.

To spell out one important example, the debates concerning sexual ethics within the gay community had parallels outside that community. In defending their particular values, both parties to such internal disputes could appeal to different moralities within the wider society. Thus, sociological research into the pre-AIDS urban gay culture has shown that a sexually 'promiscuous' lifestyle could still uphold a major cultural morality, by making friendship rather than monogamy a core ethic. Indeed, there is evidence that such gay friendship networks were more extensive and deeper than among heterosexuals (Bell and Weinberg, 1978; Berger, 1982, as discussed in another paper by Weeks, 1988). This, ironically, may have helped form the basis for the powerful gay community response to AIDS; a response which, in turn, has demonstrated to some non-gays that gay men could be 'moral' after all.

If the complexities of modern morality need careful unpacking, so too do the rather different phenomena which the term 'panic' may embrace. For a start, panic and rational anxiety need separation. It seems clear that some people were initially frightened by AIDS in ways that had nothing to do with morality and everything to do with the sheer novelty of the occasion. In the following instance, a scientist recalls working on the virus in the early days: ' . . . at that time, people who should have known better would just talk to me from the door [of the laboratory] and wouldn't come in . . . Even the professor stood at the door!' (laboratory scientist). Moreover, though some fear may have been wholly irrational, at other times, at least early on, there were grounds to be frightened. Here was a new and often fatal condition which, first identified on a small scale among gay men in the United States, suddenly appeared, already firmly entrenched, in one new population after another. Moreover, not only was it a condition which appeared to be growing rapidly in scale, it was also one about which doctors and scientists, for a time, knew relatively little and made contradictory statements to the press. In such circumstances, it seems no surprise that AIDS was popularly viewed in terms of more familiar infectious diseases and through traditional models of contagion — as the work of Warwick, Aggleton and Homans (1988) strongly suggests.

Consider another example. Nearly two-thirds of the trainee social workers interviewed in a small survey conducted in March 1985 said that they would consult a doctor immediately if they had been touched by someone with AIDS (Vass, 1986: 187). With the benefit of hindsight and a far more secure and widespread scientific knowledge base, it is easy to make stern judgments of panic. But may not such fears, however unpleasant and incorrect, have been (unfortunately) an intelligible response in the absence of both scientific consensus and major public health education?

It seems plausible to suppose that there were rational as well as irrational elements in the mix; that, faced with the apparent absence of scientific models, many people turned either to the models of folk-science or else to the non-scientific realm; or sometimes to some mixture of the two. How widespread these different reactions were, how they fitted in with different moral schema, how they were perceived by policy-makers and what their policy consequences were need further investigation.

The Role of the Mass Media

If popular reaction needs closer consideration, so too does the response of the mass media. The initial policy and scientific vacuum seems to have enabled British journalists to play an important part in the early stages of AIDS policy formation. The roles which they acted out were diverse and changed over time. Such complexities are, however, largely ignored in the literature to date, which tends to focus solely on the tabloid press. For Weeks, that press played a central part in shaping the early responses to AIDS. For Fox, Day and Klein, its influence on policy was minimal. But can ministers and civil servants have so easily brushed the tabloids aside. Even if *The Sun* and other papers did not make policy, may they not still have played a critical role both in generating a growing sense of crisis, and in focusing on issues with which ministers and their advisors had to deal, in one way or another? As one senior civil servant cited earlier put it, AIDS 'came through the media as much as anywhere.' Consider the following claims:

... *The Sun* can provoke politicians much more than *The Independent* ....
Patten tagged AIDS onto the 1986 Control of Diseases Act in response to
The Sun. (advisor to DHSS)

> . . .Television was responsible for the media explosion — but it was far more thoughtful than the tabloids. . . . The way the tabloids played it was celebrity deaths and possibility of plague. What television did was say that the government is not telling you the facts — here are the facts. It was being done on Panorama, Tomorrow's World, This Week . . . . It was the equivalent of a good article in *The Observer* on a mass basis. (gay community worker)

> . . . Graham Turner in *The Sunday Telegraph* ran a very good piece on AIDS history. It told me a lot about the gay lobby that I didn't know. (civil servant)

> . . . The government was propelled into action by the media. There were two TV programmes on it in one night, including Panorama. The next day, Newton, so it's reported, walked into DHSS and said, 'What the hell are we doing about this?' (researcher)

Given their varying markets, different sections of the media seem to have taken disparate attitudes to AIDS. If *The Times* ran a series of articles by religious leaders (reprinted in Costick, 1987), *The Guardian* was more sympathetic to gay intellectuals. Maxwell's eventual championing of AIDS may, in its turn, have produced a more sceptical view of its seriousness from the Murdoch group. Television, on the other hand, with its Reithian inheritance, seems to have set out to educate the nation.

The Image of War

If moralizing and medicalizing are not, as we have seen, the whole story, how best to capture the first few years of AIDS? Our emphasis thus far has been on the policy consequences of shock, surprise and ignorance. Another image comes to mind, just as obvious as shock, yet strangely neglected in the academic literature to date — that of war. For some social scientists, the image of war is inappropriate; both anthropomorphic and in dubious taste. Patton criticizes the 'overdrawn military metaphors' (1985: 38) used by Margaret Heckler in a speech about AIDS. Alcorn writes scathingly of the 'Cold War' approach to diseases such as cancer and AIDS (1988: 79–80). Yet one may invoke the image of war, not in a spirit of militarism, but to make the analytic point that both are emergencies of a closely related kind. Consider three events that took place immediately following the British government's decision to intervene on a major scale:

> [There was] ' . . . an amazing co-operation between the government and the BBC and ITV; a recognition — a quite courageous recognition — that if what we thought we knew was true, we had to act very fast before it was too late . . . . I can't think of any other major event in which broadcasters

voluntarily did this, outside of war ... by Autumn '87, there was a recognition that in holding that special [AIDS] week, the broadcasters had given up their editorial rights and were more or less acting as mouthpieces for the government ... We had gone down the road of becoming the COI [Central Office of Information]. (television journalist)

... The reason for this Directed Programme is that it's an emergency. It's spreading into new groups. It's a wartime situation and, like war, it produces a spirit of collaboration [between industry and academic science]. (MRC official)

... So urgent was the public concern about AIDS and so great the government's need to be seen to be acting, that less than a fortnight later (after the creation of the Whitelaw Committee) Normal Fowler, Social Services Secretary, in what *The Independent* called 'an unprecedented step', briefed the press outside Number 10 on the outcome of an AIDS Cabinet Committee meeting before the Cabinet secretary had even had time to type the minutes. (Hennessy, 1989: 359)

A long list of such events may be made. Compare the many striking parallels between the coming of AIDS and the first impact of the last World War: the initial unpredictability, the potential for massive escalation, the bitter early disputes over the reality of the danger, the eventual outbreaks on many different fronts, the considerable loss of life that then occurred, the alarm and despondency which this created, the calls for internment, the threat to conventional authority, the proclamation of local, national and international emergencies, the mobilization and coordination of science, technology, industry and the mass media, the drafting into government of external, often unconventional experts, the dynamic impact of scientific and technical innovations, the mass programmes of national propaganda, the search for an all-party, national consensus, and the way in which both emergencies linked previously unconnected groups, overrode other, conventional priorities and created a highly pragmatic social ethic.

Of course, unlike some parts of central Africa (Fleming *et al.*, 1988), in Britain the experience of AIDS has been one of local, not total, war. Problems have arisen primarily in the health and social service sectors and, even here, the impact in most parts of the country has so far been minor. Nonetheless, the parallels are real and worthy of much closer examination.

A Third Phase: The End of the Beginning

We are now in the first period of relative calm since the battle began. AIDS is not headline news in the way it once was. In no sense is the epidemic under control, but the initial 'shock' is over. Slowly, social and institutional responses have become more organized. AIDS seems well on its way to becoming less of an exception and much more like other potentially fatal conditions like cancer, heart disease or cystic fibrosis; conditions that are surrounded, buttressed and in a sense shored-off from the rest of society by the many specialist institutions that have clustered around them — charities, researchers, voluntary groups, medical and nursing specialisms, radical activists.

We would, therefore, seem to be entering a third phase, one of consolidation, normalization and (in a narrow sense) de-politicization. The rate of growth of the epidemic has slowed, firm institutional structures have been created, routine budgets have been established, staff have been appointed and policies laid down, systematic knowledge has been established and detailed plans made for further research and future services.

Moreover, with the passage of time and the passing of the immediate first shock, it now seems reasonably clear that in Britain, unlike parts of central Africa, the epidemic power of the virus *is* limited; that its rapid general spread demands specific social and biological conditions which can be found only in segments of our society. The current sense of relative calm within the United Kingdom may, therefore, rest not so much on the efforts of activists and the power of professionalism — important though both have been — but on the limitations of the virus itself. With certain terrible exceptions, we in Britain appear to have been lucky. But if HIV disease had spread throughout the whole population, could either volunteers or élites have held the liberal line? The consensus achieved in late 1986 might well have been swept aside in the onrush of the epidemic.

As it was, however, by the time our initial interviews were conducted, most of those who had been involved with AIDS for some years felt that the immediate crisis was over. Now, for the first time, they could begin to draw a little breath and look back at the hectic activity and dramatic transformations that had occurred before:

> ... The first year was completely reactive — five talks a week, going anywhere and everywhere. The philosophy was messianic zeal.... We were a small team but incredibly enthusiastic... in the end, we decided it had to stop. By that time, others were doing exactly the same thing. (gay community worker)

> ... The Advisory Group is not a force any longer. Now it's mostly done by the Department.... I don't know why I'm complaining, because I used to get phone-calls at 4.00 saying, 'We're in a panic, get down here by 4.30,' and I'd arrive to find them all wondering what to do.... There were times when I felt awfully tired, physically and emotionally. And yet I felt terribly privileged to have had a little bit of influence — though to be sure it was only a little bit of influence — to have been at the interface between medicine and politicians was terribly exciting. (clinician)

...the whole clinic loathed me then — I was telling the boss he didn't know what he was doing.... Relationships are better now. It's amazing how people turn around. I've gone from being the arch-villain... and now I'm a hero. The boss's secretary and a receptionist were sticking pins in a wax image of me! It's relatively delightful now. (clinician)

...We're past the hype bit, the papers, the television and so on and the ballyhoo around research has calmed down as people realize that only AZT helps and that has its problems. We've entered the consolidation phase. (civil servant)

There are still many unknowns and many difficult problems to be addressed. The epidemic is still unpredictable and no cures or vaccines are in sight. The majority of heterosexuals have yet to be convinced that 'it' might happen to them. Services for injecting drug users and those with STDs are often still scandalous. Housing and insurance remain apparently intractable problems. Large-scale anonymous testing has still to be tried. Government intervention has been selective, and prisons, as ever, remain a closed world. Above all, perhaps, most of those who are thought to have been infected in the first major breakouts of the virus are still in the incubation phase. The full impact of HIV disease on those who are infected and on services is yet to come. Nonetheless, as one doctor said in September 1988 to general assent from his audience: '...So, we have miles to go, but while we are clearly nowhere near the beginning of the end, we are, as Churchill said, at the end of the beginning' (American public health doctor speaking at an Anglo-American medical conference on AIDS).

References

ADLER, M. (1980) 'The Terrible Peril: A Historical Perspective on the Venereal Diseases', *British Medical Journal*, 281, pp. 206–11.

ALCORN, K. (1988) 'Illness, Metaphor and AIDS', in P. AGGLETON and H. HOMANS (eds) *Social Aspects of AIDS*. Lewes, Falmer Press.

BELL, A. P. and WEINBERG, M. S. (1978) *Homosexualities: A Study of Diversity among Men and Women*. London, Mitchell Beazley.

BERGER, R. M. (1982) *Gay and Gray: The Older Homosexual Man*. Boston, Mass., Alyson.

BERRIDGE, V. and STRONG, P. (forthcoming) 'AIDS Policies in the UK: A Preliminary Analysis'. in FEE, E. and FOX, D. (eds) *AIDS: Contemporary History*. Princeton, Princeton University Press.

BRANDT, A. (1988) 'AIDS in Historical Perspective: Four Lessons from the History of STDs', *American Journal of Public Health*. 78, 4, pp. 367–71.

COHEN, S. (1972) *Folk Devils and Moral Panics*. London, Paladin.

COSTICK, V. (ed.) (1987) *AIDS: Meeting the Community Challenge*, Slough, St Paul Publications.

DE SOLLA PRICE, D. J. (1963) *Little Science, Big Science*. New York, Columbia University Press.

FERLIE, E. and PETTIGREW, A. (forthcoming) 'Coping with Change in the NHS: A Frontline District's Response to AIDS', *Journal of Social Policy*.

FLEMING, A., et al. (eds) (1988) *The Global Impact of AIDS*. New York, Alan R. Liss.

FOX, D., DAY, P. and KLEIN, R. (forthcoming) 'The Power of Professionalism: AIDS in Britain, Sweden and the United States', *Daedalus*.

HENNESSY, P. (1989) *Whitehall*. London, Secker and Warburg.

HMSO (1987a) House of Commons, Social Services Committee. *Problems Associated with AIDS: Minutes of Evidence*. 4 February.

HMSO (1987b) House of Commons Social Services Committee. *Problems Associated with AIDS: Minutes of Evidence*. 18 February.

MCKIE, R. (1986) *Panic: The Story of AIDS*. Wellingborough, Thorson's Publishing Group.

MINER, H. (1956) 'Body Ritual amongst the Nacirema', *American Anthropologist*, 58, pp. 503–7.

MURDOCH, G. (1980) *Theories of Illness: A World Survey*. Pittsburgh, Pa., University of Pittsburgh Press.

PATTON, C. (1985) *Sex and Germs: The Politics of AIDS*. Boston, Mass., South End Press.

PORTER, R. (1986) 'History Says No to the Policeman's Response to AIDS', *British Medical Journal*, 293, pp. 1589–90.

STREET, J. (1988) 'British Government Policy on AIDS', *Parliamentary Affairs*, 41, 4, pp. 490–507.

STREET, J. (forthcoming) 'AIDS Policy Advice in the UK'. University of East Anglia.

STRONG, P. (1979) *The Ceremonial Order of the Clinic*. London, Routledge and Kegan Paul.

VASS, A. (1986) *AIDS: A Plague in Us — A Social Perspective*. St Ives, Cambridge, Venus Academica.

WARWICK, I., AGGLETON, P. and HOMANS, H. (1988) 'Constructing Commonsense: Young People's Beliefs about AIDS', *Sociology of Health and Illness*, 10, 3, pp. 213–33.

WATNEY, S. (1988) 'Moral Panic Theory and Homophobia', in P. AGGLETON and H. HOMANS (eds), *Social Aspects of AIDS*. Lewes, Falmer Press.

WEEKS, J. (1988) 'Male Homosexuality: Cultural Perspectives', in M. ADLER (ed.), *Diseases in the Homosexual Male*. London, Springer-Verlag.

WEEKS, J. (1989) 'AIDS: The Intellectual Agenda', in P. AGGLETON, G. HART and P. DAVIES (eds), *AIDS: Social Representations, Social Practices*. Lewes, Falmer Press.

WELLINGS, K. (1988) 'Perceptions of Risk: Media Treatments of AIDS', in P. AGGLETON and H. HOMANS (eds), *Social Aspects of AIDS*. Lewes, Falmer Press.

Notes on Contributors

Charles Abraham is a Lecturer in Business Studies at the Dundee Institute of Technology, and is co-director of the ESRC funded project, Young People's AIDS Relevant Cognition in Dundee and Kirkcaldy.

Dominic Abrams is a Lecturer at the Institute of Social and Applied Psychology at the University of Kent. He is co-director of an ESRC project on Young People's Socialization (16–19 Initiative) and Young People's AIDS Relevant Cognition in Dundee and Kirkcaldy. He is the secretary and treasurer of the social psychology section of the British Psychological Society and associate editor of the *British Journal of Social Psychology*. He is co-author (with Michael A. Hogg) of *Social Identifications: A Social Psychology of Inter-Group Relations and Group Processes* (Routledge, 1988).

Peter Aggleton is Head of Education Policy Studies at Bristol Polytechnic and director of the Young People's Health Knowledge and AIDS Project, the Learning about AIDS Project and the AVERT Young People and AIDS Project. He is co-director (with Geoff Whitty) of the AIDS Education Evaluation Project. His recent publications include *Nursing Models and the Nursing Process* (with Helen Chalmers, Macmillan, 1986), *Deviance* (Tavistock, 1987), *Social Aspects of AIDS* (ed. with Hilary Homans, Falmer, 1988), *AIDS: Social Representations and Social Practices* (ed. with Graham Hart and Peter Davies, Falmer, 1989) and *Health* (Routledge, 1990).

Marina Barnard is a social anthropologist working at the Social Paediatric and Obstetric Research Unit at Glasgow University. She is currently engaged in a three-year ESRC funded study looking at risks for HIV infection among injecting drug users and their sexual and social contacts.

Virginia Berridge is an historian and deputy director of the AIDS Social History Unit at the London School of Hygiene and Tropical Medicine. Her research interests have included: drugs and alcohol policy; the relationship between research and policy, the social history of medicine and newspaper history. Among her publications are *Opium and the People: Opiate Use in Nineteenth Century England* (main author, Allen Lane, 1981 and Yale University Press, 1987), and *Drug Research in Europe* (Institute for the Study of Drug Dependency, 1989).

Mary Boulton is Lecturer in Medical Sociology at St Mary's Hospital Medical School, London. Her research interests include the health beliefs and health behaviour of gay men in response to AIDS, and the sexual identity and sexual behaviour of bisexual men. She is the author of *On Being a Mother* (Tavistock, 1983) and *Meetings between Experts: An Approach to Sharing Ideas in Medical Consultations* (with D. Tuckett, C. Olsen and A. Williams, Tavistock, 1985).

Stephen Clift is Senior Lecturer in Educational Studies at Christ Church College, Canterbury and co-director of the HIV/AIDS Education and Young People Project funded by the South East Thames Regional Health Authority and AVERT.

Terry Cotton is Head of the AIDS Unit for the London Borough of Hammersmith and Fulham. He is a member of the Local Authorities Association and Royal College of Nursing Advisory Groups on AIDS. He has also been a member of various government working groups considering the implications of AIDS and the social services.

Candace Currie is Research Fellow at the Research Unit in Health and Behavioural Change, University of Edinburgh. She is principal investigator of the Scottish research team of the World Health Organization Health Behaviour in School Children Study (HBSCS). She is co-author of *Changing the Public Health* (RUHBC, John Wiley, 1989). In addition, her research interests include issues of theory and method in the study of health-related behaviour change, and media coverage of health issues.

Peter Davies is Senior Lecturer in Social Sciences at South Bank Polytechnic. He is co-director of Project SIGMA, and the author of *Key Texts in Multidimensional Scaling* (Heinemann, 1982) and *Images of Social Stratification* (Sage, 1985), and the editor of *AIDS: Social Representations, Social Practices* (with P. Aggleton and G. Hart, Falmer 1989).

Jill Dawson is a Research Officer at the University of Oxford, on a study of the behaviour of gay men in response to AIDS.

Ray Fitzpatrick is University Lecturer in Medical Sociology and a Fellow of Nuffield College, Oxford. His research interests include the health beliefs and health behaviour of gay men in response to AIDS, and the sexual identity and sexual behaviour of bisexual men. His publications include *The Experience of Illness* (with J. Hinton, S. Newman, G. Scambler and J. Thompson, Tavistock, 1984).

Graham Hart is Lecturer in Medical Sociology at University College and Middlesex School of Medicine, London. His research interests include the health beliefs and health behaviour of gay and bisexual men in relation to HIV infection and AIDS, and an evaluation of a needle exchange scheme in Central London. He has recently contributed chapters on AIDS-related issues to *Caring for Health: Dilemmas and Prospects* (Open University Press, U205, 1988) and *Reading for a New Public Health* (C. J. Martin and D. V. McQueen, eds, Edinburgh University Press, 1989). He is editor of *AIDS: Social Representations, Social Practices* (with P. Aggleton and P. Davis, Falmer, 1989).

Hilary Klee is Director of the Centre for Health Education Studies in the Faculty of Community Studies at Manchester Polytechnic. Her research into drug use and AIDS includes projects on amphetamine users, the partners of drug users and drug using prostitutes. She has also directed pilot studies that investigate the nature and extent of informal support available to people diagnosed as HIV seropositive and self-help groups for benzodiazepine dependence.

Vijay Kumari is currently working for Project SIGMA at South Bank Polytechnic and awaiting funding for a study of issues relevant to HIV transmission within the Asian community. She has previously published a report on Asians and disability and has written related articles for the Asian press.

Sandra Legg is Training Advisor (HIV) for the South East Thames Regional Health Authority and lectures in health psychology and health education at Christ Church College, Canterbury.

Neil McKeganey is a medical sociologist working at the Social Paediatric and Obstetric Research Unit at the University of Glasgow. He has conducted research on a wide range of topics, including therapeutic communities and the delivery of services to elderly people. He is co-author of *One Foot in Eden: A Sociological Study of the Range of Therapeutic Community Practice* (Routledge and Kegan Paul, 1989) and *Care of the Elderly: Policy and Practice* (with Sarah Cunningham-Burley, Aberdeen University Press, 1988). He has edited two books, *Enter the Sociologist: Reflections on the Practice of Sociology* (Avebury, 1988) and *Readings in Medical Sociology* (Tavistock, 1989).

John McLean is a Research Officer at St Mary's Hospital Medical School, London, on a study of behaviour of gay men in response to AIDS.

Deborah Marks, at the time the chapter was written, was Research Assistant on the AIDS Relevant Cognition project. She now works at Manchester Polytechnic.

Amina Memon is Research Fellow on the HIV/AIDS Education and Young People Project based at Christ Church College, Canterbury. Her main research interest is in young people's perceptions of HIV infection risk.

Hans Moerkerk is secretary of the Dutch Commission on AIDS Control.

Cindy Patton is a journalist who has been involved in AIDS organizing for seven years. She is the author of *Sex and Germs: The Politics of AIDS* (South End Press, 1985) and *Making It: A Woman's Guide to Sex in the Age of AIDS* (Firebrand Press, 1987).

Diane Richardson is a Lecturer in the Department of Sociologial Studies at Sheffield University. She is co-author of *The Theory and Practice of Homosexuality* (Routledge and Kegan Paul, 1981), and author of *Women and the AIDS Crisis* (Pandora Press, 2nd., 1989), *Feminism, Motherhood and Child Rearing* (Macmillan, 1990) and *A Woman's Guide to Safer Sex* (Pandora Press, 1990).

Lorna Ryan is Research Assistant to the HIV/AIDS Education and Young People Project based at Christ Church College, Canterbury. Her main research interests are discourse theory and media representations of prostitution and AIDS.

Zoe Schramm-Evans is a Research Associate at University College and Middlesex School of Medicine, London. She has worked for the Terrence Higgins Trust and the National AIDS Helpline as an advisor since 1986. Her research interests include the lifestyles and health behaviour of bisexual men, and she is currently concluding PhD research to be entitled 'AIDS: The Failure of Ideology'. She co-authored and edited *AIDS Help* (Thames Television, 1987) and contributed to the Terrence Higgins Trust's written submission to the Third Social Services Committee Report to the House of Commons entitled *Problems Associated with AIDS*.

David Silverman is Professor of Sociology at Goldsmith's College, University of London. He is the author of *The Theory of Organisations: A Sociological Framework* (Gower, 1970), *Qualitative Methodology and Sociology* (Gower, 1985) and *Communication and Medical Practice: Social Relations in the Clinic* (Sage, 1987). His current research interests focus on the counselling of people with HIV infection and AIDS.

Paul Simpson is a Researcher at South Bank Polytechnic. He is currently working for Project SIGMA—a longitudinal study of the behaviour of gay and bisexual men since the appearance of HIV infection and AIDS.

Russell Spears is a Lecturer at Facultit der Psychologie, Universiteit van Amsterdam, Netherlands.

David Stears is Senior Lecturer in Educational Studies at Christ Church College, Canterbury and co-director of the HIV/AIDS Education and Young People Project funded by the South East Thames Regional Health Authority and AVERT.

Philip Strong is a sociologist and director of the AIDS Social History Unit at the London School of Hygiene and Tropical Medicine. His research interests have included medical consultation, variations in clinical practice, professions and organizations and NHS management. He is the author of *The Ceremonial Order of the Clinic* (Routledge and Kegan Paul, 1979) and co-author of NHS *Under New Management* (with Jane Robinson, Open University Press, 1990). He was academic editor, deputy chair and a co-author of the Open University course (U205) *Health and Disease* (Open University Press, 1985).

Ian Warwick has been working as a researcher on the Young People's Health Knowledge and AIDS Project, and is currently Project Officer on the AVERT Young People and AIDS project at Bristol Polytechnic. As a member of the Aled Richards Trust, a community AIDS charity, he works in the Gay Mens Group and as a buddy. He is a member of 'Cultural Deviance'.

Simon Watney has been a long-term member of the Health Education Group of the Terrence Higgins Trust. He is the author of *Policing Desire: Pornography, AIDS and the Media* (Methuen, 1987; University of Minnesota, 1989). He has also co-edited with Erica Carter *Taking Liberties: AIDS and Cultural Politics* (Serpent's Tail, 1989).

Index

Index

Index

ONE WEEK LOAN

Renew Books on PHONE-it: 01443 654456
Help Desk: 01443 482625
Media Services Reception: 01443 482610

Books are to be returned on or before the last date below

Treforest Learning Resources Centre
University of Glamorgan CF37 1DL